THERE IS HOPE:

Learning to Live with HIV

THIRD EDITION

Written by Janice Ferri with Jill Schwendeman

Edited by Janice Ferri

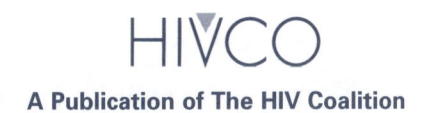

HIVCO

A Publication of The HIV Coalition

Design and Art Direction: **perolio inc**
Photography: **Jay Wolke**
Resources: **Stacy Baker**
Book Project: **Linda Davis, Marikay Belsanti**

Copyright © 1997 The HIV Coalition
All rights reserved. Printed in the United States of America.

For information regarding reproduction, please contact:

The HIV Coalition
1471 Business Center Drive, Suite 500
Mount Prospect, IL 60056
847-391-9803

Library of Congress Cataloging-in-Publication Data
Ferri, Janice.
There is Hope: Learning to Live with HIV / written by Janice Ferri with Jill Schwendeman; edited by Janice Ferri.—3rd ed.
      p.   cm.
"A publication of The HIV Coalition"
Includes bibliographical references and index.
ISBN 0-9639390-2-5 (pbk. : alk. paper)
1. AIDS (Disease)—Popular works.   I. Schwendeman, Jill
II. Title
RC607.A26F47 1997
362.1'969792—DC21

97-14113
CIP

ABOUT THIS PUBLICATION

About HIVCO

The HIV Coalition (HIVCO) is an organization of more than 500 medical and social service professionals and community members who are committed to facing and responding effectively to the epidemic of HIV disease in our communities.

HIVCO's mission is to provide programs and coordinate initiatives to meet needs in HIV care and prevention in Chicago's suburbs. The organization's principal activities include a food program serving clients in four counties, sponsorship of HIV community education programs, and networking initiatives.

About This Publication

In the early 1990s, HIVCO identified a need among newly diagnosed people with AIDS in our service area for a user-friendly guide to navigating the "red tape runaround" of government assistance programs. The scope eventually was broadened, evolving from an idea into a comprehensive "survival manual" for people living with HIV at all stages of the disease.

Extensive research with PWAs and professionals in the HIV/AIDS field shaped There Is Hope: Learning to Live with HIV into a unique amalgam of information and advice on coping with HIV, local and national resources, reprints from noteworthy publications, and first-person narratives from people living with the disease and the professionals who assist them.

With this Third Edition, There Is Hope offers expanded resource listings to enhance its usefulness to a national audience.

About the Information Contained Herein

Although great steps have been taken to ensure the accuracy of all the information presented herein, we apologize for any errors this book may contain.

Opinions expressed throughout this publication are not necessarily those of the HIVCO Board of Directors, HIVCO members, contractors, employees, or the book's authors or designer. The book is intended for information purposes only, and is not an endorsement of, or for, any medical treatment, institution, or product. Contents of this book should not be construed as legal, medical, or nutritional advice or opinion on any specific fact or circumstance. The reader is urged to consult a doctor or lawyer concerning the reader's own situation and any specific questions the reader may have. Under no circumstances should the information in this book be construed as a substitute for the advice of a professional who has been informed of your individual situation and needs.

July, 1997
The HIV Coalition

© HIVCO 1997

ACKNOWLEDGMENTS

We are greatly indebted to the following HIVCO friends, organizations, and colleagues for lending their time, expertise, and support in creating the Third Edition of this book:

Nancy Abraham

Kathleen J. Ahler

ACLU Foundation, Inc. National Prison Project

AIDS Alternative Health Project

AIDS Legal Council of Chicago

AIDS Project Los Angeles

Juan Alegria

American Dental Association

Scott Anderson

Stacy Baker

Carrie Barnett

Rick Bejlovec

Nina Beaty

Emily Berendt

Sharon Berry

Rex M. Best

Better Existence with HIV (BEHIV)

Dan Bigg

Bill Black

Body Positive

Sandi Boyd

Carlos Chavez

Cook County Department of Public Health

Gene Coughlin

Chad Davis

Kathy Doyle and Doyle Research Associates

Ann Dunmore

Thomas Dunning

Shelly Ebbert

Per Erez

Evanston Health Department

Evanston Public Library Information Center

Ronald Falen

John Fortunato

Susan M. Gall

Gay Men's Health Crisis

Bo Gyung

Susan Harris

C. J. Hawking

Diane Hayes

Tiger Heise

Hemlock Society

Hemophilia of Georgia

Hemophilia Foundation of Michigan

Ronald Hirsch, M.D.

HIV Talk Radio Project

Horizons

Howard Brown Health Center

Illinois Department of Children and Family Services

Illinois Department of Public Aid

Illinois Department of Public Health

Impact AIDS

Indi-indexers

Angela John

Daniel Johnson, M.D.

Julie Justicz

Thomas Klein, M.D.

Lambda Rising Books

Derek Libbey

LifeSource

Roberta Luskin-Hawk, M.D.

Noreen Luszcz

Kate Mahoney

Annie Martin

Michelle Mascaro

Phillip Matthews

Midwest AIDS Training and Education Center

Howard Mirsky

Russell Mills

Elizabeth Monk

National Association of People with AIDS (NAPWA)

National Hemophilia Foundation

Judith Nerad, M.D.

Bill Northrup

Joan Palmer

PATH

Pediatric and Adolescent HIV Care Team, University of Chicago Children's Hospital

People Like Us Books

People with AIDS Coalition

Sharayn Perez

Pets Are Wonderful Support (PAWS)

Rae Pistone

POZ

Project Inform

Allen Reed

Joan Reilly

Felicia Rodriguez

Dion A. Richetti, D.C.

Justine Ritchie

Mary Romeyn, M.D.

Richard R. Roose

Greg Rose

Jessica Rucker

Walt and Terry Rucker

San Francisco AIDS Foundation

Search for a Cure

Seyfarth, Shaw, Fairweather & Geraldson

Eric Secoy

Kim Stieglitz

Deborah Steinkopf

James Sullivan, M.D.

Test Positive Aware Network (TPAN)

Kathy Thill

Tucson AIDS Project

Charles Van Sant

Steve Wakefield

Mildred Williamson

Judy Wittman

Harvey Wolf

Ram Yogev, M.D.

Marianne Zelewsky

…and the men and women who have so generously shared their personal stories of living with HIV and AIDS in order to help others learn to do the same.

Book Funders
Special thanks to our funders for their support of this book:

The Abbott Fund

Abbott Laboratories

John S. Baran Fund

Blue Cross/Blue Shield of Illinois

Bristol-Myers Squibb

Chicago Department of Public Health

Glaxo-Wellcome Foundation

Merck & Company Human Health Division

Nestle Clinical Nutrition

Pharmacia & Upjohn

Roche Pharmaceuticals

Schaumburg (Illinois) Township

Statscript Pharmacy

Tenneco Packaging

CONTENTS

	Page
About This Publication	iii
Acknowledgements	iv
Introduction	x

Part 1: Questions and Answers about HIV — 1
- Where can I get more information? — 7
  1. Using a Phone — 8
  2. Using a Computer and Modem — 11
  3. Using a Fax Machine — 14
  4. HIV Care Consortia — 15
  5. Local Health Departments — 16
  6. Libraries and Booksellers — 17
  7. Books, Publications, and Videos — 18
  8. Media — 20
  9. Local AIDS Service Organizations — 20
  10. HIV/AIDS Education and Advocacy Organizations — 21
  11. Resources for Women — 22
  12. Resources for Children — 25
  13. Resources for Teens — 27
  14. Resources for Gay and Bisexual Men and Youth — 28
  15. Resources for People of Color — 29
  16. Resources for Family, Friends, and Caregivers — 31
  17. Resources for Professionals — 33

Part 2: Voices of Hope — 34
- You Are Not Alone — 35
- Changes That Have Come from AIDS — 39
- The Effect of an AIDS Diagnosis on My Life — 42
- Treat Yourself Right! — 43
- Positively Positive — 44
- Surviving and Thriving with AIDS — 47
- What Does It Take to Be a Long-Term Survivor? — 48

Part 3: First Steps — 50

1. Taking Charge — 52
   - My Suggestions for Those Diagnosed with AIDS — 55
   - Taking Charge as a Person of Color — 57

2. Finding and Working with a Doctor — 63
   - Coping with an Insensitive or Rejecting Doctor — 63
   - Why You Need an HIV Specialist — 63
   - Characteristics of the "Ideal" HIV Specialist — 64
   - Finding the *Right* HIV Specialist — 65

- Streamlining Your Care 65
- Physician Referral Services 66
- Local Hospitals and HIV Clinics 66
- Narrowing Down Your Options 71
- Working with a Doctor 72
- The "Baseline" Exam 72
- Regular Health Monitoring: The Basics 73
- Monitoring Immune Strength and HIV: T Cell Counts and Viral Load Testing 73
- Patient Rights and Responsibilities 75
- Finding and Working with a Dentist 77
- Dental Referral Services 77

3. Exploring the Range of Treatments
   - Mainstream Approaches 78
     - Antiretroviral Drugs and Combination Therapies 78
     - Immunomodulators 84
     - Prevention and Treatment of Opportunistic Infections 86
     - Clinical Drug Trials 89
     - Clinical Trials Information 91
     - Paying for Treatment 92
     - Patient Assistance Program Resources 97
     - Pharmacies and Buyers' Clubs 97
   - "Complementary" or "Holistic" Approaches 98
     - Dovetailing with the Mainstream 98
     - AIDS Fraud Is Dangerous! 99
     - Complementary Treatment Resources 101
   - Learning More about Drugs, Trials, and Treatments 103

4. Telling Others
   - Whether to Tell 107
   - When to Tell 107
   - How to Tell 109
   - Telling Your Employer 110
   - Working with Your Child's School 112
   - Personal Perspectives on Telling 115
   - Talking with Your Children 121
   - A Note to Teens 123
   - Surviving the Company Blood Drive 124
     - Blood Donation or HIV Test? 125
     - Home Testing for HIV 125
     - Needle-Free HIV Testing 127

Part 4: Learning to *Live* with HIV   **128**

- Nutrition   130
  - Nutrition Assistance   133
- Food Safety   135
  - Food Safety Resources   136
- Exercise   136
  - Exercise Resources   137
- Rest and Relaxation   137
- Emotional Support   137
  - Support Groups and Mental Health Services   146
- Spiritual Support   149
  - Spiritual Support Resources   153
- Sex   155
  - Safer Sex Resources   160
- HIV in Newborns and Children   162
- Having Children   164
- Alcohol and Other Drug Use   166
  - Syringe Exchange Programs   168
  - Finding Chemical Dependency Treatment and Support   171
- HIV and Homelessness   176
- HIV in Prison   177
  - Prisoner Resources   179
- Hygiene   181
- Pets   182

Part 5: Getting Through the Runaround   **186**

1. Insurance   188
   - Health Insurance   188
   - Disability Insurance   198
   - Life Insurance   199
   - Insurance and Benefits Information   202

2. Government Assistance Programs   203
   - Case Management   203
     - Finding a Case Manager   207
   - Going It Alone: A Few Pointers for Navigating the System   212
   - Lessons from the Front Lines   213
   - Social Security Administration Programs   216
   - Illinois Department of Public Aid Programs   220
     - Cash Programs   220
     - Other Illinois Programs   221
   - Housing and Rental Assistance   223
   - Housing, Food, Transportation, and Other Resources   225

3. Financial Planning	232
4. Your Legal Rights	233
• Finding and Working with an Attorney	234
• Legal Assistance	238

Part 6: Prepared for Whatever Comes — 242
- Life Planning with HIV or AIDS: Wills,
  Living Wills, and Powers of Attorney — 244
- A Matter of Letting Go — 252
- On Surrender — 255
- A Taste of Heaven — 256
- Hospice Care — 260
  Hospice and Other Resources — 262
- On Saying Goodbye — 268
- Epilogue — 271

Appendices — 272
Appendix A: Needs Assessment Form — 273
Appendix B: Appointment Form — 274
Appendix C: Health Record — 275
Appendix D: Record of Contacts Related to HIV — 276
Notes — 321-23

Resources Index — 279

Index — 297

Note: When they appear in quotes ("Elizabeth"), the names of the men and women whose personal stories and opinions appear herein have been changed for reasons of privacy. If not (Steven), that person's real name was used with permission.

When I left that doctor's office, I felt there was absolutely no hope for anything, that I was going to die from this, and that none of my questions were answered. I remember walking down Lincoln Avenue crying, thinking it was the end for me. I would never be able to see my grandchildren grow up.

"ELIZABETH"

My hematologist is not a personality doctor. He kind of looked at me with a blank face when he delivered the news. He had nothing to offer me, nothing to give me. Imagine being pulled over by a cop and you've got an open bottle of wine, a handgun, and a lit joint in your mouth. That's the feeling you get—you're just panicked. It's like all the blood goes zhoop! and drains right out of your face.

ADAM

I just sat there in the examining room staring straight ahead. I knew I'd better not try to talk too much as I felt the lump in my throat and the moistness in my eyes. My doctor asked if I was all right and I lied and said, "Yes." I remember being glad on the way home that it was a sunny day, and I had good reason to be wearing sunglasses.

STEVEN

When I found out about my mom, it was really scary. We were staying with her roommate, and I came home from school and she said Mom was in the hospital. My sister didn't cry, but I started bawling. I tried to look away from her as much as I could.

PATRICK (AGE 11)

"Your test came back positive."

Five of the scariest words in the English language—especially if you don't really understand what "testing positive for HIV" means.

When some people first hear the news, a million questions race through their minds. Others are too numb to think of any questions or even hear much of what the doctor or counselor is saying. After the initial shock wears off, most people want two things: information and hope. This book was written to provide both for people who have recently tested positive for HIV or been diagnosed with AIDS.

Though it may not feel like it right now, confirming your HIV status was a very wise move. There's no more worrying or wondering. Now you can begin to take steps that may help you live longer and stay healthier. Finding out as much as possible about your condition is the first, most important of these measures.

One of the biggest problems in writing about HIV is that there's so much information out there. Countless books, newsletters, articles, pamphlets, and documentaries have been produced on the subject. Researchers are making new discoveries all the time. No one publication can address every issue or answer every question—so we won't even try. What we *will* do is give you an overview of HIV disease, introduce you to some men and women who are living with it, and point you in the direction of resources that can help you learn to do the same.

Some of this information may be hard for you to deal with. HIV touches every aspect of a person's life. It's not at all uncommon to feel overwhelmed at first. You may decide you only want to read a little bit at a time, and that's okay. Just take in what you can handle and leave the rest for later. Put the book away. It'll be there when you need it.

If you were to read only this introduction and never look at this book ever again, we'd like you to walk away with four key messages:

1) You are not alone, and help is available.

2) There is hope; you *can* have a future. More and more, AIDS is being viewed as a chronic, manageable health problem. While HIV is life-threatening, it is not necessarily a death sentence.

3) Your life will never be the same—but that doesn't have to be all bad. Think of yourself as simply having a different set of potentials now.

4) The person you'll have to rely on most in learning to live and cope with this disease—is *you*.

For some people, testing positive is the worst thing that could ever happen to them. For others, impossible as it sounds, it could turn out to be one of the best.

Life is what you make of it. So is HIV.

I remember this doctor was looking for a really nice way to put, "You have AIDS." He asked me if I knew what it was. Soon as he did that, I knew what was coming next. I kinda got, like, a rush. It was a weird feeling. I don't know what he said after that, I didn't hear much of it. I was devastated.

GEORGE

I was sitting there in the doctor's office with my lover on the other side of the room, and the doctor turns to him and says, "Mike, good news—you're okay." And I knew, instantly, that I wasn't. It's like the room got 500 feet long, and I knew that Mike was going to go. My lover was going to leave me.

CHARLIE

Once those words came out—"You're positive"—I didn't hear a thing the guy said, and I didn't care. I was totally in a state of shock. I thought, "I am going to die." That's all.

"LUIS"

All I could think about was my son. What was going to happen to him—that he was not going to have any parents.

"MARIE"

PART 1

Questions and Answers about HIV

What is HIV; how is the virus transmitted; what does an HIV-positive test result mean; how does HIV harm the body; what's the connection between HIV and AIDS; how much time do I have before I get sick; how can I keep track of how HIV is affecting me; what about the new wonder drugs; what if I already have AIDS; illness and life expectancies; symptoms to watch for; information for mothers and mothers-to-be; T cells; where to get more information:

1. Using a Phone
2. Using a Computer and Modem
3. Using a Fax Machine
4. HIV Care Consortia
5. Local Health Departments
6. Libraries and Booksellers
7. Books, Publications, and Videos
8. Media
9. Local AIDS Service Organizations
10. HIV/AIDS Education and Advocacy Organizations
11. Resources for Women
12. Resources for Children
13. Resources for Teens
14. Resources for Gay and Bisexual Men and Youth
15. Resources for People of Color
16. Resources for Family, Friends, and Caregivers
17. Resources for Professionals

What is HIV?

"HIV" stands for Human Immunodeficiency Virus.

H → **Human.** It affects only humans, male and female.
I → **Immunodeficiency.** It creates a deficiency in the immune system.
V → **Virus.** A virus is an organism that can cause disease.

Many people also refer to HIV as the "AIDS virus."

How is the virus transmitted?

HIV lives in blood and other body fluids that contain blood or white blood cells. People have gotten HIV through:

- unprotected sexual intercourse with an HIV-infected person. This includes vaginal or anal intercourse, and oral sex on a man or woman without a condom or other barrier. Intercourse while a woman is having her period, or during outbreaks of genital sores or lesions (caused by herpes and other sexually transmitted diseases) can increase the risk of HIV transmission.
- sharing drug injection equipment (needles and/or works); or being accidentally stuck by needles or sharp objects contaminated with infected blood.
- infected blood used in transfusions, and infected blood products used in the treatment of certain diseases and disorders (like hemophilia), before March, 1985. (Since 1985, federally mandated screening of the blood supply has reduced the risk of transmission through this route to 1 in 500,000.)
- pregnancy, childbirth, and/or breast feeding, where the virus is passed from mother to child.
- transplanted organs from infected donors. (Routine screening of organ donors also began in 1985.)

HIV and AIDS are *not* transmitted through casual contact (that is, where no blood or body fluids are involved). HIV is what gets passed from person to person. People don't "catch AIDS"; they "become infected with HIV."

What does an "HIV-positive" test result mean?

A positive test result means your body has been infected by the human immunodeficiency virus—and that you are capable of transmitting it to others. The test did not look for the actual virus itself, but found evidence of it in your blood in the form of antibodies. There's no way to tell from this result who gave you the virus, how long you've had it, or when it will begin to affect your health.

You may see or hear the results called "HIV-positive," "HIV+," "HIV-antibody positive," or "seropositive for HIV." These terms all mean the same thing. People who have been infected with the human immunodeficiency virus are said to have "HIV disease." Although the virus itself is not a disease, it progressively damages the body's immune system. This puts you at risk for developing illnesses you wouldn't otherwise get.

At this time, doctors don't know of any way to rid the body of HIV. Once you've been infected, you have it for life.

How does HIV harm the body?

Viruses tend to be specialists. They zero in on a few particular types of cells in the body and move in. HIV is best known for targeting the T cells of the immune system. However, it can also attack cells of the brain, nervous system, digestive system, lymphatic system, and other parts of the body.

The immune system is made up of specialized cells in the bloodstream that fight off invading germs to keep the body healthy. The "T4" cells (also known as "helper-T" or "CD4" cells) are the brains of the operation. These white blood cells identify invaders and give orders to other cells, such as CD8 or "attacker" cells, which battle various bacteria, viruses, cancers, fungi, and parasites that can make a person sick.

Like all viruses, HIV is interested in only one thing: reproducing itself. Once it has attacked and moved into a T cell, it converts that cell into a miniature virus factory. Eventually, there are so many new virus particles in the cell that the T cell explodes, scattering HIV back into the bloodstream. The virus then moves on to fresh T cells and repeats the process. Over time, HIV can destroy virtually all of an infected person's T cells in this manner.

Then what happens?

With fewer and fewer "helpers" to rely on for warnings, the "attacker" cells become powerless. They can no longer recognize and fight off common organisms that would not present a problem to a healthy immune system. These organisms may be lying dormant in the body already, or they may enter from outside. The immune system's weakness gives them the opportunity to wake up, multiply, and cause illness. Thus, we call these illnesses "opportunistic infections." People with fully functioning immune systems are almost never troubled by these particular infections—but those with damaged immune systems are highly vulnerable to them.

So what's the connection between HIV and AIDS?

When a person with an HIV-weakened immune system comes down with one or more of these rare opportunistic infections, or has a T cell count below 200 or 14%, that person may be diagnosed by a doctor as having AIDS. "AIDS" stands for "Acquired Immune Deficiency Syndrome." The "syndrome" part means that AIDS is not a single disease but a collection of diseases. The Centers for Disease Control (CDC) has put together a list of 37 "AIDS-defining illnesses" in adults. Diagnosis of AIDS in children involves a list of slightly different ailments.

It is important to note that *not all people with HIV have AIDS*. In fact, only about 36% of the 2 million people in the U.S. now estimated to be infected with HIV have progressed to that stage of the disease. AIDS can be thought of as the most severe form of HIV disease. It is not yet known whether everyone living with HIV will go on to develop AIDS, or if HIV is the only factor that causes it. Many experts describe AIDS as "the tip of the iceberg," since there are several people with HIV for every person with AIDS.

How much time do I have before I get sick?

There is no blanket answer to that question because no two people are alike. Everyone with HIV will have a different experience.

A few people (described by doctors and researchers as "non-progressors") won't have any HIV-related symptoms at all. They may only come down with an AIDS-defining illness years down the road—if ever. In fact, there is evidence that a sizeable percentage of these people may never advance in their disease (although they remain infected and capable of transmitting the virus to others). Others ("typical progressors"—the majority of people with HIV) will face a series of non-life-threatening symptoms as the virus gradually weakens their immune system. Symptoms (which may include rashes, fungal infections, or fatigue) won't appear on any set schedule or in any particular order. After some years, they will tend to develop "full-blown" or "classic" AIDS. Still other people with HIV ("rapid progressors") will develop much more serious, life-threatening problems, such as cancers or pneumonia, a relatively short time after becoming infected.

Experts now say the *average* length of time between infection with the virus and diagnosis of the first serious AIDS-related illness is about ten years. Women, infants, and the elderly seem to become ill sooner. For women and the elderly, it may be because they tend to be diagnosed later in the course of their illness.

Keep in mind that these "predictions" apply to the group of HIV-infected people as a whole. You as an individual may have a very different outlook. A lot can depend on your general state of health at the time you got the virus, how long you've had it—and how aggressively you decide to fight it. Only time will tell what your own experience will be.

How can I keep track of how HIV is affecting me?

Once you get established with a doctor, you will undergo periodic tests to monitor the strength of your immune system, including the

Live fifteen more years and, if history is a teacher, you'll live to see a cure. No disease has not been conquered when it's being researched this aggressively.

MARTELLI

If you give up hope, you're giving up the best medicine available! The new drugs are great, but they can't supplant the will to survive.

WOOD

number of T cells in your blood. The two most important types of T cells are the CD4 "helper" and CD8 "attacker" cells. An adult with a healthy immune system would expect to have a total T cell count between 800 and 1500 cells per cubic milliliter (ml^3) of blood, with twice as many CD4 as CD8 cells.

An HIV-infected person with a T cell count of 500 or whose T cell count is moving quickly toward that number might want to think about starting a combination of antiviral drugs. Those whose T cell counts are around 200 usually are advised to add preventive treatments for opportunistic infections. You and your doctor can discuss these and other treatment options together and decide on a plan that meets your individual needs.

Keep in mind that T cell counts are neither exact nor unchanging. Your counts may go up and down over time in response to illness, stress, pregnancy, new medications, or many other factors. T cell counts may also vary from day to day or at different times of day. Not everyone experiences a steady downward decline. Ultimately, the approximate number of T cells you have at any given time is much less important than your general state of health. You may have 400 T cells and feel lousy, or 10 T cells and feel great.

Your doctor will also keep track of your "viral load," or the amount of virus that's in your bloodstream. Viral load tests measure virus particles that are "free floating"—not yet attached to cells. Patients with higher viral loads tend to progress more quickly in their disease than patients with lower viral loads. As a result, many researchers believe that the best opportunity to lengthen your life may be early on, before you show symptoms.

Like T cells, viral load counts vary over time. Try not to let an unexpected or disappointing test result shake you up too much. What is important is your overall clinical picture, and what strategies you and your doctor plan for improving it.

What about the new "wonder drugs"? Could they be a cure?

HIV is a "retrovirus," meaning it uses the genetic material within your body (most often, inside T cells) to churn out more copies of itself. Antiretroviral (or antiviral) drugs (such as AZT, ddI, d4T, and others) work by preventing the virus from reproducing itself using your cells.

In 1996, two new classes of drugs, called non-nucleoside reverse transcriptase inhibitors and protease inhibitors, were approved for use by the U.S. Food and Drug Administration. These drugs also interrupt the creation and release of the newly formed virus into the bloodstream, especially when used as a "cocktail" in combination with the earlier drugs.

For some people who've tried them, results have been dramatic. Individuals who were close to death have regained their health and can once again lead active lives. Their viral loads have dropped in some cases to the point of being undetectable.

Many have called this exciting news "the end of AIDS," or at least a sign that a cure is around the corner. Unfortunately, the new drugs don't appear to work equally for everyone. Some patients continue to have high levels of HIV in their blood. Others can't tolerate the side effects and must stop taking the drugs. Still others "crash" after awhile—that is, they experience a brief period of apparent success followed by a setback. Protease inhibitors can quickly become ineffective, especially if doses are not taken faithfully on a rigorous schedule. Some of the medications also require severe dietary restrictions. Many doctors will prescribe these drugs only to patients whom they feel are capable of coping with these very complicated regimens.

The new drugs also are expensive, and often aren't covered by insurance or state drug assistance programs. You should also be aware that, even in the best-case scenario, where the drugs produce a drop in viral load to undetectable levels, patients taking them are still infected with HIV. Protease inhibitors and other drugs available as this book is being published do not eradicate HIV from the body. Reduced viral loads indicate only that HIV is now below measurable levels in the bloodstream. It may be "hiding" in the lymph system or in some other site within the body.

If you decide to try protease inhibitors despite these challenges, it is important to take them exactly as directed and never skip or miss a dose. These drugs may work best and can be less problematic to take when used early in the course of the disease, suppressing HIV when it is first establishing itself in the body. Work closely with your doctor to control troublesome side effects and monitor how the virus is responding.

What if I already have AIDS?

If you've already been diagnosed with AIDS, you may be sick now, but that doesn't mean you'll stay sick. With proper treatment, you could feel fine again (although you will, medically speaking, still have AIDS). Average life expectancy for people with AIDS varies widely. There are people who have lived at this stage of the disease as long as 17 years. Until long-term clinical trials are done, we will not know how long current treatments can keep patients alive and healthy.

The key thing to remember is, *an HIV-positive test result or diagnosis of AIDS does not mean that your life is over!* There are preventive measures you can take to help increase your chances for staying well. With good medical care and a positive mental attitude, you may "survive and thrive" for years to come. You may even be fortunate enough to one day witness the development of a cure.

That sounds almost too good to be true. Doesn't AIDS kill you?

While the virus itself does not cause death, the infections it allows are often fatal. About two-thirds of the Americans diagnosed with AIDS since its discovery in the early 1980s have died.

> *The people who are passive seem to spend a lot of time and energy confronting this virus and hating it but not <u>doing</u> anything about it. They can't face the fact that it's real. So maybe you can't stop it, but you can do lots of things to moderate it, slow it down, modify the form it takes.*
>
> CHARLIE

This lady came on the TV and said her hands hurt — and then, my hands started to hurt! That happens to me a lot these days. You have to be very careful not to let things make you feel sick when you're not.

"LUIS"

It used to be every little thing that happened to me—whether my eye blinked, or I got fuzzy vision, or a pain in my back—I was always ready to panic: "Oh, I'm dying, it's AIDS-related!" Today, if there's nothing wrong, I don't look for it to be wrong.

GEORGE

However, many passed away in the first few years of the pandemic, before doctors really knew what AIDS or HIV was. Back then, people with AIDS were told that nothing could be done and there was no hope. In the past decade, much has changed. Advances in knowledge, drugs, and treatment strategies have had a great impact on life expectancy. Just as important, the *quality* of life for people with AIDS has steadily improved.

What symptoms or illnesses should I be watching out for?

As mentioned, the CDC has drawn up a specific list of AIDS-defining illnesses. Doctors use this list to make a diagnosis of AIDS in their HIV-infected patients who become ill.

The most common AIDS-related illness is *Pneumocystis carinii pneumonia* ("PCP," for short). The first symptoms are a dry cough and unusual shortness of breath. The bad news about PCP is that it's one of the most deadly opportunistic infections you're likely to face. The good news is, it often can be prevented. Your doctor can prescribe medication to be used on a regular basis that can reduce your chance of getting PCP. This is known as "prophylactic treatment."

Kaposi's sarcoma (or "KS") is a rare form of cancer that occurs most commonly in men. Those who get it may notice pink, brown, or purplish spots or lesions on their skin, or in their nose or mouth. KS also may show up internally. The external lesions can often be successfully removed, and the disease is treatable with radiation and chemotherapy.

There are 35 other AIDS-defining illnesses and conditions on the CDC list. You can ask your doctor to tell you more about them. *Only a licensed medical practitioner is qualified to make a diagnosis of AIDS.*

In general, if you notice any of the following symptoms in an extreme, chronic, or unexplainable form, it *may* signal an HIV- or AIDS-related condition:

- night sweats or fever
- cough, shortness of breath, tightness or pressure in the chest
- loss of appetite
- fatigue
- weight loss
- diarrhea
- pain or difficulty swallowing
- headaches
- confusion or forgetfulness
- change in vision
- swollen glands
- sores or whitish patches in the mouth
- specific women's health problems, such as pelvic inflammatory disease, chronic yeast infections, and cervical abnormalities
- any new skin condition (rash, hives, lump, lesion, sore, spot, or growth).

The key words to remember here are "extreme," "chronic" (meaning it won't go away), and "unexplainable." Every symptom on the list could just as easily apply to some other condition that may have nothing to do with HIV or AIDS. A person with one or more of those symptoms could have a plain old touch of the flu. Try to resist the temptation to panic at every little twinge or "blah" day; it doesn't necessarily mean you now have AIDS, or that the end is near. If there's any doubt in your mind, ask your doctor.

What if I'm pregnant or have children?

If you are a mother or are about to become one, you may feel an additional burden in response to the news that you're HIV-positive. It's natural for your mind to race through terrible questions: are my children infected? If they are, will I see them die? What will happen to them if I die first? What will they think of me? How can I forgive myself if I'm the one who gave them HIV? Facing your own illness may seem easy next to the possibility of watching your children suffer or die.

To ease your mind of these worries, you'll want to gather lots of information. If you're pregnant now, you'll need to decide whether you want to proceed with the pregnancy. That decision, as well as the decision to undergo treatments during pregnancy, is yours alone. Read as much as you can, consult an obstetrician who is experienced with HIV, and speak with a supportive partner, family member, or friend. Try to stay calm and trust yourself, and follow the course of action you feel most comfortable with.

If your answer is yes, you do want to proceed with the pregnancy—learn what steps can be taken to help protect your health and your baby's. As a mother or mother-to-be, it's more important than ever to seek out early medical care.

Don't assume any child born to you will be HIV-infected. Clinical trials have shown that the antiviral drug AZT can reduce the risk of HIV transmission from mother to child more than threefold. When the drug is administered to the mother during pregnancy and delivery, and to the newborn during the first six weeks of life, the baby's risk of becoming infected can be as low as 1 in 12. By controlling the level of HIV in the mother's blood before childbirth, the risk can be brought even lower. Other studies suggest that changes in nutrition may help prevent the spread of HIV to newborns.

Where can I get more information about HIV and AIDS?

The best place to go for advice about living with HIV is your own doctor. However, if she or he is not an HIV specialist, you both may benefit from further reading or consultation. (Besides, no one person— your doctor included—can be expected to know everything.) There are many excellent information sources and publications available free or at low cost from around the country. We've listed a few of the best-known ones following.

There are times, being out in the suburbs, that I sort of feel isolated—like I'm only one of a few people who have HIV. Just having someone with you when you get the diagnosis, and that first week afterward to say, "You know what? It stinks, but you are not the only person." I wish I'd had that.

SANDI

You should start looking for resources quickly. Don't wait! Because I'm one who waited, and now I'm being faced with having to hurry up and get a place to live, and realizing that I'm not going to go back to work.

SONIA

1. USING A PHONE

No matter where you are, you needn't feel isolated. Telephone hotlines give people living in small towns and rural areas access to the same high-quality information and support available in large urban areas. They're easy to use and a great way to begin scoping out the services in your town. (To save on long-distance charges, seek out the hotlines with toll-free numbers.)

In Illinois and elsewhere, the state HIV/AIDS hotline may be the first resource you'll want to check out. They have up-to-date listings of local HIV-related medical, legal, case management, support group, and testing services. If you live in an area where there are few resources available, state hotlines often can be an enormous help. Whether you're trying to get a flu shot, treatment for a substance abuse problem, or low-cost counseling, your state hotline can probably point you in the right direction with one free call. *When in doubt about where to go, phone the state hotline.*

Be aware that hotlines are often staffed by volunteer personnel. While most of these men and women have received some sort of training, and in fact may be experts in some areas, you may reach someone who is not fully equipped to answer your particular question. Don't be afraid to ask if there is anyone else there who is an expert, or if there is a time you can call back and talk to someone who knows more about the subject you're interested in. The hotline people won't be offended; in fact, they will often refer you to other information sources they feel can better serve you. You may also get different answers or advice depending on which service you call.

National AIDS/STD Information and Referral Hotlines

CDC National AIDS Clearinghouse
800-458-5231—English/Spanish
800-243-7012—Hearing-impaired TTY/TDD
9 a.m.-7 p.m. Mon-Fri
(Eastern time)
• Questions answered and publications mailed confidentially, free or low-cost. Reference specialists do free database searches and make referrals on any aspect of HIV/AIDS.

CDC National AIDS Hotline
800-342-2437—English
800-344-7432—Spanish
800-243-7889—Hearing-impaired TTY/TDD
• 24-hour toll-free hotlines providing confidential information, referrals, and educational materials to all.

National STD Hotline
800-227-8922
8 a.m.-11 p.m. Mon-Fri
(Eastern time)
• Provides confidential information, referrals, and educational materials in English and Spanish on many sexually transmitted diseases.

Gay Men's Health Crisis (New York)
212-807-6655—General Information and Crisis Line
212-337-3504—Legal Services Information Line
212-807-7519—Financial Information Line
212-337-1526—Ombudsman Information Line
• Resources open to all. All aspects of HIV/AIDS, including referrals and educational materials.

National Native American AIDS Hotline
800-283-2437
• Telephone assistance available 8:30 a.m.-5 p.m. Mon-Fri (Pacific time).

People with AIDS Coalition, Inc.
50 West 17th Street, 8th Floor
New York, NY 10011
212-647-1415
212-647-1419—FAX
800-828-3280—Hotline,
10 a.m.-6 p.m. Mon-Fri
(Eastern time)
• Toll-free hotline is staffed exclusively by people with HIV/AIDS. Provides peer counseling, treatment information, and referrals. Request their monthly magazine, "Newsline" in English, and quarterly magazine, "SIDAhora" in Spanish and English (produced by and for Latinos affected by HIV/AIDS). English/Spanish.

Project Inform
1965 Market Street, Suite 220
San Francisco, CA 94103
415-558-8669
800-822-7422—Hotline,
9 a.m.-5 p.m. Mon-Fri,
10 a.m.-4 p.m. Sat
(Pacific time)
• National HIV/AIDS treatment information and advocacy organization. Publishes the journal, "P.I. Perspective." Not a crisis line. Mailing service and national speakers program. English/Spanish.

Teens Tap AIDS Hotline
800-234-TEEN (234-8336)
4-8 p.m. Mon-Fri
(Central time)
• Nationwide AIDS hotline by teens, for teens. Provides information, education, and referrals. Sponsored by Good Samaritan Project of Kansas City.

Finding Other National Hotlines

AIDS Hotlines and Service Organizations
http://www.thebody.com/hotlines.html
• Provided by The Body, this Internet site has a listing of national hotlines, state hotlines, and AIDS service organizations. The Body's own Web page <http://www.thebody.com/cgi-gin/body.cgi> may also be of interest. (See Section 2, "Using a Computer and Modem," for more information on accessing the Internet to get information.)

National Association of People with AIDS (NAPWA)
Fax Information Line
202-789-2222—FAX
• Through this fax information service, you can get a list of national HIV/STD hotlines. Be sure to call from the handset of a fax machine and follow the voice instructions. (See the section on "Using a Fax Machine" for further instructions on using a fax information service.)

Illinois AIDS Information and General Referral Hotline

Illinois AIDS Hotline
800-243-2437—Hotline staffed 8 a.m.-11 p.m., 7 days/week
800-782-0423—Hearing-impaired TTY/TDD
• Referrals to HIV and general health and social services throughout Illinois. Up-to-date information on HIV transmission, HIV counseling and testing sites. Offers information, risk reduction, and support resources. English/Spanish.

Chicago Area AIDS Information and Referrals

AIDS Foundation of Chicago Information Line
411 South Wells, Suite 300
Chicago, IL 60607
312-922-2322
312-922-2916—FAX
312-922-2917—Hearing-impaired TTY/TDD
• Information on AIDS-related education, health care, and social services. Up-to-date information on the latest clinical trials and new programs for HIV-affected persons.

State Hotlines

Alabama AIDS Hotline
800-228-0469—AL only

Alaska HIV/AIDS Hotline
800-478-2437—AK only
907-276-4880—Nationwide

Arizona AIDS Hotline
800-352-3792—Nationwide

Arkansas AIDS Hotline
Call: CDC National AIDS Hotline
800-342-2437—English
800-344-7432—Spanish
800-243-7889—Hearing-impaired TTY/TDD

Northern California Trilingual AIDS Hotline
800-367-2437—Northern California only
415-863-2437—Nationwide
415-864-6606—Hearing-impaired TTY/TDD

Southern California HIV/AIDS Hotline
800-922-2437—Southern CA only
800-553-2437—Hearing-impaired TTY/TDD

Colorado AIDS Hotline
303-782-5186—Denver only
800-252-2437—CO only

Connecticut HIV/AIDS Hotline
800-203-1234—CT only
203-240-9119—Nationwide

Delaware AIDS Hotline
800-422-0429—DE only

District of Columbia AIDS Information Line
202-332-2437—Hotline

Florida AIDS/HIV Hotline
800-352-2437—FL only
800-545-7432—FL only Spanish
800-243-7101—FL only Haitian/Creole

Georgia AIDS Information Line
800-551-2728—GA only
404-876-9944—Nationwide

Hawaii STD/AIDS Hotline
800-321-1555—HI only
808-922-1313—Nationwide

Idaho AIDS Foundation Hotline
800-677-2437—ID only

Illinois AIDS Hotline
800-243-2437—IL only
800-782-0423—IL only Hearing-impaired TTY/TDD

Indiana HIV/AIDS Hotline
800-848-2437—IN only
317-639-5937—Nationwide
800-972-1846—IN only Hearing-impaired TTY/TDD

Iowa HIV/AIDS Hotline
800-445-2437—IA only
515-242-5150—Nationwide

Kansas
Call: CDC National AIDS Hotline
800-342-2437—English
800-344-7432—Spanish
800-243-7889—Hearing-impaired TTY/TDD

Kentucky HIV/AIDS Hotline
800-338-2437—KY only
800-840-2865—Nationwide

Louisiana HIV/AIDS Hotline
504-944-2437—New Orleans area only
504-944-2492—Hearing-impaired TTY/TDD
800-444-7993—Central LA only
800-992-4379—Nationwide

Maine AIDS Hotline
800-851-2437—ME only
800-775-1267—Nationwide

Maryland AIDS Hotline
410-945-2437—Baltimore area only
410-333-2437—Baltimore area only Hearing-impaired TTY/TDD
800-322-7432—VA and Metro DC
800-638-6252—MD only English/Spanish
301-949-0945—Hispanic AIDS Hotline

Massachusetts AIDS Hotline/AIDS Action Hotline
800-235-2331—MA only
617-536-7733—Nationwide
617-437-1672—Hearing-impaired TTY/TDD

Michigan AIDS Hotline
800-872-2437—MI only
800-332-0849—MI only Hearing-impaired TTY/TDD
800-826-7432—MI only Spanish
800-750-8336—Teen Line
800-522-0399—Health care workers

Minnesota AIDS Line
612-373-2437—Minneapolis area only
800-248-2437—MN only

Mississippi AIDS Hotline
800-826-2961—MS only

Missouri AIDS Information Line
800-533-2437—Nationwide

Montana AIDS Hotline
800-233-6668—MT only
800-675-2437—Eastern MT only
800-663-9002—Western MT only

Nebraska AIDS Hotline
800-782-2437—Nationwide

Nevada AIDS Information Line
800-842-2437—NV only

New Hampshire AIDS Hotline
800-752-2437—NH only

New Jersey AIDS Hotline
800-624-2377—NJ only
201-926-8008—Hearing-impaired TTY/TDD

New Mexico AIDS Hotline
800-545-2437—NM only

New York State AIDS/HIV Hotlines
800-233-SIDA—Albany only
800-872-2777—NY only (live counseling)
800-541-2437—NY only (tape system)
800-633-7444—NY only (treatment info)
800-233-7432—NY only Spanish Hotline

North Carolina HIV/AIDS Hotline
800-289-2437—Nationwide

North Dakota AIDS Hotline
800-472-2180—ND only
701-224-2376—Nationwide

Ohio AIDS Hotline
800-332-2437—OH only
800-332-3889—OH only Hearing-impaired TTY/TDD

Oklahoma AIDS Hotline
800-535-2437—OK only

Oregon AIDS Hotline
503-223-2437—Portland area (voice line and Hearing-impaired TTY/TDD)
800-777-2437—Area codes 503, 206, and 208 only

Pennsylvania AIDS Hotline
800-662-6080—PA only

Puerto Rico
Linea de Informacion SIDA y Enfermedades de Transmision Sexual
Puerto Rico Department of Health
800-981-5721—PR only
787-765-1010—Nationwide

Rhode Island Project AIDS Hotline
800-726-3010—Nationwide

South Carolina HIV/AIDS Hotline
800-322-2437—SC only

South Dakota AIDS Hotline
800-592-1861—SD only

Tennessee AIDS Hotline
800-525-2437—TN only

Texas AIDSLINE
800-299-2437—TX only

Utah AIDS Information Hotline
800-366-2437—UT only
801-487-2100—Nationwide

Vermont AIDS Hotline
800-882-2437—VT only

Virgin Islands AIDS Hotline
809-773-2437—Nationwide

Virginia STD/AIDS Hotline
800-533-4148—VA only
800-322-7432—VA only
Spanish Hotline
804-487-2323—Nationwide

Washington HIV/AIDS Hotline
800-272-2437—WA only

West Virginia AIDS Hotline
800-642-8244—WV only

Wisconsin AIDS Hotline
414-273-2437—Hotline

Wyoming AIDS Hotline
800-327-3577—Nationwide

Crisis, Emergency Referral, and Support Lines

Connection Crisis Intervention and Referral Services
PO Box 906
Libertyville, IL 60048
847-362-3381
847-362-8783—FAX
847-367-1080—24-hour crisis and referral service
800-310-1234—Teen Line

• Trained crisis workers can help with a wide range of emergency and basic needs beyond HIV. Telephone support and referrals for depressed and suicidal individuals. Referrals to assistance programs, general social services, and mental health agencies in the Chicago metropolitan area. Prevention information to those with HIV and their caregivers. No fees.

National Runaway Switchboard
800-621-3230
• 24-hour hotline providing crisis intervention and referrals for youths age 12 to 18. Multilingual (using translators).

Parental Stress Services
600 South Federal Street,
Suite 205
Chicago, IL 60605
312-427-1161
312-427-3038—FAX
312-427-1102—Enrollment in groups/classes
10 a.m.-2 p.m. Mon-Fri (Central time)
312-3PARENT (372-7368)—24-hour Parental Stress Hotline
312-427-1102—Hearing-impaired TTY/TDD
• 24-hour hotline offers support, problem-solving, and referrals. Parent education classes, parent support, and children's groups. HIV-affected families welcome. English/Spanish.

Ravenswood Community Mental Health Center Crisis Line
773-769-6200
• 24-hour crisis line for emotional and psychological emergencies. English/Spanish.

Talkline Help Lines
PO Box 1321
Elk Grove Village, IL 60009
847-228-6400—Talkline for adults
847-228-8336—Teen Line (ages 13-19)
847-228-5437—Kids' Line (12 and under)
847-981-1271—Administrative
847-228-3461—FAX
• Telephone helplines provide 24-hour crisis intervention, emotional support, information and referrals. Teen line is staffed by teen volunteers. Serves northwest suburban Cook County and some DuPage County areas.

911
If you are in immediate danger from others or may harm yourself, call 911 (in areas with this service).

2. USING A COMPUTER AND MODEM

The Internet can be a great source of up-to-the-minute HIV/AIDS information. Resource listings, treatment and clinical trial alerts, articles and essays, discussion groups, and more are accessible by computer twenty-four hours a day, often in a very user-friendly format. Most Web sites (areas you visit on the Internet) also allow you to download information, so you can capture it on your hard drive and read or print it out at your leisure.

The only real downside to using the Internet is the need for access to a computer, modem, and communications software or subscription to an online service provider—as well as the need for some knowledge of computers and the Internet. If you are not "online" (hooked up to the Internet) at home, you might know of a friend or family member who is. Alternatively, some libraries, social service agencies, and health care providers (such as Howard Brown Health Center in Chicago) offer free Internet access, as well as advice on how to navigate online. Some employers also provide Internet access at work.

There are literally thousands of different HIV/AIDS resources available in cyberspace. The listing below is meant to provide you with some of the most useful sites. If you don't know where to start, two of the best general sources of information are "The Body: A Multimedia AIDS and HIV Resource" and "The HIV InfoWeb" (see below for Internet addresses). Other excellent sites include the "AIDS Education Global Information System," the "America Online AIDS and HIV Resource Center," "Gay Men's Health Crisis on the Web," and "NOAH: New York Online Access to Health AIDS Information Page." More specialized information is available at other sites.

To explore a number of different AIDS sites, you might check out "Marty Howard's HIV/AIDS HomePage," and the "Yahoo AIDS/HIV Search Site"—one of several areas with a "search engine" to help you find information on a particular topic. Just type in a word or topic (like "fever" or "protease inhibitors"), and the program directs you to Internet areas that match your interest.

Sites on the Internet are constantly growing and changing. New sites appear while others disappear. If you can't connect to a particular site listed here, don't give up! There are plenty of other resources out there.

In addition to static Web sites, you can "chat live" online with other HIV-positive people from around the U.S. Some of these interactive forums take on the flavor of 'round-the-clock support groups, with a bonus of added anonymity. You can also get on e-mail lists to receive daily updates on HIV-related topics. America Online and other services like it are great places to make valuable, one-on-one connections with other people who are going through many of the same experiences you are.

Using the Internet to get information can be one more way for you to take charge—to become more educated about HIV/AIDS and learn how to take better care of yourself. If you're an Internet "newbie" or beginner, try not to be intimidated by all the technical jargon. With a little practice, you'll soon be "surfing the 'Net" like a pro.

America Online (AOL)

America Online AIDS and HIV Resource Center
• Accessible via keyword "AIDS" or "HIV" (without the quotation marks) if you have AOL. This area provides connections to "The Positive Living Forum," web sites featuring HIV/AIDS information, and more. For an online chat room and support area, go to the "Positive Living Room" within the "Positive Living Forum."

World Wide Web Sites

ACT UP: Real Treatments for Real People
http://www.aidsnyc.org/rtrp/index.html
• Nutritional information, including a guide to micronutrients and vitamins. Provides contact numbers if you have more specific questions.

AIDS Daily Summary
http://www.cdcnac.org/summary/html
• The CDC National AIDS Clearinghouse compiles breaking HIV/AIDS news from a daily media sweep of more than 700 sources. Articles come from newspapers, magazines, wire services, and periodicals focusing on AIDS-related issues. Includes a search engine.

AIDS Education Global Information System (AEGIS)
http://www.aegis.com/
• Contains the world's largest collection of HIV-related documents, along with an online library of journals, a newsline, and more. Includes a search engine and links to other sites.

AIDS Hotlines and Service Organizations
http://www.thebody.com/hotlines.html
• Provided by The Body, this site lists prominent service organizations, national and state hotlines, and more. The Body's own Web page <http://www.thebody.com/cgi-gin/body.cgi> may also be of interest.

AIDS Legal Council of Chicago
http://www.thebody.com/alcc/alccpage.html
• The Council provides legal services to financially needy people in the Chicago area who are affected by HIV. Various legal information and forms are available at this site.

AIDS Research Information Center (ARIC)
http://www.critpath.org/aric/aricinc.htm
• ARIC is a private, nonprofit AIDS medical information service committed to making complex medical information understandable to the average person. Issues of ARIC's newsletters and excerpts from other publications are accessible through this site.

The AIDS Treatment Data Network
http://www.aidsnyc.org/network/index.html
• Good information source on treatments and clinical trials. Contains glossaries of drugs and opportunistic infections, issues of their newsletter, "Treatment Review," and more.

The Body: A Multimedia AIDS and HIV Resource
http://www.thebody.com/cgi-bin/body.cgi
• An excellent site offering HIV/AIDS information and support resources. Topics include AIDS Basics, Safer Sex, Treatments, Antiviral Medications, Infections/Complications, Research, Experimental Drugs, and Alternative Medicine. Quality of life issues are also addressed, including Diet & Nutrition, Mental Health, Financial & Legal Issues, and more. Get online support and post messages in "Connecting to Others." Links to other sites.

Centers for Disease Control and Prevention (CDC) National AIDS Clearinghouse
http://www.cdcnac.org
• Geared toward individuals, professionals, and community groups, the CDC National AIDS Clearinghouse facilitates the sharing of HIV/AIDS resources, published information, and trends. Includes a search engine and links to other sites.

CDC National AIDS Clearinghouse AIDS Info
http://www.cdcnac.org/aidsinfo.html
• A thorough compilation of HIV/AIDS fact sheets.

CDC National AIDS Clearinghouse Gopher Site
gopher://cdcnac.aspensys.com:72/11/0
• Provides access to a wealth of general and specialized HIV/AIDS information (though not as user-friendly as other CDC sites).

Closing The Gap
http:www.omhrc.gov/ctg/ctg-aids.htm
• Offers a newsletter from the U.S. Department of Health and Human Services Office of Minority Health. Topics include "Facing AIDS Among Minorities" and "Minority Health Perspectives."

Critical Path AIDS Project
http://www.critpath.org/
• Access to information on mainstream and alternative treatments, clinical trials, research, and more. Specific links for women, minorities, and youth.

The Food & Drug Administration (FDA) HIV and AIDS Page
http://www.fda.gov//oashi/aids/hiv.html
• Information on approved HIV/AIDS therapies, clinical trials, articles and brochures. Links to other sites.

Gay Men's Health Crisis (GMHC) on the Web
http://www.gmhc.org/
• A good source of information on the basics of HIV/AIDS, safer sex, living with AIDS or HIV, and more. Also includes an "AIDS Library" of useful facts and newsletters. Links to other sites.

The HIV/AIDS Treatment Information Service (ATIS)
http://www.hivatis.org/
• ATIS is a coordinated Public Health Service project sponsored by seven public agencies, including the CDC, NIAID, and the National Library of Medicine, among others. The site provides information about federally approved treatment guidelines for HIV and AIDS, as well as the CDC's "AIDS Daily Summary." English/Spanish. Links to other sites.

The HIV Coalition (HIVCO)
http://www.hivco.com
• Includes excerpts from HIVCO's book, There Is Hope: Learning to Live with HIV (Third Edition).

The HIV InfoWeb
http://carebase2.jri.org/infoweb/
• One of the best resources available on the Internet. A service of JRI Health Information Systems, the HIV InfoWeb provides information on treatments, clinical trials, newsgroups, and legal resources. Includes a search engine and links to other sites.

The Journal of the American Medical Association (JAMA) HIV/AIDS Site
http://www.ama-assn.org/special/hiv/hivhome.htm
• An interactive collection of useful and high-quality resources for physicians and other health professionals, patients, and the public. Includes support group information, a glossary, and more. Links to other sites.

Marty Howard's HIV/AIDS HomePage
http://www.smartlink.net/~martinjh/
• Compiled by an individual, this is an exhaustive list of HIV/AIDS-related links. Includes new HIV/AIDS sites, alternative thinking sites, news and newsgroup sites, Social Security information, and more. You can also auto-subscribe to many HIV/AIDS-related e-mail lists via this page.

The National Institute of Allergy and Infectious Disease (NIAID) Gopher Site
gopher://odie.niaid.nih.gov/11/aids
• An extensive listing of publications and other information from the government's key HIV/AIDS research institute. General AIDS information, a glossary of AIDS-related terminology, NIAID AIDS-related press releases, and more. Links to other sites.

National Library of Medicine (NLM) AIDS Information Gopher Resource
gopher://gopher.nlm.nih.gov/11/aids
• Provides access to AIDS-related information available from the NLM, including the Guide to NIH AIDS Information Resources, the monthly AIDS Bibliography, and the online databases AIDSLINE, AIDS-TRIALS, AIDSDRUGS, DIRLINE, and HSTAT. Links to other sites.

NOAH: New York Online Access to Health AIDS Information Page
http://www.noah.cuny.edu/aids/aids.html—English
http://www.noah.cuny.edu/spaids/spaids.html—Spanish
• Extensive, detailed information on opportunistic infections, drugs, nutrition, treatments, clinical trials, and more. Specific information pertinent to women, youth, and race issues. Includes a search engine and links to other sites.

Women Alive
http://www.thebody.com/wa/wapage.html
Created by and for women living with HIV/AIDS, this site includes articles from the organization's newsletter, "Women Alive: Involvement Is Power, Awareness Is Life."

Yahoo AIDS/HIV Search Site
http://www.yahoo.com/Health/Diseases_and_Conditions/AIDS_HIV/
Provides a strong search engine for HIV/AIDS information and resources.

3. USING A FAX MACHINE

If you have access to a fax machine, you can receive up-to-date documents on a variety of topics within minutes. Automated fax information services are easy to use and available 24 hours a day. (Call at night to save on long-distance charges.) Simply call the service from your fax machine telephone and follow the recorded instructions. The system will ask you to enter your fax number and the number of the document you want, using the number keys on your dial pad. The system will then automatically fax your order to you. Your first call should be to order a directory of all the information you can get through the automated fax service. Once you get the directory, choose the items you want to have faxed to you and call the service back.

If you don't have a fax machine at home, or feel uncomfortable receiving HIV-related faxes at work, there are other options. Don't be afraid to ask the staff at your doctor's office, library, or local AIDS service organization to get fax information for you. You could also ask a friend, partner, or family member who has a fax at home or at work.

Automated Fax Information Services

NAPWA Fax
National Association of People with AIDS
202-789-2222—FAX
• An amazing selection of more than 400 HIV/AIDS publications available by fax. NAPWA fax documents are grouped into four English catalogs: 1) Living with HIV (including information about medical treatments, alternative therapies, clinical trials, nutrition, safety, benefits, legal information, prescription buyers' clubs, and more); 2) HIV/AIDS News; 3) AIDS Service Organizations (including information about lobbying, policies, AIDS funding, and national organizations); and 4) NAPWA information. A Spanish catalog is also available.

National AIDS Treatment Information Project
800-399-AIDS—FAX
• Very current, easy-to-understand information available toll-free. Fact sheets can help people with HIV understand medical conditions, common symptoms, the latest treatments, and the meaning of many tests that doctors order. Because the service is fairly new, everything has been written since 1995. To order the entire set, enter #1156. The voice instructions for using this fax service are in English or Spanish, but the faxes come through in English only.

U.S. Centers for Disease Control and Prevention (CDC)
404-332-4565—CDC Fax Information Service
800-458-5231—National AIDS Clearinghouse Fax Service (NAC FAX)
• Offers HIV-related fax documents produced by the CDC and other sources. The Fax Information Service Disease Directory (document "000004") lists fax documents on HIV/AIDS, as well as other diseases such as hepatitis, tuberculosis (TB), and cytomegalovirus. NAC FAX offers a wider selection of Clearinghouse materials, but only on AIDS. Follow the voice prompts to request the NAC FAX directory. Most fax documents are in English only, but the CDC Clearinghouse will mail free brochures in Spanish.

4. HIV CARE CONSORTIA

Throughout Illinois, you can easily find AIDS services in your area by calling your region's HIV Care Consortia. The State of Illinois currently funds eleven Consortia that provide a wide range of HIV/AIDS services based on community needs throughout the State. When you call, ask to speak to the HIV Care Coordinator or a case manager.

The Illinois consortia are:

Adams County Health Department
333 North 6th Street
Quincy, IL 62301
217-222-8440, ext. 138
217-222-8508—FAX
• Serves Adams, Brown, Calhoun, Greene, Jersey, Pike, Schuyler, and Scott Counties. Provides case management, dental, housing, primary care, mental health, nutrition, transportation, and utilities assistance.

AIDS Foundation of Chicago
411 South Wells, Suite 300
Chicago, IL 60607
312-922-2322
312-922-2916—FAX
312-922-2917—Hearing-impaired TTY/TDD
• Serves Cook County. Provides case management, home health, primary care, housing, mental health, substance abuse counseling, and nutrition.

Champaign-Urbana Public Health District
710 North Neil Street
Champaign, IL 61824
217-352-7961
217-352-0126—FAX
• Serves Champaign, Coles, Ford, Iroquois, Vermilion, Edgar, DeWitt, Douglas, Piatt, and Livingston Counties. Provides case management, dental, housing, primary care, mental health, nutrition, legal assistance, and utilities assistance.

Heartland Human Services
1108 South Willow
PO Box 1047
Effingham, IL 62401
217-342-7058
217-342-6716—FAX
• Serves Clark, Clay, Crawford, Cumberland, Edwards, Effingham, Fayette, Jasper, Jefferson, Lawrence, Marion, Moultrie, Richland, Shelby, Wabash, and Wayne Counties. Provides case management, housing, primary care, transportation, and utilities assistance.

Jackson County Health Department
415 Health Department Road,
PO Box 307
Murphysboro, IL 62966
618-684-3143, ext. 168
618-687-1255—FAX
• Serves Alexander, Franklin, Gallatin, Hamilton, Hardin, Jackson, Johnson, Massac, Perry, Pope, Pulaski, Saline, Union, White, and Williamson Counties. Provides case management, dental, housing, primary care, mental health, nutrition, transportation, and utilities assistance.

Peoria City/County Health Department
2116 North Sheridan Road
Peoria, IL 61604
309-679-6013
309-685-3312—FAX
• Serves Peoria, Tazewell, McLean, Mason, Woodford, Marshall, Stark, Knox, Putnam, Fulton, and LaSalle Counties. Provides case management, dental, housing, primary care, mental health, nutrition, transportation, and utilities assistance.

Rock Island County Health Department
2112 25th Avenue
Rock Island, IL 61201
309-793-1955, ext. 302
309-794-7091—FAX
• Serves Bureau, Hancock, Henderson, Henry, McDonough, Mercer, Rock Island, and Warren Counties. Provides case management, dental, housing, primary care, mental health, nutrition, transportation, and utilities assistance.

St. Clair County Health Department
#19 Public Square, Suite 150
Belleville, IL 62220
618-233-7703, ext. 401
618-233-7713—FAX
• Serves St. Clair, Madison, Monroe, Bond, Randolph, Washington, and Clinton Counties. Provides case management, dental, housing, primary care, nutrition, transportation, and utilities assistance.

Southern Illinois University School of Medicine
PO Box 19230—MC1311
Springfield, IL 62794
217-782-7683
217-788-5504—FAX
• Serves Sangamon, Macon, Montgomery, Christian, Logan, Morgan, Macoupin, Cass, and Menard Counties. Provides case management, dental, dentures, oral surgery, housing, primary care, mental health, transportation, nutrition, legal assistance, substance abuse counseling, and utilities assistance.

Will County Health Department
501 Ella Avenue
Joliet, IL 60433
815-727-5062
815-727-8484—FAX
• Serves Kane, McHenry, DuPage, Will, Lake, Kendall, Kankakee, and Grundy Counties. Provides case management, dental, primary care, housing, transportation, nutrition, and utilities assistance.

Winnebago County Health Department
401 Division Street
Rockford, IL 61104
815-962-5092, ext. 253
815-962-5161—FAX
• Serves Winnebago, Jo Daviess, Stephenson, Boone, Carroll, Ogle, DeKalb, Lee, and Whiteside Counties. Provides case management, dental, home health, housing, primary care, mental health, nutrition, transportation, legal assistance, substance abuse counseling, and utilities assistance.

Outside Illinois
If you live in a state other than Illinois, contact:

CDC National AIDS Hotline
800-342-2437—English
800-344-7432—Spanish
800-243-7889—Hearing-impaired TTY/TDD
• 24-hour toll-free service with a database of over 19,000 organizations that can help people in any U.S. state or territory identify state and local resources. Because many state hotlines have restricted hours and may not have Spanish-speaking staff, the National AIDS Hotline is an excellent "first stop" for people needing information and support.

5. LOCAL HEALTH DEPARTMENTS

Many local health departments provide free anonymous and confidential HIV testing. This service may be useful if you want a confirmatory test or want your partner, spouse, or children to be tested. Many health departments also have numbers you can call during business hours to ask questions about HIV and AIDS. Additional HIV/AIDS services offered by health departments may include case management, partner notification, medical care, dental services, support services, and physician referral.

To find the nearest health department or services you need, consult your local phone directory, or call:

Illinois AIDS Hotline
800-243-2437—8 a.m.-11 p.m., 7 days/week
800-782-0423—Hearing-impaired TTY/TDD
English/Spanish.

6. LIBRARIES AND BOOKSELLERS

Libraries

Gerber Hart Gay & Lesbian Library and Archives
3352 North Paulina Street
Chicago, IL 60657
773-883-3003
773-883-3078—FAX
• Offers a large selection of materials on HIV/AIDS. Archival material collected from Chicago-area HIV/AIDS organizations. Membership required to check out items, but anyone can use the library's resources.

Sulzer Regional Library
4455 North Lincoln Avenue
Chicago, IL 60625
312-744-7616
312-744-2899—FAX
312-728-2062—Hearing-impaired TTY/TDD
• North regional branch of Chicago Public Library offers special collection with books, articles, clippings, and brochures on medical and social issues related to HIV/AIDS.

Test Positive Aware Network
1258 West Belmont
Chicago, IL 60657
773-404-8726
773-472-7505—FAX
773-404-9716—Hearing-impaired TTY/TDD
• Extensive on-site resource center.

Vida/SIDA
2703 West Division Street
Chicago, IL 60622
773-278-6737
773-278-6753—FAX
• STD/HIV prevention project and alternative health clinic. Library, condom distribution, acupuncture and chiropractic services, and peer education training. Public Aid accepted. English/ Spanish.

Bookstores and Mail Order

Amazon.com Books
http://www.amazon.com
• Huge selection of HIV-related books available for purchase on the Internet. You can search by topic, title, or author, so it's easy to find what you need. They can get many hard to find or out of print books.

Lambda Rising Books
1625 Connecticut Avenue NW
Washington, DC 20009
202-462-6969
800-621-6969—Mail orders
• Gay and lesbian bookstore with wide range of AIDS-related books, videos, and magazines. Confidential mail order shipped anywhere in the world. Some publications in Spanish.

Lambda Rising Bookstore Online
via America Online
Keyword: Gaybooks
• If you have AOL access, Lambda offers an easy and confidential way to browse hundreds of HIV-related books. A wide range of books for gay men, people of color, women, families, and others affected by HIV. Gives a description of the book and picture of the cover. HIV/AIDS videos include documentaries, dramas, and educational titles.

People Like Us Books
3321 North Clark Street
Chicago, IL 60657
773-248-6363
• Gay and lesbian bookstore carrying large selection of books on HIV/AIDS.

Pride Agenda
1109 Westgate
Oak Park, IL 60301
708-524-8429
• Gay and lesbian bookstore carrying large selection of books on HIV/AIDS.

Unabridged Books
3251 North Broadway
Chicago, IL 60657
773-883-9119
• Gay and lesbian bookstore carrying large selection of books on HIV/AIDS.

Women and Children First
5233 North Clark Street
Chicago, IL 60640
312-769-9299
312-769-6729—FAX
• Feminist, children's, and lesbian specialty bookstore with large selection of books on HIV/AIDS in their Health section. Carries

books for children affected by HIV/AIDS. Large selection of books on grief; small selection of meditation tapes.

7. BOOKS, PUBLICATIONS, AND VIDEOS

Books

Early Care for HIV Disease (Second Edition)
Baker, Ronald, Jeffrey Moulton, and John Tighe
San Francisco AIDS Foundation
Mail order: Lambda Rising Books, 800-621-6969
• Practical information about early HIV care, written in plain language. Explains what people with HIV can do to stay healthy.

The Essential HIV Treatment Fact Book
Douglas, Paul Harding and Laura Pinsky
PB Company, 1992
• An invaluable guide and reference book for people at all stages of HIV infection.

The Guide to Living with HIV Infection
John, G. Bartlett and Ann K. Finkbeiner
Baltimore: Johns Hopkins University Press, 1991
• A complete resource to help people deal with medical and emotional problems surrounding HIV. Available in Spanish.

HIV Positive: Working the System
Rimer, Robert and Michael Connally
Alyson Publications, 1993
Mail order: Lambda Rising Books, 800-621-6969
• This practical, lively guide tells how to make the medical system work for you.

Immune Power: A Comprehensive Treatment Program for HIV
Kaiser, Jon
St. Martin's Press, 1993
Mail order: Impact AIDS, 505-995-0722
• Skillful integration of nutritional and psychological support and medical therapies. Offers a comprehensive plan for treatment.

No Time to Wait: A Complete Guide to Treating, Managing, and Living with HIV
Siano, Nick
Bantam Books, 1993
• Contains a clear description of HIV disease and its stages, and offers advice on choosing doctors and medical care.

Surviving AIDS
Callen, Michael
New York: HarperPerennial, 1990
• Long-term survivor and AIDS activist Callen offers his personal philosophy of living, along with other essays on surviving the disease.

Surviving and Thriving with AIDS: Collected Wisdom, Volume Two
Callen, Michael, Editor
Mail order: People with AIDS Coalition, Inc., 212-647-1415
• An informative, sometimes radical, always inspirational anthology of articles and personal stories written by people living with HIV and AIDS.

Take Control: Living with HIV and AIDS
Clum, Nathan
AIDS Project Los Angeles, 1996
Mail order: AIDS Project Los Angeles, 213-993-1600
• Comprehensive "how to" guide. Excellent Appendices.

Note: Additional publications are listed throughout this book by topic.

Videos

"Active Duty: Lending Support to PWAs"
Mail order: Howard Brown Health Center, 773-871-5777
• A 60-minute documentary by Chicago filmmaker Ron Pajak on Howard Brown Health Center's PWA buddy program. This video is helpful to primary caregivers or those close to someone with AIDS. It is available for $49.95, or can be previewed for a $5.00 charge.

"Caring for Infants and Toddlers with HIV Infection," and "Caring for School-Aged Children with HIV Infection"
Mail order: Child Welfare League of America, 800-407-6273
• Compassionate videos address rewards and fears of caring for children with HIV. Highlights many issues of daily living, medical care, day care, and school.

"Common Threads: Stories from the Quilt"
Available at video rental stores
• 1989's Academy Award-winning documentary gives an overall history of the HIV pandemic and the Names Project AIDS Memorial Quilt, as well as moving stories from people affected.

"Eating Defensively: Food Safety for Persons with AIDS"
Mail order: National AIDS Information Clearinghouse
800-458-5231—English/Spanish
800-243-7012—Hearing-impaired TTY/TDD

"HIV/AIDS Clinical Trials: Knowing Your Options"
Mail order: CDC National AIDS Clearinghouse
800-458-5231—English/Spanish
800-243-7012—Hearing-impaired TTY/TDD

"Living Proof"
Mail order: Lambda Rising Books, 800-621-6969
• A documentary by Gay Men's Health Crisis about gay men and lesbians living with HIV and in recovery.

"Living with Loss: Children with HIV"
Mail order: Child Welfare League of America, 800-407-6273
• Explores positive ways to cope with loss for families and others caring for children with HIV/AIDS.

"Nutrition and HIV"
Available for viewing at:
Test Positive Aware Network (TPAN or TPA)
1258 West Belmont
Chicago, IL 60657
773-404-8726
773-472-7505—FAX
773-404-9716—Hearing-impaired TTY/TDD
• A short video stressing the important role nutrition plays in managing HIV.

"Silverlake Life: The View from Here"
Available at video rental stores, or through TPA's resource center
• Award-winning documentary of a gay couple's experiences with HIV.

"Sun Chi: Techniques of Relaxation and Positive Imagery"
Mail order: Lambda Rising Books, 800-621-6969
• A self-care video for people with HIV and other illnesses. Teaches the basic principles of tai chi, positive thinking, and relaxation.

"Thinking about Death"
Mail order: Lambda Rising Books, 800-621-6969
• People with HIV and their loved ones talk about mortality, mourning, and loss from different spiritual perspectives.

"What about My Kids?"
Mail order: Gay Men's Health Crisis, 212-337-1950
• Guides parents through the process of arranging guardianship of their children. (Note: Legal explanations from service providers are specific to New York.)

"Work Your Body"
Mail order: Gay Men's Health Crisis, 212-337-1950
• Shows how people with HIV can take steps to stay healthy.

Organizations Offering Additional Publications

CDC National AIDS Clearinghouse
800-458-5231—English/Spanish
800-243-7012—Hearing-impaired TTY/TDD
9 a.m.-7 p.m. Mon-Fri (Eastern time)
• Ask for the free consumer guides, "Understanding HIV" (good for people recently diagnosed with HIV), and "HIV and Your Child." Easy-to-read booklets in the "Help Yourself" series cover common HIV-related infections and wellness. English/Spanish.

Gay Men's Health Crisis
129 West 20th Street
New York, NY 10011
212-807-6655
212-337-1975—FAX
10 a.m.-9 p.m. Mon-Fri,
12 noon-3 p.m. Sat
(Eastern time)
• Ask for their free catalog of educational materials and books.

Impact AIDS, Inc.
440 Cerrillos Road, #F
Santa Fe, NM 87501
505-995-0722
10 a.m.-4 p.m. Mon-Fri (Mountain time)
• Ask for their free catalog of educational materials and books.

Test Positive Aware Network
1258 West Belmont
Chicago, IL 60657
773-404-8726
773-472-7505—FAX
773-404-9716—Hearing-impaired TTY/TDD
• Offers bi-monthly publication, "Positively Aware," and the "Chicago Area HIV/AIDS Services Directory." Extensive on-site resource center.

8. MEDIA

The HIV Talk Radio Project
180 North Michigan Avenue,
Suite 405
Chicago, IL 60601
312-541-TALK (541-8255)
312-541-8258—FAX
• Weekly 30-minute talk show, "Aware: Positive Health Talk Radio," providing information on HIV and wellness, social, medical, legal, and health care topics. Airs weekly in Chicago, St. Louis, Detroit, Cleveland, Kansas City, South Bend, Los Angeles, and Philadelphia. Chicago stations and times: WEDC, 1240 AM, Mondays at 7 p.m. WNUA, 95.5 FM, Sundays at 7:30 a.m.; WLUP, 97.9 FM, Sundays at 4:30 a.m.; WKQX, 101.1 FM, Sundays at 1:30 a.m.; and WLUW, 88.7 FM, Saturdays at 6 p.m. and Tuesdays at 9 a.m.

LesBiGay Radio
WNDZ, 750 AM
1246 West Pratt Boulevard,
Penthouse
Chicago, IL 60626
773-973-3999
773-973-3230—FAX
• Daily "drive time" radio programming for Chicago, surrounding Illinois counties, southern Wisconsin, and northwest Indiana. Gay and lesbian-oriented news and programs include "Positive Living" (Living with HIV) on Wednesdays and "Great Sex!" (safer sex and relationships) on Fridays.

9. LOCAL AIDS SERVICE ORGANIZATIONS

These comprehensive organizations are excellent places to begin learning about local services and living with HIV. All offer information, education, and support to persons at all stages of HIV.

Chicago-Area AIDS Service Organizations

Better Existence with HIV (BEHIV)
PO Box 5171
Evanston, IL 60204
847-475-2115
847-475-2820—FAX
• Individual and group counseling for people living with HIV and their partners and families. Offers a wide range of services, including support groups, case management (including DORS), domestic assistance, a buddy program, financial assistance with rent and utilities, a food pantry, community education and outreach. "Safe Start" program assists homeless persons with an AIDS diagnosis who have a mental illness and/or use substances. Serves northern Chicago and north/northwest suburbs. Free. English/Spanish.

Community Response
225 Harrison Street
Oak Park, IL 60304
708-386-3383
708-386-3551—FAX
• Comprehensive support services for people with HIV/AIDS and those close to them. Provides food, long- and short-term housing assistance, case management, mental health counseling, health and nutrition teaching, peer-led support groups, volunteer services, and companions. Free. English/Spanish.

Cook County HIV Primary Care Center
1835 West Harrison Street
CCSN 1268
Chicago, IL 60612
312-633-3005
312-633-3002—FAX
• Provides medical care, HIV counseling and testing, education and prevention programs, case management, substance abuse and mental health treatment, pastoral care, clinical trials, housing referrals, as well as financial assistance and help with food/transportation. Offers legal assistance through AIDS Legal Council's on-site project. Other services available through the Cook County Hospital Women and Children's HIV Program. Free. English/Spanish.

Hemophilia Foundation of Illinois
332 South Michigan Avenue,
Suite 1720
Chicago, IL 60604
312-427-1495
312-427-1602—FAX
• Hemophilia Foundation of Illinois offers education and counseling for those with hemophilia. Video and reading library. HIV case management, financial counseling, and DORS. Summer camp for boys. English/Spanish.

National Hemophilia and AIDS/HIV Network for the Dissemination of Information (HANDI)
800-42HANDI (424-2634)–
National information line
(9 a.m.-5 p.m. Mon-Fri,
Eastern time)
• Offers information over the phone or by mail on hemophilia and HIV/AIDS as it relates to hemophilia. English/Spanish.

Howard Brown Health Center
945 West George Street
Chicago, IL 60657
773-871-5777
773-871-5843—FAX
• Howard Brown Health Center offers primary care for HIV, outpatient health services including STD and HIV testing on a sliding scale, and social services including counseling, case management, support groups, prevention programs, alcohol/drug abuse counseling, and referrals for legal and other assistance. Women's program offers a health clinic for women, counseling, seminars, and support groups. "Stop AIDS" is a program of Howard Brown. English/Spanish.

Test Positive Aware Network (TPAN or TPA)
1258 West Belmont
Chicago, IL 60657
773-404-8726
773-472-7505—FAX
773-404-9716—Hearing-impaired TTY/TDD
• Self-help organization with resources, referrals, and numerous peer support groups for people with HIV/AIDS, including a group for people newly diagnosed. Peer support, buddy programs, legal clinic, social events, exercise/stress reduction activities. Publishes the bimonthly journal, "Positively Aware," and "The Chicago Area HIV/AIDS Services Directory," Chicago's most comprehensive listing of service agencies. Extensive on-site library of HIV-related books, newsletters, periodicals, and video/audio tapes. Free. English/Spanish.

Outside Illinois

If you live outside the Chicago area, call your local or state HIV/AIDS hotline to find the service organization nearest you.

10. HIV/AIDS EDUCATION AND ADVOCACY ORGANIZATIONS

American Red Cross/ Mid-America Chapter
43 East Ohio Street
Chicago, IL 60611
312-440-2000
312-440-5216—FAX
• Educational services and programs, brochures, and community presentations. HIV/AIDS instructor training for language-specific and culturally sensitive presentations. Also offers HIV/AIDS in the workplace programs. Serves Cook and surrounding Illinois counties; call for referrals to other Illinois chapters. English, Spanish, American Sign Language.

CAVDA — Citizens AIDS Project
PO Box 31915
Chicago, IL 60631
847-398-3378
847-398-7309—FAX
• Education about AIDS and sexually transmitted diseases.

Circle of Hope
PO Box 1152
Woodstock, IL 60098
815-334-9116—Voice/FAX
• Community education and advocacy by and for persons impacted by HIV/AIDS in northern Illinois.

HIV-Positive Action Coalition (HIVPAC)
700 West Bittersweet Place, Suite 207
Chicago, IL 60613
773-871-0130 or 773-871-3475
e-mail: arossi@interaccess.com
• Coalition of HIV-positive people for political action at the local, state, and national levels. Advocacy and education for HIV-positive people.

Illinois Department of Public Health
160 North LaSalle Street, 7th Floor South
Chicago, IL 60601
312-814-4846—Chicago
312-814-4844—Chicago FAX
217-524-5983—Springfield
217-524-6090—Springfield FAX
800-547-0466—Hearing-impaired TTY/TDD
• Information and educational materials on living with HIV, AIDS-related services, and transmission prevention. Referrals to local educational programs throughout Illinois. English/Spanish.

National Association of People with AIDS (NAPWA)
1413 K Street NW
Washington, DC 20005
202-898-0414
202-898-0435—FAX
202-789-2222—NAPWA Fax (automated fax information service)
• Serves as a national resource and voice for people affected by HIV/AIDS. Public policy and advocacy programs, national HIV-positive speakers' bureau, and extensive information and referral program. NAPWA Fax

offers hundreds of up-to-date fax documents on a range of topics. English/Spanish.

Stop AIDS
945 West George Street
Chicago, IL 60657
773-871-5777—Main number (call for other locations)
773-871-5843—FAX
• Prevention education, outreach, safer sex discussions, workshops, and testing buddy program. Prevention programs for substance users and persons in recovery. Lesbian and bisexual women's programs. A program of Howard Brown Health Center. English/Spanish (Mexican, Puerto Rican).

The HIV Coalition (HIVCO)
1471 Business Center Drive, Suite 500
Mount Prospect, IL 60056
847-391-9803
847-391-9839—Hand-to-Hand Food Line
847-391-9826—FAX
• Provides programs and coordinates initiatives to meet needs in HIV care and prevention in Chicago's suburbs. Serves as a clearinghouse and referral service for suburban HIV support groups, services, and education programs. Publishes There is Hope: Learning to Live with HIV. Coordinates the Suburban HIV/AIDS Roundtable, a networking and education forum. Educational programs and quarterly newsletter. Hand-to-Hand Food Program distributes non-perishable food to people with HIV/AIDS living in suburban Cook, Lake, McHenry, and Kane Counties. English/Spanish.

Test Positive Aware Network
1258 West Belmont
Chicago, IL 60657
773-404-8726 (call for meeting location and times)
773-472-7505—FAX
773-404-9716—Hearing-impaired TTY/TDD
• Self-help organization provides a wide range of HIV-related educational and advocacy programs. Bimonthly publication, "Positively Aware," resource directory, on-site resource center. English/Spanish.

11. RESOURCES FOR WOMEN

ADD—Residence for Women
5517 North Kenmore, 3rd Floor
Chicago, IL 60640
773-271-3418
773-271-3550—FAX
• Residential aftercare facility for recovering female alcoholics and substance abusers. Length of stay is three months to one year. Minimum clean time prior to admission is five days. Counseling, AA meetings, referrals, and risk reduction education. Offers outpatient aftercare counseling to women who were previous clients. Public Aid accepted. English/Spanish.

Chicago Women's AIDS Project
5249 North Kenmore Avenue
Chicago, IL 60640
773-271-2242
773-271-2618—FAX
• Counseling, case management, financial assistance referrals, support groups for women, and individual counseling for children and teens of parents living with HIV/AIDS. Also offers child care, second-hand clothing, buddies, social events, massage therapy, speakers bureau, peer advocacy, and STD/HIV prevention programs. Free.

Children's Memorial Hospital
2300 Children's Plaza
Chicago, IL 60614
773-880-3718
• HIV counseling and testing, clinical trials, in/outpatient medical care, outpatient medical/OB-GYN care for mothers of HIV-positive children. Multi-disciplinary medical team with referral to specialty clinics as needed. Public Aid accepted. Multilingual.

Cook County Hospital Women and Children's HIV Program
1835 West Harrison Street
CCSN 1200
Chicago, IL 60612
312-633-5080
312-633-4902—FAX
• Provides inpatient and outpatient care for HIV-positive adults and children, including chemical dependency counseling and clinical trials. Educational counseling, peer education, and training on HIV/AIDS for adults and adolescents, as well as psychosocial services and legal assistance. On-site child care available. English/Spanish.

Gateway Foundation—South
2615 West 63rd Street
Chicago, IL 60629
773-476-0622
773-476-0859—FAX
• Women's group, outpatient substance abuse treatment, and basic aftercare. Accepts pregnant women. Public Aid accepted.

Genesis House
911 West Addison Street
Chicago, IL 60613
773-281-3917
773-281-0961—FAX
• Provides food, clothing, counseling, case management, and risk reduction education to women who have been or are involved in prostitution. On-site residence program for women who have gone through a detox program and are in recovery.

**Genesis House—
West Side Satellite**
743 South Sacramento
Chicago, IL 60612
773-533-8701
773-533-8705—FAX
• Provides food, clothing, counseling, case management, detox and treatment, and risk reduction education to women who have been or are involved in prostitution. Free medical care and HIV testing.

Haymarket House
108–120 North Sangamon
Chicago, IL 60607
312-226-7984
312-226-0638—FAX
• Provides substance abuse detox, case management, residential and outpatient services for women, prenatal/postnatal counseling, education, and HIV test counseling. English/Spanish.

Howard Brown Health Center—Women's Program
945 West George Street
Chicago, IL 60657
773-871-5777
773-871-5843—FAX
• Women's health clinic offers general check-ups, blood tests, HIV testing, breast exams, counseling for individuals and couples, support groups, substance abuse treatment, education, and workshops for those contemplating parenthood. Public Aid accepted. English/Spanish.

Lutheran Social Services of Illinois
1144 West Lake Street
Oak Park, IL 60301
708-445-8341
708-445-8351—FAX
• "Second Family" program assists HIV-positive parents in making long-term plans for their children. Prospective adoptive "second families" trained and licensed. Support group for Gay/Lesbian parents affected by HIV, and case management for parents. "Positive Care" program places state wards with HIV/AIDS, and works with families in reuniting children with their parents. The program also offers medical care, parenting classes, and support groups. English/Spanish. Free.

Planned Parenthood, Chicago Area
14 East Jackson Boulevard, 10th Floor
Chicago, IL 60604
312-427-2276
312-427-2275—Hotline
312-427-0802—FAX
• Provides family planning and gynecological services. STD testing and treatment, HIV testing for women and male partners of clients, birth control/counseling services and referrals, and abortion services and counseling. Seven locations throughout the Chicago area. Spanish-speaking staff at some locations. Public Aid accepted.

WATCH Program
5841 South Maryland Avenue
Chicago, IL 60637
773-702-4317
• Offers OB/GYN, perinatal care, and some adult clinical trials for HIV-positive women. Also offers case management, transportation assistance, and support groups for women. Public Aid accepted. English/Spanish.

Women and Infants Transmission Study (WITS)
Department of Pediatrics
(M/C 856)
840 South Wood Street
Chicago, Illinois 60612
312-996-5510
312-996-7479—Information and enrollment appointment
312-996-5327—FAX
• WITS is a medical research project focused on perinatal transmission of HIV. HIV-positive pregnant women between the ages of 15–44 are eligible to participate in WITS. Participants need not have medical insurance; all study visits and exams are free. Participants receive comprehensive medical care and social support, including prenatal care, delivery, and postpartum care, as well as specialty pediatric care for their infants at the University of Illinois. Also offers other adult and pediatric clinical trials. Call for eligibility and enrollment information.

Publications for and about Women

"LAP Notes"
(Lesbian AIDS Project)
Gay Men's Health Crisis
129 West 20th Street
New York, NY 10011
212-337-1950
212-337-1975—FAX
• The only national newsletter by and for lesbians living with HIV and AIDS. Covers medical issues, safer sex, legal issues, substance use, lesbians in prison, recovery, and resources.

Until the Cure
Kurth, Ann
New Haven: Yale University Press, 1993
• A guide to the medical and social treatment of women with HIV.

"WISE Words"
(Women's Information Service and Exchange)
125 Fifth Street NE
Atlanta, GA 30308
404-817-3441
800-326-3861
(Noon-5 p.m. Tue-Fri)
404-815-7755—FAX
• Monthly newsletter focused on current treatment and research issues for HIV-positive women.

Women and HIV/AIDS
Bere, Marge and Sunanada Ray
Harper San Francisco, 1993
• A comprehensive and accessible international resource book providing information, action, and worldwide contacts pertinent to HIV and women. Good material on reproductive health and sexual relationships.

"Women Alive"
1566 Burnside Avenue
Los Angeles, CA 90019
Los Angeles, CA 90026
213-965-1564
213-965-9886—FAX
800-554-4876—Peer support hotline staffed by HIV-positive women
11 a.m.-6 p.m. Mon/Wed/Fri (Pacific time)
• Quarterly national publication by and for women living with HIV/AIDS. Call for a free sample copy, confidentially mailed. Free to those who cannot afford to pay.

"WORLD"
(Women Organized to Respond to Life-Threatening Diseases)
PO Box 11535
Oakland, CA 94611
510-658-6930
510-601-9746—FAX
• Monthly newsletter with a wide range of articles about women and HIV, including personal stories in every issue. Medical information, parenting and disclosure issues, legal issues, substance abuse and recovery. Call for a sample copy or to subscribe. Free or sliding scale subscriptions for HIV-positive low-income women or women in prison.

Video

"It's Like This..." (1996)
Mail order: RFMH/HIV Center, 212-740-0046
• Story of Gladys, a pregnant woman who learns she is HIV-positive. She lives with her boyfriend, who later tests positive. She learns to cope with many issues around her diagnosis, including telling her sons and family members.

Using a Computer and Modem

Women Alive
http://www.thebody.com/wa/wapage.html
• Created by and for women living with HIV/AIDS, this site includes articles from the organization's newsletter, "Women Alive: Involvement Is Power, Awareness Is Life."

NOAH: New York Online Access to Health AIDS Information Page
http://www.noah.cuny.edu/aids/aids.html
• Extensive, detailed information on opportunistic infections, drugs, nutrition, treatments, clinical trials, and more. Specific information pertinent to women. Some information is available in Spanish <http://www.noah.cuny.edu/spaids/spaids.html>. Includes a search engine and links to other sites.

Using a Fax Machine

NAPWA Fax
National Association of People with AIDS
202-789-2222—FAX
• Publications on women's issues and resources available by fax, including information about sex, nutrition, mother-to-child transmission, and medical problems for women with HIV. Request the "Living with HIV" catalog of fax documents in English. A Spanish catalog is also available. You must be at a fax machine to use the NAPWA Fax service.

12. RESOURCES FOR CHILDREN

Ascension Respite Care Center
1133 North LaSalle Street
Chicago, IL 60610
312-751-8887
312-751-3904—FAX
• Serves families of HIV-affected individuals. Provides in-home and on-site care for HIV-positive children and preschool for children ages 2–5 when regular school is not in session. Also offers case management, individual counseling for family members, mother's support groups, and food pantry.

Camp Getaway
4753 North Broadway, Suite 800
Chicago, IL 60640
773-334-5333
773-334-3293—FAX
• Interfaith and intercultural outdoor respite experience for HIV-impacted families. Sponsored by AIDS Pastoral Care Network.

Children's Home and Aid Society of Illinois—Viva Family Center
2516 West Division Street
Chicago, IL 60622
773-252-6313
773-252-6866—FAX
• Individual, group, and family counseling, and support services for children and their families living with HIV/AIDS. Also offers social activities and psychosocial counseling. Serves Chicago's west side. Free. English/Spanish.

Children's Memorial Hospital
2300 Children's Plaza
Chicago, IL 60614
773-880-3718
312-880-4620—Hemophilia Treatment Center
312-880-3053—FAX
• HIV counseling and testing, clinical trials, in/outpatient medical care, outpatient medical/OB-GYN care for mothers of HIV-positive children. Multi-disciplinary medical team with referral to specialty clinics as needed. Hemophilia Treatment Center manages children with hemophilia and other coagulopathies. Public Aid accepted. Multilingual.

The Children's Place
3059 West Augusta Boulevard
Chicago, IL 60622
773-826-1230
773-826-0705—FAX
• Temporary residential home for children from birth–5 years. Children's play group (ages 2–5), summer camp for HIV-positive or HIV-negative children (ages 6–12), individual counseling, and support groups for children. Respite care. Services available to natural or foster parents and siblings. English/Spanish.

Cook County Hospital Women and Children's HIV Program
1835 West Harrison Street
CCSN 1200
Chicago, IL 60612
312-633-5080
312-633-4902—FAX
• Provides inpatient and outpatient care for HIV-positive adults and children. Educational counseling, peer education and training on HIV/AIDS for adults and adolescents. Also provides psychosocial services, chemical dependency counseling, legal assistance, and clinical trials. On-site child care available. English/Spanish.

University of Illinois at Chicago Hospital HIV/AIDS Project
Family Center for Immune Deficiency (FCID)
840 South Wood Street,
Room Red-5
Chicago, IL 60612
312-996-8337
312-413-1421—FAX
312-413-2562—Hearing-impaired TTY/TDD
• Outpatient clinic for adults and children with HIV/AIDS in the Chicago area. Clinical trials, adult support group, social services, and nutrition. Dental and inpatient care offered through UIC.

Hemophilia Foundation of Illinois
332 South Michigan Avenue,
Suite 1720
Chicago, IL 60604
312-427-1495
312-427-1602—FAX
• HIV case management, education, and counseling for persons with hemophilia. Financial counseling and DORS. Summer camp for boys. Video and reading library. English/Spanish.

Illinois Department of Children and Family Services (DCFS)
750 West Montrose Avenue
Chicago, IL 60613
773-989-5884
773-989-3478—FAX
• Support services for HIV-affected families, children, and youth. Referrals and help in accessing foster care, child day care, and respite care. "Permanency Planning" program helps HIV-positive parents plan for the care of their children. Provides family presentations, counseling, legal services, homemaker, and early

intervention services. Free. English/Spanish.

Jewish Children's Bureau of Chicago "Take Five" Programs
5150 Golf Road
Skokie, IL 60077
847-568-5100
847-568-5125—FAX
• In-home respite care program for HIV-positive, disabled, chronically and terminally ill children ages birth–21 years.

Kaleidoscope-Star Program
1279 North Milwaukee Avenue, Suite 250
Chicago, IL 60622
312-278-7200
312-278-5663—FAX
• Child welfare agency providing services to HIV-affected children and their families. Foster care, independent living programs for adolescents ages 18–21, and in-home services for families in need. Support groups for foster parents of HIV-positive children. English/Spanish.

Lutheran Family Mission
4945 West Division Street
Chicago, IL 60651
773-287-2921
773-287-5181—FAX
• Home-based day care for HIV-affected children at various locations in Chicago. Free to natural or foster families/relatives. English/Spanish.

Lutheran Social Services of Illinois
1144 West Lake Street
Oak Park, IL 60301
708-445-8341
708-445-8351—FAX
• "Second Family" program assists HIV-positive parents in making long-term plans for their children. Prospective adoptive "second families" trained and licensed. Support group for Gay/Lesbian parents affected by HIV, and case management for parents. "Positive Care" program places state wards with HIV/AIDS and works with families in reuniting children with their parents. The program also offers medical care, parenting classes, and support groups. English/Spanish. Free.

Make-A-Wish Foundation
640 North LaSalle Street, Suite 289
Chicago, IL 60610
312-943-8956
312-943-9813—FAX
• Charity providing special wishes to children who have a life-threatening illness. There are Make-A-Wish chapters across the country.

National Pediatric HIV Resource Center (NPHRC)
15 South Ninth Street
Newark, NJ 07107
800-362-0071—Resource Center, 9 a.m.-5 p.m. Mon-Fri (Eastern time)
201-485-2752—FAX
• Consultation, technical assistance, and training for professionals caring for children, youth, and families affected by HIV. English/Spanish.

Starlight Foundation
30 East Adams
Chicago, IL 60603
312-251-7827
312-251-7825—FAX
• Nonprofit organization granting special wishes to seriously ill children. Provides entertainment in pediatric facilities.

Wyler Children's Hospital of the University of Chicago
5841 South Maryland Avenue (MC 6054)
Chicago, IL 60637
773-702-3853
773-702-1196—FAX
• Services for HIV-infected children and teens include a pediatric clinic for comprehensive medical care, case management, clinical trials, mental health counseling for caregivers and patients, transportation, child care, information and referrals.

Publications for and about Children

Child Welfare League of America
440 First Street NW, 3rd Floor
Washington, DC 20001
800-407-6273–Mail Order
202-638-4004–FAX
• Publications and videos for parents, foster parents, and others caring for children with HIV. The booklet, "Caring At Home: A Guide for Families" shows families how to cope with the daily emotional, psychosocial, and physical needs of medically fragile children. To protect family privacy, this publication does not use the word "AIDS." Videos include, "Caring for Infants and Toddlers with HIV Infection," and "Caring for School Aged Children with HIV Infection."

CDC National AIDS Clearinghouse
800-458-5231—English/Spanish
800-243-7012—Hearing-impaired TTY/TDD
9 a.m.-7 p.m. Mon-Fri (Eastern time)

- Ask for the free booklet, "HIV and Your Child: Consumer Guide," an excellent resource for parents and caregivers of children with HIV. Covers ways to keep your child healthy, immunizations, working with a doctor, giving medicines to babies, telling your child about HIV infection, and getting family support. English/ Spanish.

Illinois Department of Public Health—HIV/AIDS Section
527 West Jefferson
Springfield, IL 62761
217-524-5983
217-524-6090—FAX
800-547-0466—Hearing-impaired TTY/TDD
- Coloring and activity books to help children learn about AIDS. Free.

Children and the AIDS Virus
Hausherr, Rosemarie
New York: Clarion Books, 1989
Mail order: Clarion Books, 800-225-3362
- Award-winning book introduces the story of AIDS to schoolchildren. A compassionate book for children, parents, and teachers.

Losing Uncle Tim
Jordan, Mary Kate
Chicago: Albert Whitman
Paperback, 1989
- Realistic story about a boy who learns his uncle has AIDS, and how the boy comes to terms with losing him.

My Brother Has AIDS
Davis, Deborah
Mail order: Lambda Rising Books, 800-621-6969
- When her older brother returns home because he is dying of AIDS, 13-year-old Lacy deals with changes in her family life, in relationships with classmates, and in her commitment to her swimming team.

My Dad Has HIV
Alexander, Earl, Sheila Rudin, and Pam Sejkora
Fairview Press
Mail order: Lambda Rising Books, 800-621-6969
- Story of a 7-year-old girl whose father has HIV. Presented in a sensitive and hopeful way for children ages 5–8.

What's a Virus, Anyway? The Kids' Book About AIDS
Que es un Virus?: Un Libro para Ninos Sobre el SIDA
Fassler, David and Kelly McQueen
Mail order: Lambda Rising Books, 800-621-6969
- A simple introduction to help adults talk about AIDS with children 4–10. English/Spanish.

13. RESOURCES FOR TEENS

Chase House—North
1133 North LaSalle
Chicago, IL 60610
312-751-8887
312-751-3904—FAX

Chase House—South
2555 East 73rd Street
Chicago, IL 60649
773-374-0422
773-374-0370—FAX

Chase House—West
1657 North Karlov
Chicago, IL 60639
773-486-9479
773-486-1240—FAX
- All three Chase House locations offer family support services for HIV-impacted families. Youth/teen and family counseling, day and respite care.

Chicago Adolescent HIV Network (CAHN)
1900 West Polk Street,
Room 701
Chicago, IL 60612
312-633-7438
312-572-3813—FAX
- Provides comprehensive health care and support to HIV-positive youth ages 12–18. The Network is a consortium of four area hospitals: Cook County Hospital, Northwestern Memorial Hospital, Rush Presbyterian–St. Luke's, and University of Chicago Hospital. Serves the Chicago Metropolitan area.

Illinois Department of Children and Family Services (DCFS)
750 West Montrose Avenue
Chicago, IL 60613
773-989-5884
773-989-3478—FAX
- Group home for HIV-positive adolescents ages 13–18 who are wards of the state. Support services for HIV-affected families and youth. Free. English/Spanish.

The Night Ministry
1218 West Addison Street
Chicago, IL 60613
773-935-8300
773-935-6199—FAX
- Shelters for youth ages 14–21 and their children, nighttime street outreach and ministry service. Free.

Project VIDA
2659 South Kedvale Avenue
Chicago, IL 60623
773-522-4570
773-522-4573—FAX
• Counseling for HIV-positive youth and families. Peer educators and resource center. English/Spanish.

Teen Living Programs
3179 North Broadway
Chicago, IL 60657
773-883-0025
773-883-1218—FAX
• Crisis intervention and shelter for youth; transitional living program for homeless youth, foster care placement, life skills education, and substance abuse services.

Travelers & Immigrants Aid—Neon Street Center
4822 North Broadway, 2nd Floor
Chicago, IL 60640
773-271-6366
773-271-8810—FAX
• Multi-service drop-in center for homeless youth ages 13–21. Open 7 days/week. Housing, food, counseling, education, and outreach. Free.

Wyler Children's Hospital of the University of Chicago
5841 South Maryland Avenue (MC 6054)
Chicago, IL 60637
773-702-3853
773-702-1196—FAX
• Comprehensive medical care and social services for HIV-infected teens. Case management, clinical trials, counseling for caregivers and patients, transportation, child care, information and referrals.

Publications for Teens

Growing Up Positive: Stories from a Generation of Young People Affected by AIDS
Lucas, Ian
Mail order: Lambda Rising Books, 800-621-6969
• Real experiences of young people and their families, and how they've grown up having to face the realities of living with HIV and AIDS.

Teens with AIDS Speak Out
Kittredge, Mary
Englewood Cliffs, NJ: Julian Messaer Paperback, 1991
• True-life stories from HIV-positive teens on coping with the disease.

14. RESOURCES FOR GAY AND BISEXUAL MEN AND YOUTH

Aunt Martha's Youth Services
Matteson, IL
708-747-2701, ext. 573
9 a.m.-5 p.m. Mon-Fri
• Social support, HIV prevention education and referrals for gay, lesbian, bisexual, and questioning youth. Call for meeting locations and times.

Gay Men's Health Crisis
129 West 20th Street
New York, NY 10011
212-337-1950
212-337-1975—FAX
• Information, referrals, educational materials, videos, and other resources for gay and bisexual men.

Horizons Community Services
961 West Montana
Chicago, IL 60614
773-472-6469
773-472-6643—FAX
773-929-4357—Lesbian/gay Helpline, 6-10 p.m. daily
773-871-8873—24-hour Anti-violence Crisis Hotline
773-327-4357—Hearing-impaired TTY/TDD hotline
• Offers services and referrals for gay, bisexual, and lesbian adults and youth, including persons with questions and concerns about HIV/AIDS. Offers individual and group psychotherapy services on a sliding scale. Provides short-term counseling for PWAs, their lovers, or the couple together. English/Spanish.

Howard Brown Health Center
945 West George Street
Chicago, IL 60657
773-871-5777
773-871-5843—FAX
• Howard Brown Health Center offers gay-friendly primary care for HIV, outpatient health services including STD and HIV testing on a sliding scale, social services including counseling, case management, support groups, prevention programs, alcohol/drug abuse counseling, and referrals for legal and other assistance. English/Spanish.

Men's Network—Heart of Illinois HIV/AIDS Center
PO Box 1649
Peoria, IL 61656
309-671-8418
• Peer support, health education and advocacy for central Illinois gay and bisexual men. Referrals to HIV/AIDS services.

National Hotline for Gay and Lesbian Youth
Indianapolis, IN
800-347-TEEN (347-8336)
7 p.m.-10 p.m. Sun-Thu,
7 p.m.-midnight Fri-Sat
• Telephone support, information, and referrals for gay, lesbian, bisexual, transgender, and questioning youth. Not HIV specific; not a crisis line.

OUTpost
Champaign, IL
217-239-4688
6-9 p.m. Mon-Fri, 1-4 p.m. Sat
• Referrals to other programs in central Illinois.

Pride Youth
LINKS North Shore Youth Health Service
Evanston and Palatine, IL
847-441-9880
6-10 p.m. Mon-Thu
• Social support, HIV prevention education, and referrals for gay, lesbian, bisexual, and questioning youth. Call for meeting locations and times.

Prism Youth Network
Oak Park Area Lesbian and Gay Association
Oak Park, IL
708-FUN-FIND (386-3463)
• Social support, HIV prevention education and referrals for gay, lesbian, bisexual, and questioning youth. Call for meeting locations and times.

Review
PO Box 7406
Villa Park, IL 60181
630-629-6946
• Meetings and telephone support for adult men who are married or in straight relationships and who are also attracted to other men. Serves men who question their orientation, as well as those who identify as gay, bisexual, or heterosexual. Peer HIV risk reduction information. Telephone information and referrals for female partners of gay and bisexual men.

Test Positive Aware Network
1258 West Belmont
Chicago, IL 60657
773-404-8726
773-472-7505—FAX
773-404-9716—Hearing-impaired TTY/TDD
• Self-help support and information groups for gay men and couples. Also offers self-help support groups for straights.

Windy City Rainbow Alliance of the Deaf
PO Box 138543
Chicago, IL 60613-8543
773-275-1715
773-275-0513—FAX
312-738-9755—Hearing-impaired TTY/TDD
• Social support for deaf gay men. Not HIV specific.

Many other resources, publications, and Web sites specific to gay and bisexual men are listed throughout this book by topic.

15. RESOURCES FOR PEOPLE OF COLOR

AIDS Pastoral Care Network/ Equipo de Cuidado Pastoral Contra el SIDA
4753 North Broadway, Suite 800
Chicago, IL 60640
773-334-5333
773-334-3293—FAX
• Direct spiritual support services include pastoral care and counseling, support groups, bereavement support, and pastoral support in various institutions. Offers faith-based domestic assistance to clients through the "Communities of Care" program. Outreach and education efforts include education for clergy and congregation of all faiths with specialized services in African-American and Latino communities. Quarterly newsletter, "The Spirit." English/Spanish.

American Indian Health Service
838 West Irving Park Road
Chicago, IL 60613
773-883-9100
773-883-0005—FAX
• Community health services center for Native Americans. Primary medical and dental care, transportation, and advocacy. After school program for Native American children.

Asian American AIDS Foundation
4750 North Sheridan Road, Suite 429
Chicago, IL 60640
773-989-7220
773-989-7769—FAX
• Case management, housing (Asian House), home health care, cultural food service, group support, AIDS prevention materials, referrals. Free. Multilingual (Asian languages).

Association House of Chicago
2150 West North Avenue
Chicago, IL 60647
773-276-0084
773-276-7395—FAX
• Foster care, emergency food/ shelter/clothing, and legal services.

Residential and addiction recovery programs for the economically, mentally, and/or physically disabled. Shelter for women. English/Spanish.

Brother to Brother
Mount Sinai Family
Health Centers
5401 South Wentworth Avenue
Chicago, IL 60609
773-288-6900
• Support groups, prevention education, and referrals for African-Americans, primarily men who have sex with men. HIV primary care clinic and case management.

Children's Home and Aid Society of Illinois— Viva Family Center
2516 West Division Street
Chicago, IL 60622
773-252-6313
773-252-6866—FAX
• Individual, group, and family counseling, and support services for children and their families living with HIV/AIDS. Also offers social activities and psychosocial counseling. Serves west side of Chicago. Free. English/Spanish.

Comprension y Apoyo a Latinos en Oposicion al Retrovirus (CALOR)
2015 West Division Street
Chicago, IL 60622
773-235-3161
773-772-0484—FAX
• Case management and support groups for Spanish-speaking persons with HIV. Information on HIV-related issues, alternative therapies, and benefits. Free. English/Spanish.

El Rincon Community Clinic
1874 North Milwaukee Avenue
Chicago, IL 60647
773-276-0200
773-276-4226—FAX
• HIV counseling and confidential testing, methadone treatment for heroin addiction, support groups, and workshops. Public Aid accepted. English/Spanish.

Erie Family Health Center
1701 West Superior Street
Chicago, IL 60622
312-666-3488
312-666-5867—FAX
• Confidential HIV counseling and testing. HIV primary care, case management, and referrals. Public Aid accepted. English/Spanish.

Minority Outreach Intervention Project (MOIP)
1579 North Milwaukee Avenue, Suite 314
Chicago, IL 60622
773-276-5990
773-276-3002—FAX
• Offers peer support groups and prevention education for HIV-positive African-American men. Case management services to African-American and Latino gay and bisexual men who are HIV-positive or at risk. Free. English/Spanish.

People with AIDS Coalition, Inc.
50 West 17th Street, 8th Floor
New York, NY 10011
212-647-1415
212-647-1419—FAX
800-828-3280—Hotline
• Request the quarterly magazine, "SIDAhora" in Spanish and English (produced by and for Latinos affected by HIV/AIDS). English/Spanish.

Project VIDA
2659 South Kedvale Avenue
Chicago, IL 60623
773-522-4570
773-522-4573—FAX
• Counseling for HIV-positive youth and families. Peer educators and resource center. English/Spanish.

Stop AIDS— African-American Program
1718 East 75th Street
Chicago, IL 60649
773-752-7867
773-752-9695—FAX
• HIV counseling and testing, education and outreach to African-American communities. Safer sex discussions, workshops, and testing buddy program.

Stop AIDS—Latino/a Program
1352 North Western Avenue
Chicago, IL 60622
773-235-2586
773-235-2662—FAX
• Offers HIV/AIDS education and outreach to Latino communities. Safer sex discussions and workshops. English/Spanish (Mexican, Puerto Rican).

Test Positive Aware Network
1258 West Belmont
Chicago, IL 60657
773-404-8726
773-472-7505—FAX
773-404-9716—Hearing-impaired TTY/TDD
• Self-help support groups, including programs for African-Americans ("Brothers United in Support") and Latinos. Information and resources for men and women of color.

Travelers & Immigrants Aid
208 South LaSalle Street
Chicago, IL 60604
312-629-4500
• Legal services for new immigrants and persons seeking asylum. Administrative office provides referrals to comprehensive HIV services available in other locations. English/Spanish.

Vida/SIDA
2703 West Division Street
Chicago, IL 60622
773-278-6737
773-278-6753—FAX
• STD/HIV prevention project and alternative health clinic. Library, condom distribution, acupuncture and chiropractic services, and peer education training. Public Aid accepted. English/Spanish.

Publication

La Guia Para Vivir Con La Infeccion VIH
(Third Edition, 1996)
Bartlett, John and Ann Finkbeiner
Johns Hopkins University Press
Mail order: Lambda Rising Books, 800-621-6969
• Revised and updated Spanish-language edition of Guide to Living with HIV Infection. Explains available treatment, offers advice on coping with HIV, and addresses financial and legal concerns. New sections on drugs, special considerations for women, viral load testing, opportunistic infections, and prevention.

Using a Computer and Modem

Closing the Gap
http:www.omhrc.gov/ctg/ctg-aids.htm
• Offers a newsletter from the U.S. Department of Health and Human Services' Office of Minority Health. Topics include "Facing AIDS among Minorities" and "Minority Health Perspectives."

The HIV/AIDS Treatment Information Service (ATIS)
http://www.hivatis.org/
• Web site providing treatment information, the CDC's AIDS Daily Summary, and links to other HIV/AIDS Web sites in Spanish.

Test Positive Aware Network
http://www.tpan.com
• Site includes full listings from the "Chicago Area HIV/AIDS Services Directory," including many agencies serving African-Americans, Latinos, Asians, and other communities of color. Site organizes listings of references and resources in Spanish.

Using a Fax Machine

NAPWA Fax
National Association of People with AIDS
202-789-2222—FAX
• Receive by fax a telephone list of national organizations serving African-Americans, Hispanics/Latinos, Native Americans, Asian-Pacific Islanders, and other minority groups. Request the "Living with HIV" fax catalog of fax documents in English. A Spanish catalog is also available. You must be at a fax machine to use the NAPWA Fax service.

16. RESOURCES FOR FAMILY, FRIENDS, AND CAREGIVERS

Support Groups

AIDS Care Network
221 North Longwood,
Suite 105
Rockford, IL 61107
815-968-5181
815-968-3315—FAX
• Support groups for HIV-positive individuals, their families and friends.

AIDS Support Coalition
PO Box 1548
Crystal Lake, IL 60039
815-459-1985
• Support groups and services for HIV-positive individuals, their families and friends in McHenry County.

Bethany Ministries
Deerfield & Wilmot Roads
Deerfield, IL 60015
847-945-1678
847-945-9511—FAX
• Non-denominational support group for families and friends of those with HIV/AIDS.

Center for New Beginnings
10300 West 131st Street
Palos Park, IL 60464
708-923-1116
708-923-6524—FAX
• Individual and group support for bereavement and for persons affected by HIV/AIDS. Serves Chicagoland area.

**Children's Home and
Aid Society of Illinois—
Viva Family Center**
2516 West Division Street
Chicago, IL 60622
773-252-6313
773-252-6866—FAX
• Individual, group, and family counseling, and support services for children and their families living with HIV/AIDS. Also offers social activities and psychosocial counseling. Serves Chicago's west side. Free. English/Spanish.

Family AIDS Support Network
1258 West Belmont
Chicago, IL 60657
773-404-1038
773-472-7505—FAX
773-404-9716—Hearing-impaired TTY/TDD
• Support groups for families, caregivers, partners, and friends of those with HIV. Provides family members for speaking engagements and educational programs. A program of Test Positive Aware Network. Free. English/Spanish.

Northwest Community Hospital
Joshua Ministries Support Group/Positive Approach
To Health (PATH)
800 West Central Road
Arlington Heights, IL 60005
847-618-4255
847-618-7739—FAX
• Support groups for HIV-positive persons, as well as their families, friends, and caregivers. Bereavement group for persons who have lost loved ones to AIDS.

P-FLAG (Parents, Families, Friends of Lesbians & Gays)
773-472-3079—Chicago area
202-995-8585—National referrals and resources

• Support groups for parents, families and friends of gays and lesbians, including education and advocacy. Not affiliated with any political, ethnic, or religious organization. Chapters across the U.S.; five Chicago-area locations.

Publications and Books for Family, Friends, and Caregivers

<u>AIDS Care At Home: A Guide for Caregivers, Loved Ones, and People with AIDS</u>
Greif, Judith and Beth Ann Golden
Wiley & Sons
Mail order: Lambda Rising Books, 800-621-6969
• Guide to giving quality home care in a comfortable environment. Practical advice on daily routines and common concerns. (On America Online, use keyword: Gaybooks to access Lambda Rising's complete online selection of publications for caregivers of people with AIDS.)

<u>The Caregiver's Journey: When You Love Someone with AIDS</u>
Pohl, Mel, M.D. and Kay Deniston, Ph.D.
Harper San Francisco, 1991
• Comprehensive resource for caregivers helping people with AIDS.

<u>For Those We Love: A Spiritual Perspective on AIDS</u>
Cleveland: Pilgrim Press, 1991
• Focuses on caregiving, friends and family, and grieving from a pastoral care perspective. Developed by the AIDS Ministry Program of the Archdiocese of Saint Paul in Minneapolis.

<u>When Someone You Know Has AIDS</u> (Revised Edition)
Leonard J. Martelli, with
Fran D. Peltz, C.R.C. and
William Messina, C.S.W.
Crown Publishers
Mail order: Lambda Rising Books, 800-621-6969
• Comprehensive advice on everything from dealing with fear and grief to managing medical, legal, and financial issues.

Gay Men's Health Crisis
129 West 20th Street
New York, NY 10011
212-337-1950
212-337-1975—FAX
• Request the brochure, "When a Friend Has AIDS" (Spanish version: "Cuando un Amigo Tiene SIDA").

Impact AIDS, Inc.
440 Cerillos Road, #F
Santa Fe, NM 87501
505-995-0722, 10 a.m.-4 p.m. Mon-Fri (Mountain time)
• Low cost publications include, "Caring for a Loved One with AIDS," "Living with Dementia: A Guide for the Family," "The AIDS Family Guide," and "AIDS Caregiving: Lessons for the Second Decade."

**CDC National
AIDS Clearinghouse**
800-458-5231—English/Spanish
800-243-7012—Hearing-impaired TTY/TDD
9 a.m.-7 p.m. Mon-Fri
(Eastern time)
• Request the free U.S. Department of Health and Human Services brochure, "Caring for Someone with AIDS."

17. RESOURCES FOR PROFESSIONALS

CDC National AIDS Clearinghouse
800-458-5231—English/Spanish
800-243-7012—Hearing-impaired TTY/TDD
9 a.m.-7 p.m. Mon-Fri (Eastern time)
• Medical professionals should call for clinical references, "Evaluation and Management of Early HIV Infection: Clinical Practice Guideline" or "Managing Early HIV Infection: Quick Reference Guide." Produced by the Agency for Health Care Policy and Research. Free.

Gay and Lesbian Physicians of Chicago
PO Box 14864
Chicago, IL 60614
312-670-9630
• Referral service for gay- and lesbian-friendly physicians and dentists in the Chicago metropolitan area. Free.

Illinois State Medical Society
20 North Michigan Avenue, Suite 700
Chicago, IL 60602
312-782-1654
312-814-4500—FAX
• Educational seminars and materials on HIV/AIDS for physicians.

Impact AIDS
440 Cerrillos Road, #F
Santa Fe, NM 87501
505-995-0722
505-995-0780—FAX
• Publishes The HIV Medical Manual of HIV related symptoms and treatment. Written for health care professionals, as well as others who must understand and explain complex medical information to people with HIV and their families. 1996. Also offers a range of other books for professionals, caregivers, and clients.

Midwest AIDS Training and Education Center (MATEC)
808 South Wood Street
Chicago, IL 60612
312-996-1373
312-413-4184—FAX
• Offers training for health care providers in all aspects of HIV disease. Resources and consultation for training workshops for health professionals throughout Illinois. Clinical training programs and clinical conference calls for physicians.

National Minority AIDS Council
1931 13th Street NW
Washington, DC 20009
202-483-6622
202-483-1135—FAX
• Offers technical assistance and resources to help minority organizations provide comprehensive HIV/AIDS services. Free. English/Spanish.

National Pediatric HIV Resource Center (NPHRC)
15 South 9th Street
Newark, NJ 07107
800-362-0071—Resource Center
201-485-2752—FAX
9 a.m.-5 p.m. Mon-Fri (Eastern time)
• Consultation and technical assistance and training for professionals caring for children, youth, and families affected by HIV. English/Spanish.

National HIV Telephone Consultation Service Warmline
800-933-3413
10:30 a.m.-8 p.m. (Eastern time)
• Consultation service for physicians and other medical professionals on the clinical management of people with HIV disease. Referrals to other physician consultation services around the country.

Book

The Medical Management of AIDS (Fifth Edition)
Sande, Merle A., and Paul A. Volberding, Editors
W.B. Saunders Company, 1996
Mail order: W.B. Saunders Company, 800-245-8744
• State-of-the-art clinical reference on all aspects of HIV care, including adult, pediatric, and obstetric patients.

PART 2

Voices of Hope

- You Are Not Alone
- Changes That Have Come from AIDS
- The Effect of an AIDS Diagnosis on My Life
- Treat Yourself Right!
- Positively Positive
- Surviving and Thriving with AIDS
- What Does It Take to Be a Long-Term Survivor?

You Are Not Alone
by Jim Lewis and Michael Slocum

Maybe you tested HIV-positive very recently, or maybe you've known for some time but this is the first time you have reached out for information or support. You need to know that YOU ARE NOT ALONE. There are an estimated 2 million people who are HIV-positive in the United States, including more than 45,000 living in the Chicago area.

Testing positive for HIV does not necessarily mean you have AIDS, but HIV is probably the greatest threat to your life you have ever faced. This virus may remain inactive in your body for a long time, but it may not. If you are healthy now, you may still go on to develop some sort of health problems related to HIV. You may develop AIDS.

There remain many uncertainties surrounding HIV, and although there is currently no cure for HIV infection, there are treatments. You need to learn what information is available and work to make informed choices about your health.

A Brighter Outlook

Many HIV-positive people now live fulfilling and happy lives. Many are healthy and show no symptoms of disease. Many have chosen to take certain treatments and drugs that show promise to preserve and lengthen their lives. So, as serious as this is, THERE IS HOPE! You do not have to look at testing HIV-positive as though you've just been given a death sentence.

It's a good thing you finally found out! As upsetting as testing positive may have been for you, you're better off knowing, so you can learn about this virus and decide what you want to do about it. The fact that you cared enough about yourself to get the HIV test and the fact that you are reading this book shows that you are concerned about your health. So give yourself some credit. You have taken important first steps to take care of yourself and your family, and you should be proud.

Years ago, those who tested HIV-positive had few places to turn for support. These people felt like they were hanging in limbo. Fortunately, much has changed. We know more about HIV now, and many organizations and networks have formed around the world to offer support and information to people living with this virus.

I think you should title the book, "There Is Hope," because there is. When I was first diagnosed with AIDS, from that point to where I am now, I am so relieved! I thought back then I was going to die right away, because of what I saw on TV and heard from other people. I heard the worst stuff about AIDS, and it's not true. Now that I have it and am going through it, I know different. It is a bad disease, but it's not going to kill you yet. Especially if you take care of yourself and if you have a good doctor. Someone who will give you hope.

"LUIS"

When I found out I was positive, I was really angry because I had worked very, very hard to change my life. I really felt I had escaped this disease. I had quit doing drugs and gotten my GED. I went to college; I went to insurance school and became an insurance agent. I had even managed to save up some money—which is almost gone now—to open up my own insurance agency. At first, I felt it was unfair for this to happen to a person who had really worked to change her life. I felt betrayed.

"SONIA"

Many people have already faced the questions inherent in living with HIV, and many more people will follow. You don't have to face this by yourself. There are many hands reaching out to assist you. Remember, *you are not alone!*

Your Emotional Health

Finding out you're infected with HIV is usually overwhelming. Even if you had suspected for some time that you were infected, actually discovering that you are infected can be a very traumatic experience.

Testing positive for HIV has led some people to quit their jobs and quickly write out their wills and say goodbye to their friends and family, only to find out that they are not sick and may live for years to come. It's common to perceive these test results as an immediate death sentence. This is simply not true.

Feelings, Fears, and Facts

What you are feeling now is perfectly normal. Anger, fear, guilt, confusion, numbness, depression—all are completely natural reactions to the kind of news you've heard.

If you've known for even several weeks, you may find yourself having a normal kind of day, then suddenly you remember that you are HIV-positive. It is very common for this kind of realization to "hit you in the face" out of nowhere, over and over again. You are not going crazy if this happens to you. It's happened to all of us. Your moods may swing from profound sadness one moment to extreme anger the next. That's normal, too.

While there are many ways of dealing with all these feelings, the first step in getting through this kind of emotional turmoil is to acknowledge what you are feeling.

One common reaction is numbness—you don't seem to be feeling anything at all. Don't be surprised if you find yourself going through the day in a state of shock. Allow yourself to feel nothing. All of your other feelings will probably come rushing in soon enough. This is one way that your mind "turns off" to allow you to cope with a problem.

If you are feeling angry, that's fine. You have every right to be angry and a lot to be angry about. This little virus is threatening your very existence, and possibly that of your entire family. It's okay to express this anger, as long as you don't hurt yourself or those around you. If you are feeling fearful, acknowledge your fears. You are thinking about things that would make anyone fearful. YOU ARE ALLOWED TO FEEL THE WAY YOU ARE FEELING! Don't be hard on yourself or think that you "have to be strong." You don't have to *be* anything.

Fear of Sickness and Dying

Almost everyone is afraid of getting sick or dying. If you are young, you may never have had to face the death of someone close to you. If you're a parent, your worst nightmare is probably the thought of your child dying. Often we think of dying as something that happens when we are old.

You may have never really considered the possibility of your own death. Now suddenly you are faced with HIV and your mortality becomes very real. You may be very afraid of pain, or afraid that an illness may make you unattractive to others. You may be afraid of hospitals.

Your reaction to the idea of getting sick or dying could go one of two ways. You may decide you're definitely going to live and that there is no way that this virus is ever going to "get you." This is a form of what is called *denial*—refusing to face some of the possibilities of living with HIV.

If you find yourself feeling this way, try to keep in mind that having hope to go on with your life is good. However, it can become dangerous if it keeps you from seeking essential medical care or prevents you from taking care of yourself.

The other way you might choose to deal with the subjects of sickness and dying is by deciding that you absolutely are going to die of this and there is nothing you can do about it. If you go this way, you may find yourself fantasizing about your own sickness and death at the hands of HIV or AIDS.

You need to keep in mind that there are many people who are HIV-positive who are living productive, happy lives, and you can be among them if you choose. It's good to face up to the possible consequences of this infection, but not to the point that living today becomes less important than what you fear may happen in the future. It may help to remind yourself that EVERYONE will die someday, but that doesn't prevent them from living today.

Starting Over

One of the truths of testing HIV-positive is that once you know, you can never *not know* again. For bad or for good, your life will always be different in some ways.

You may be experiencing great feelings of loss about this. You may feel that certain areas of your life are now in the hands of doctors, insurance companies, or symptoms. This can make you feel as though you have less control over your own life and may cause you incredible anxiety.

Know this: you don't have to give up control of your life. By arming yourself with information and deciding what is right for you, you will soon realize that you are still the same person you were. It is YOUR life, YOUR body, YOUR health, and no matter how well-meaning your family, friends, or even your doctor may be, they have no right to take control over your life. Allow yourself to take time to decide what you want to do, then do it.

Times of Change

You may find that many priorities in your life are changing rapidly. If you are considering making major changes in your life, just make sure you think them through carefully.

With HIV, there is a tremendous loss of things that have helped you define yourself. All your experience, education, career, employment, development—it's vulnerable. You can really get down. But then you have to get yourself up and say, "I'm not dead yet—I have to get myself together!"

When you meet someone, the first thing they ask is what kind of work you do. For me, the illness has meant that I'm going to have to reinvent myself and my image of what my life is and where my self-worth is.

WOOD

Many HIV-positive people have made huge changes in the way they live. Many have broken bad habits such as drinking too much or smoking. Some have gotten out of bad relationships or quit jobs they really hated. Facing the possibility of getting sick or dying actually has made many of our lives better because it has made us take action in areas we have previously ignored. Mortality can be a great motivator!

Blame, Guilt, and Grief

Some people blame themselves for being HIV-positive. This kind of guilt and self-hate can be very destructive. Regardless of how you were infected, whether by sexual contact, drug use, blood transfusion, or some other way, you probably did not intentionally go somewhere to get yourself infected with HIV—so why beat yourself up? You are facing enough right now that you don't need to be punishing yourself for testing HIV-positive.

Grief, or extreme sadness, is one of the emotions that most HIV-positive people face at some point. You may be grieving for yourself facing the possibility of your own death. For many of us, this virus is not only affecting our lives, but the lives of those we love. Many have lost friends and loved ones to HIV, or have many people in their lives who are also HIV-positive.

If you sense this grief within you, you should allow yourself to express it in some way. You might try writing down how you feel, or if you can, allowing yourself to cry. These feelings are valuable and normal, and ignoring them will not make them go away.

Positive Self-Image

You may also feel that you are now damaged in some way—that no one will want to touch you or love you or that you are less than desirable because you are HIV-positive. You may feel that you will never be able to love again, that no one would want to be with you if they knew that you are HIV-positive.

You are still a valuable person, capable of giving and receiving love. You can make your own decisions, relax, and enjoy each day. This may be a struggle and you may have to find new ways of coping with daily life, but it's worth it.

Getting Support

Many of us have been raised with the idea of "rugged individualism," that we must face things on our own, that this is what "strength" is all about. Asking for help or reaching out for support are often considered weaknesses. Consequently, a very common response to testing HIV-positive is withdrawal. We isolate ourselves, hiding the news of our HIV status. This can be very painful.

Your life doesn't have to be gloom and doom. It's possible to have a very positive attitude as a person living with HIV; thousands are doing it right now. But it's much more difficult to get on with your life and live happily if you're trying to do it alone.

There is no need for you to handle this all by yourself, and it's probably a mistake to even try. You are not the only person facing this. There are a number of organizations and individuals ready to assist you. Learn who they are and what they offer. Start making decisions about the kind of support you need or want.

Strength from Others

Just hearing how someone else has adjusted to testing HIV-positive can be enough to help you realize that life is still good, and that you can still have love and laughter. And you just might be surprised to learn how your own sharing can help others. Those of us dealing with HIV and AIDS share many issues together and each voice can be a source of support.

Support groups are a powerful means of learning to cope with this new beginning. There are mixed groups, as well as groups tailored to gays, lesbians, straight people, parents, teens, people of color, substance abusers, and others. If there's no support group in your city, you may be just the person to get one going! You could always talk to your physician or a local AIDS organization to get the ball rolling.

Just remember that those thousands of people living successfully with this virus are individuals who've reached out to get the help they needed. Wherever you are, you can find support or the means to help you create it. It just doesn't make sense for so many of us to face the same issues without sharing and supporting each other.

Adapted with permission from "The Body Positive", a monthly newsletter published by Body Positive, an HIV information and peer-support organization in New York City. For subscription information, write: Body Positive, 19 Fulton Street, Suite 308B, New York, NY 10038. Or call 212-566-7333. Reduced or free subscriptions available for people with HIV.

Changes That Have Come from AIDS
Contributed by George

I have AIDS, and because of that I've been able to make a lot of positive changes in my life. Not to say I'm glad I have AIDS—I'm not. But it's made a big difference for me in a lot of ways.

I'm a recovering heroin addict. Until a couple of years ago, I'd been on and off heroin for about twenty years. I can't count the number of times I tried to get off drugs in institutions and hospitals. But all my attempts to stop using them failed.

Five or six years ago, I decided I really ought to get tested for HIV because people around me were literally dropping dead. I finally had to ask myself, "How could I *not* have it?" 'cause I was sharing needles with all these people. And I started coming down with these different things—I had thrush in my mouth, I'd always be tired. But I kept putting off the test. I guess I was still in denial, and I figured things like the fatigue might just as well be from the drug use.

Of course, back then, nothing really mattered to me anyway, except getting more and better drugs. My whole life was surrounded around that, from morning 'til night. I didn't worry about any of my responsibilities, including my children. I didn't worry about making the rent or the phone bill or the car payment. It was kind of like tunnel vision: all I saw and all I'd make out of anything was ways and means to get more drugs. When I had them, I was pretty content. When I didn't, I was miserable, and I'd do whatever I had to to get more—sell things, steal things—which puts you into prison and stuff.

Then I came down with a certain kind of meningitis, which automatically told the doctors I had AIDS. I was devastated. I figured even if I had gotten the virus, I had maybe ten more years. The way they told me was, "Time's up, it's too late. You've already got AIDS."

My immediate response was to go out and party and drink and use all the drugs I could get my hands on. Not really trying to kill myself, but just keeping on with the lifestyle I was already living. You know, a drug addict really don't care for much anyway. Now I hear this, and it gave me that much less to really shoot for in straightening out. I figured well, this is it, George. You fucked up. Now you're gonna die.

The party lasted about two and a half years. Then I got seriously ill with PCP. Since my insurance had run out in New York State, this drug program flew me here to Chicago to get treated. I got cleaned up then, they successfully detoxed me. I don't think I was really expected to live through that.

When I did, it just kind of made me really appreciate being alive. I think for the first time in my life, I really faced death. I guess I always knew some day I was gonna die, but until then I never really felt or believed it.

And that was the turning point for me. Most stories you hear, it's people who go downhill from the time they found out they had AIDS. My life actually went the other way around. I had been using drugs for over twenty years, and now suddenly, I wasn't.

I'm in recovery; I work a 12-step program. I'm still tempted sometimes, but up till now I've done real well. I think being one way for so long, and then seeing what life was really supposed to have been like through all that time—that motivates me. And having AIDS motivates me, because I couldn't live too long abusing drugs and alcohol. All that keeps me pretty much in check, as far as getting back into the old ways.

I kind of regress sometimes. I'll wake up in the morning and wonder, "Is this the day?" But I try to stay away from that kind of thinking. I try to wake up and see the sun, and think about all the things I have going for me. I haven't really been sick that much. I can use my hands and my legs. I can see. I have AIDS, but there's people in a lot worse physical shape than me who *don't* have AIDS.

A lot's changed for me, dealing with this disease—just even accepting that I *have* it. The worst part of having AIDS was what I did to myself mentally, in the beginning. I scared the life out of myself. My attitude sucked. I kinda quit living, tried to drown things in the drugs. I thought, "Why should I look for a relationship, or buy a new home? 'Cause I'm just gonna die anyway."

Because of that negative attitude, sure enough—that's what happened. I was terribly lonely. I didn't own anything and didn't care to. I was getting down to the bottom.

Now today, a couple of years later, because of the way I feel, I'm in a relationship. In fact, six months ago, I got married. I met her in the hospital, she was a nurse where they detoxed me.

My wife's a pretty special person. I haven't met a lot of people like her. I didn't think there would be people out there who'd be willing to get in bed with a person who had AIDS when they didn't—but there are. She's a recovering addict herself, so she's been able to help me a lot with my heroin addiction.

This whole new lifestyle of being in recovery, staying drug-free, has made it easier to live with AIDS. Just realizing who I am and why I'm here. I'm not going anywhere that everyone else isn't coming along with me. There are people out there who are gonna die ahead of me who don't have AIDS. In the end, we're all leaving this planet as we know it. Death is the very last part of living; it's part of life. If it wasn't AIDS, it'd be something else.

There were plenty of times in my twenty using years when I probably didn't even care if I died, but now I really do. Now, I value every day that's given to me. I value my family, different relationships. Things I took for granted mean so much more to me now.

Like I said before, AIDS isn't a blessing; I'm not glad I have it. But in my case it's really turned my life around. In the event I didn't ever get it, and kept on using, there's a good chance I'd be dead from that now anyway—from an overdose, or with a bullet in me. Strange as it sounds, AIDS could have *added* time for me, given the way I was living before. It's been five years now, and counting, since I was first diagnosed.

The *quality* of my life has gotten so much better, too. I do some things now, they shouldn't really be new to me, not at forty years of age, but they *are* new. I eat three meals a day. I sleep eight hours every night. I take all my prescription medicines religiously. I wash my body. I try to do things I should have been doing but I wasn't. I'm more cautious—if I get a little cut, I wash it, bandage it; I kind of baby myself. Maybe that's been to my advantage, too.

My only regret is, I wish I would've gone for emotional help sooner. I wasted almost two and a half years, half the time since I've known I had AIDS. Now it's gone. I wish I'd known then what I know now, in terms of how important having a good attitude is.

If I could sit someone down and tell them what to do when they first find out they're HIV-positive or have AIDS, I'd say: take it easy. Slow down. Don't panic. If you're already in the hospital, don't make a bad situation worse. If you're just HIV-positive and not sick yet, continue on with your life. Easier said than done, I know, 'cause I didn't do it myself at first. But go slow, it might not be that tragic. When you first find out, you think you're gonna die next week, next month. You might not die for another twenty years—they don't know. "They" don't really know much of anything, come to think of it. Remember that.

The Effect of an AIDS Diagnosis on My Life
Contributed by Gail

I am a 35–year–old suburban heterosexual female who is *living* with AIDS. I say living because, for the very first time, that is exactly what I am doing. I am living my life to the very fullest my health will permit and am making the very best out of each and every *single day* I am here. After battling and beating Hodgkin's disease 10+ years ago, someone suggested that I must have dealt with my mortality at that time. That is entirely untrue.

There was a definite "light at the end of the tunnel" for me at that time—a cure—and I never doubted for a minute that I would and did achieve it. Unfortunately, I was transfused during that battle…

Having AIDS is a battle like no other. It has taught me what is truly important in this life, and the preciousness of each and every moment we have to enjoy it.

I am living moment to moment right now and enjoying it immensely. I don't look more than a day or so ahead because my future is very uncertain. However, I feel blessed with a very positive attitude and I do all I can to share that attitude with those like myself who are HIV-positive or have AIDS.

I get so much out of each and every day, and even though I had to leave my job of eleven years, I have the luxury right now of not having to work. Yet, there are still not enough hours in the day to do all that is important to me.

I started a support group with a local suburban hospital and have named it "PATH—Positive Approach To HIV." PATH, along with writing many, many letters for more funding, education, and just about everything associated with HIV, keeps me very busy and extremely fulfilled.

I have a tremendous inner peace with myself and this brings me my most happiness. I also have the love of a wonderful family and some very dear friends. At times, it isn't always easy having AIDS, but in many ways I feel truly blessed for all the knowledge I have obtained with it. I have also developed much respect and tremendous compassion for gay men.

To sum up my feelings in a paragraph: for all that I have been through in my thirty-five short years, and all the pain I have endured, I would not trade my life with anyone. There have been too many moments and too much love and happiness I wouldn't ever want to give up.

This article first appeared in the March, 1991 issue of the HIVCO newsletter. The PATH organization Gail helped found is still going strong in northwest suburban Arlington Heights, with active support groups for HIV-positive persons, their families, friends, and caregivers. PATH also offers a bereavement group for persons who have lost loved ones to AIDS. Call 847-618-4255 for more information.

Treat Yourself Right!
Contributed by Steven

I was tested five times for HIV. Four times I was elated to hear my doctor say the results were negative. The fifth time, my luck ran out.

I never asked the question, "Why me?" but rather said, "Why *not* me?" I never had any bitterness or anger; just the immediate disappointment of perhaps not being able to realize some long-standing goals and desires. I resolved this by simply deciding to push up the time frame in which to achieve them—acknowledging I might not have as much time to bring them to fruition, but never assuming they wouldn't be realized.

It's a waste of time and energy to worry about when you got this virus, or how you got it, or who you *got* it from, because it's not going to change the fact that you've got it. It could be someone you had sex with in 1980. It could've been an IV needle you shared in 1984, that's now showing up. You just don't know. A lot of people torture themselves over this, but it's a waste of time. At some point, everyone goes through this: "Did I do something wrong? Am I a shameful, disgusting person?" Trouble is, some people stay on it for the rest of their lives, and that's not healthy. Take yourself off the hook!

There are many different ways to deal with the reality of HIV and AIDS. Some people try to deny it, until that's no longer possible. Some turn to drugs or alcohol and take a destructive course. Too many choose to give up without a fight and die prematurely.

Still others manage to find positive ways to cope with the ups and downs of this disease. They aren't afraid to ask for help or draw on the strength of others. They realize it's time to start taking better care of themselves. I've personally found that helping others learn to adjust and cope gives me great pleasure, as well as great strength and courage. I also try to be good to *me* and not deny myself the things in life I want—knowing full well that life is tentative with or without HIV!

I decided this winter I was going to have a fur coat. I went to a sale with the intention of buying one—but then I thought, "Why just be good to me? Let's be REAL good to me"—and bought three! Another time, a friend said he couldn't see why I was buying new stereo components when the system I have sounds great. I told him, "Because I *want* to." When there are suddenly a lot of new "have to's" in your life, the "want to's" become very precious.

HIV changes your whole perspective about what is really important. Enjoying life becomes more critical, instead of hassling about this or that. Learning to roll with the punches helps. That doesn't mean rolling over, however. I remain firm and strong in my standards and principles. I take responsibility for the choices I make—some easy, others very difficult—but all, ultimately, mine.

Every time I look out my living room window at Lake Michigan and the high-rises along Sheridan Road, it reminds me of how much I love Chicago and life itself. I have no immediate plans or desires to die. It's not that I'm afraid to die—I'm just not tired of living yet!

Positively Positive
Contributed by Edward Rothas

Dedicated to Mike, Paul, Lamar, Carol, and all of those who have suffered so that I may live.

My name is Ed, and I am thirty-six years old. I have been living with HIV for over eleven years. The purpose of my writing this is to share my experience, strength, and hope with as many people as possible. Because whether you know it or not, we are *all* living with the reality of HIV.

Everyone knows somebody with HIV, although they may not realize it. You can't look at a person and tell if they have HIV or AIDS. Often, people don't get tested before they are hospitalized, or they get sick with this disease even while denying they are at risk. This is the "It Can't Happen to Me" syndrome. But believe me, it can.

Even though I was an IV drug abuser and had risky sexual relationships, I did nothing to protect myself from becoming infected. All I cared about was the pleasure of using drugs and having sex. Besides—none of the people I used drugs with or had sex with *looked* like they were "sick." I associated having HIV with looking sick, and therefore didn't think it would ever touch me. Well, so much for my thinking.

I was arrested on drug charges in the State of Georgia in 1985. I was sentenced to prison, and during the initial intake process was forced to take a blood test. I knew I was at risk for HIV, but I was still in denial. The prison people told me to assume that I was HIV-negative if I didn't hear the results within two weeks. Two weeks went by and I was not contacted, so I believed I was negative. The thought never crossed my mind again until the following week, when two prison officials came to my cell along with two officers in biohazard-type space suits. They informed me that my HIV test was positive. The officers then proceeded to gather all of my belongings and bedding to be taken out and burned. I was told that I would die within five years, and then led out to a segregation area with all the other inmates who were either HIV-positive or had AIDS.

There were ninety people in this special HIV unit. By being segregated in one block, the whole prison knew that we were PWAs (persons

With AIDS). There was a "C" on the uniforms we wore, designating our cell block. So while walking down the corridors, on the way to the infirmary or chow hall, any people we passed, inmates and guards, would shrink away from us—pressing themselves against the opposite wall out of fear and ignorance. They would make all kinds of comments and assumptions concerning our sexual preference. You know the ones: faggots, queers, sissies. They would also tell us to stay the fuck away from them because they didn't want the shit we got. So little was known about the disease at that time, and there was no education about it, even from the prison doctor.

I think the unknown scared me more than anything. I remember thinking that the "C" on our uniforms stood for "contagious." I knew then how lepers must have felt, how gay people are discriminated against—treated like low-lifes, talked about, put down, and even physically hurt. It's sad that there are so many uncaring, unloving, uneducated people when it comes to this disease.

After I learned my diagnosis, the next two weeks were hell. I didn't want to believe it at first. I couldn't sleep. I remember feeling numb, walking around in a daze. I'd never felt so alone in my life. Besides being segregated and discriminated against, all I thought of was that I was going to die alone in prison. Talk about being scared! The way we were treated just fed into that fear. I still have flashbacks to the day I was told, and all that happened afterward. I can still see the terror on the faces of the people in the same situation.

I think that as a result of being diagnosed I was put up for parole early, since I was incarcerated on a non-violent offense. I was released two weeks later.

Upon returning to my home in a small Georgia town, I was visited by a woman from the Department of Public Health. She asked me if I was aware of the fact that I was infected. She then asked what that meant to me and I replied, "That I'm dying." I recall still feeling that initial shock. I guess she could tell I was scared and didn't know what my diagnosis really meant. She had me come to her office and talked to me about HIV, explaining what she knew about it. She also told me of the resources available to me as far as financial and emotional support. Of course, thinking that I was dying, and being afraid, I relied on my "fuck it and run" response. I figured what the hell, I'm dying anyway—might as well go out with a bang. So I instantly started scamming and thinking how I was going to get messed up on drugs. I don't remember much of what the lady told me that day, except that there were other people in my situation and that there was a support group meeting the next evening, and that she would pick me up if I wanted to go. I said YES.

And so I went to my first support group. About twelve other PWAs were in attendance—even a couple of sisters from a convent. I don't remember much from that first group except that I shared my experience of what happened in prison, and I was scared, and I cried my eyes out. I remember feeling empty and spiritually dead. I kept thinking, "Why me? How could God let this happen to *me?*" I was wallowing in self-pity and sensed this was a punishment from God. I was dwelling on all the negatives of my perception of this disease, and how I would be treated as a leper until I died.

Afterward, all those people in the support group came to give me a big hug. This was the first physical contact I'd had with other people in a long time. Their sensitivity was overwhelming. I could feel their compassion when I spoke.

Through my experience in prison, I had lost all confidence in God and in other people. I thought I'd never be happy again. I couldn't understand why God put this dreaded disease in so many good people. It wasn't until I met people who were educated about and living with AIDS that some of that confidence and trust was restored.

At present I have a love/hate relationship with my disease. There are days when I'm not doing so well, when the disease reminds me of its presence. And there are days when I'm glad that it's shown me how to live for the moment and enjoy today. HIV has also taught me to love all people, regardless of race, religion, or sexual preference. Most of all, it's taught me to love *myself*.

On April 14, 1996, I was asked to speak of my experiences at the "AIDS, Medicine & Miracles" conference in Denver. The time of my talk correlated almost to the minute with the revelation of my diagnosis ten years earlier. Today, I am happy about being able to feel as hopeful as I do. This disease has opened many doors and has brought a lot of loving, caring people into my life. It also has given me a new perspective and a goal of helping others every day.

Education lets people make responsible choices in life. I pray every day for the people who still use IV drugs or have unprotected sex. Seeing just how far education goes to reduce the stigma attached to AIDS allows me to do everything that God intended for me to reach as many people as possible. My devastating experiences in prison motivated me to become active in reforming some of the prison rules regarding the treatment of HIV-positive inmates. I've raised money for AIDS research, spoken out at conferences—whatever I can do to help others understand what it is like to deal with this on a daily basis. And I've found *that* keeps me going! It diverts my thoughts away from what the disease is doing to me and makes me stronger. Dwelling on my declining health and surrounding myself with pity and anger only makes me more depressed and more ill.

From AIDS, I have learned that love replaces fear. I have learned to trust in God, in other people, and in myself. Accepting my diagnosis has given me hope and helped me stop seeing this as a death sentence. It has also brought me to a place in my spiritual growth where I have an awesome God who has given me faith, and the knowledge that everything will come together for good. Most of all, AIDS has taught me to be kind, loving, and compassionate, and to respect ALL people.

Today, people can't tell I have AIDS by looking at me. I'm healthier in body, mind, and spirit than I've ever been in my life. I am grateful for the loving and understanding people God has put in my life, and I'm grateful for the chance He's given me to help others. Even with this disease, I know that people love and accept me unconditionally, just the way I am.

Surviving and Thriving with AIDS
by Michael Callen, Editor

Surviving and Thriving with AIDS: Collected Wisdom, Volume Two

I have become more convinced, as a result of my own experience with AIDS and from my interviews with about twenty-five other long-term survivors, that there is a bi-directional mind-body connection which some day we may be able to pin down scientifically. I think the body needs to receive a "live" message. The mind needs to tell the body to fight—that life is precious and worth living. The mind is a great, largely untapped pharmacy and we've got to find creative ways to mine it. Joy juice is what the body needs to live. And hope is like the air that we breathe; without it, we wither and die.

• • • • •

In the first years of AIDS, I had a pretty simplistic notion of hope. I thought that if one believed hard enough in the possibility of survival—if you were a "fighter"—you could beat AIDS. Then some of the bravest and best—fighters who had believed as much as I had that they'd beat this thing—fell to AIDS. I have refined my belief: having hope won't guarantee that you'll survive AIDS, but not having hope seems to guarantee that you'll succumb quickly.

Although I'm winded from years of more or less peacefully co-existing with AIDS, I must now readjust to the possibility of lymphoma (and to the reality of KS). Even in dark moments, when doubt and hopelessness threaten to consume me, I am aware of an almost palpable will to live. The preciousness and exhilaration of living overwhelm. The hysterical *joie de vivre* of Julia Child cooking videos, my cookie cutter collection, the imminent release of Streisand's next album, and the secure sensation of my lover coming to bed sometimes make me want to weep with joy. I should miss them so, if I died.

In the end, I'm convinced that it's as rational to have hope as it is to give up. If 85% of people diagnosed with AIDS are dead after five

> *When people are first diagnosed, whether it's HIV or AIDS, I think it's important for them to know they're not going to die in a couple of weeks. That if they take care of themselves, they can live a long time. I plan to.*
>
> "ELIZABETH"

years, then 15% are still alive. I intend to remain among that prophetic minority.

From the articles "AIDS 201" and "Surviving and Thriving with AIDS," both by Michael Callen. ©1988, People with AIDS Coalition. Reprinted with permission.

What Does It Take to Be a Long-Term Survivor?

In the past, the CDC has defined a "long-term survivor" as a person who lived at least three years after an AIDS diagnosis (or T cell count below 200). However, new treatments are improving the odds that people with AIDS can live long and healthy lives. Because these treatments are so new, health officials are not yet able to offer an accurate definition of a long-term AIDS survivor.

Despite this ambiguity, becoming a "member of the club" remains a challenge. As Lew Katoff, former Director of Client Services for New York's Gay Men's Health Crisis, noted in a speech before the VII International AIDS Conference:

> *Living with AIDS can be among the most stressful of human experiences. All activities of daily life are profoundly affected by loss of stamina, aggressive and toxic treatments, and the ever-present possibility of new life-threatening infections. Living with AIDS requires extraordinary adaptations. Most difficult of all, the longer one survives after a diagnosis of AIDS, the more likely one is exposed to these challenges.*

Lew Katoff's speech was adapted for publication in the October, 1991 issue of "Positively Aware."

Universities and AIDS service organizations around the country are studying long-term survivors (or HIV "non-progressors") to see if they are different in some way from people who developed symptoms much earlier or haven't lived as long. Thus far, researchers have found that attitude seems to be a key ingredient to longevity among people with AIDS.

Taken together, the results of several prominent studies have shown that the majority of long-term survivors:

1) *Are realistic*—they understand and accept their diagnosis. They take steps to educate themselves about HIV/AIDS and keep abreast of the latest medical advances.

2) *Are life-oriented*—willing to learn to live with their condition instead of waiting to die from it. They reject the idea that AIDS is a "death sentence" and refuse to give up without a fight.

3) *Are proactive*—taking charge of their own life and health. They refuse to be helpless or hopeless and do not wait for others to take care of their problems for them. Instead, they learn to handle things themselves. Long-term survivors tend to be assertive—they

can say no when the situation calls for it. They make decisions based on what they believe is best for them, rather than on what others want or think is best.

4) *Are skilled medical consumers*—developing an active partnership with their doctor, in which both have an equal say in how the illness is managed. They are not afraid to ask questions, decline treatments they're not comfortable with, ask for additional opinions, and even change doctors if they don't feel they're getting the care they need or want.

5) *Are analytical*—able to weigh the pros and cons of an issue and make informed choices after evaluating all the facts at their disposal.

6) *Are self-aware*—able to recognize and interpret the signals their bodies are sending them and communicate that information effectively to their health care providers.

7) *Are optimistic*—feeling strongly that life is worth living, and that good times lay ahead. They continue to pursue work and other activities they find personally meaningful to the full extent their health permits. There is a sense of "unfinished business," of unrealized hopes and dreams that must be fulfilled. Long-term survivors tend to feel their lives, and sometimes even the disease itself, have purpose.

8) *Are flexible*—willing to make adjustments in personal habits, fitness level, or health choices to better combat the disease.

9) *Are veteran copers*—often having previous experience in overcoming obstacles or difficult situations.

10) *Are accepting of their own limits*—willing to ask for and receive outside support. Many also find value in giving support to others through volunteering, education, advocacy, and activism.

PART 3

First Steps

1. Taking Charge
    - "My Suggestions for Those Diagnosed with AIDS"
    - "Taking Charge as a Person of Color"

2. Finding and Working with a Doctor
    - Coping with an Insensitive or Rejecting Doctor
    - Why You Need an HIV Specialist
    - Characteristics of the "Ideal" HIV Specialist
    - Finding the *Right* HIV Specialist
    - Streamlining Your Care
    - Narrowing Down Your Options
    - Working with a Doctor
    - The "Baseline" Exam
    - Regular Health Monitoring: The Basics
    - Monitoring Immune Strength and HIV: T Cell Counts and Viral Load Testing
    - Patient Rights and Responsibilities
    - Finding and Working with a Dentist

3. Exploring the Range of Treatments
    - Mainstream Approaches
      Antiretroviral Drugs and Combination Therapies
      Immunomodulators
      Prevention and Treatment of Opportunistic Infections
      Clinical Drug Trials
    - Paying for Treatment
    - "Complementary" or "Holistic" Approaches
    - Learning More about Drugs, Trials, and Treatments

4. Telling Others
    - Whether to Tell
    - When to Tell
    - How to Tell
    - Telling Your Employer
    - Working with Your Child's School
    - Personal Perspectives on Telling
    - Talking with Your Children
    - A Note to Teens
    - Surviving the Company Blood Drive

If you've recently tested positive for HIV or been diagnosed with AIDS, it's only natural to wonder what you can do about it. In fact that's a very healthy sign. It means you want to get a handle on this thing—find some way to control it instead of letting it control you.

The good news is, to some extent you can control it. As little as ten years ago, there were few treatments available to slow down the virus or prevent infections. Now, doctors have a number of good tools to help you live longer and stay healthier, with more in development all the time.

The not-so-good news is, HIV disease can be very unpredictable—and it's hard to fight what you can't foresee. Michael Callen, a nationally renowned AIDS activist and long-term survivor who inspired many others, described it this way:

> *I thought I'd made a separate peace with AIDS, but it's continually negotiating in bad faith. AIDS is a wily adversary. One cannot turn one's back for an instant. The moment you feel you've wrestled it to the ground, it slithers out from under you, to return in another form at another time in whatever way you'd least expect.*

From Surviving and Thriving with AIDS: Collected Wisdom, Volume Two.
©1988, People with AIDS Coalition. Reprinted with permission.

Squaring off against HIV means preparing for the battle of your life. There are several steps you can take *right now* to fight this disease and live better in the process. They include:

1) Taking charge of your own life and health;

2) Finding the right doctor and learning to work together effectively;

3) Exploring the range of treatments;

4) Deciding whether, when, and how to tell others; and

5) Learning to live with HIV (emphasis on *living*).

The first four of these steps are discussed in this section. "Learning to Live with HIV" comprises Part 4 of this book.

The first day I was sitting there bawling my eyes out, and then after that it was like—well, what do I do now?

CHARLIE

When I first found out I was positive, I wondered what was going to happen. I kept looking for some assurances that maybe the situation wasn't completely hopeless, but there wasn't anything out there back in 1985. More than anything, I wanted to know what I could do.

"PAUL"

After I calmed down a bit, I wondered how I could live longer. Was there a diet or anything I should follow? That was the biggest thing—just the fact that I wanted to live longer.

"ELIZABETH"

"AIDS" is just a word but it comes with a lot of decisions. Each day, a different one comes up.

"LUIS"

> *I've seen a lot of people, myself included, who go through a phase of a lot of confusion. You want to know what to do now, how do you handle this, how do you begin to approach it and integrate it into your life? You're at sea for awhile, trying to figure it all out. It was worse a few years ago when there was less information; your doctor would tell you, "Well, go home, take care of yourself, and when you start getting sick, come see me." You were just kind of thrown out there.*
>
> *Now, a lot's changed. There <u>are</u> things you can do. You just have to make up your mind to do them.*
>
> "GARY"
>
> *I have HIV but it doesn't have me! True, I know it is inside me, doing something all the time—trying to break down my immune system, trying to make me weak and sick. But I'll just keep building myself back up over and over again, until maybe the virus will realize it doesn't have a chance, because I know I will never give up. It's just a virus and only has the power that I give to it. HIV cannot control my thoughts—they are my own.*
>
> SHARI

Why go through all this? Perhaps the best answer comes from a person with AIDS quoted in Peter A. Hendrickson's book, <u>Alive & Well: A Path for Living in a Time of HIV</u>, who said:

> *There's a chance that doing these practices will cure AIDS, that I'll lead a full life and become completely healthy. There's a second chance that these practices will lengthen my life until a medical solution becomes available. The third possibility is that I will live my fixed amount of time, but that that amount of time would be much happier and more fulfilling as a result of living this way. With any of these three outcomes, I'm much better off pursuing the self-healing process.*

New York: Irvington Publishers, Inc., 1990.

If *you're* ready to begin that process…read on.

1. TAKING CHARGE

No matter what type of personality you have, finding out you have this virus can knock the wind out of you. If you're used to being in charge, HIV may seriously undermine your confidence. If, on the other hand, you've spent your life drifting along rather passively, it can feel like one more unfair thing conspiring against you.

Taking charge of your life and health is one of the most important first steps in learning to live with HIV. If being in control came easily to you before your diagnosis, with time and support it should again. You already have the inner resources to deal with this from a position of strategy and strength. You'll just have to develop a new set of tactics.

If you've never thought of yourself as being in control of your life, the command to "start now" might sound very intimidating. It would be very easy and comfortable to just continue in your pattern of letting things happen around you and to you. The thought of letting others take care of you and handle things for you during this frightening time may seem tremendously appealing.

The trouble with this passive way of thinking is that it shuts you out of the process. Once you turn your care over to others, it's very difficult to take it back. You become an outsider in the decisions that are made about *your* life and *your* body! If down the road you become uneasy or dissatisfied with the way your illness is being handled, you'll have a much harder time making changes than if you had a clear, active role right from the start.

Fortunately, taking charge is something you *can* learn. It may not be easy. There may be times when you'll be tempted to just give in and let others take over for you. By resisting these urges and staying involved, your chances for survival will be that much greater.

Taking charge means learning to:

1) *Put yourself first.* Decide once and for all that you're the single most important person in your life. Sometimes, this will mean

putting your needs ahead of others', uncomfortable as that might make you. Still, this is no time to "settle." Your health and quality of life are simply too important now.

Putting yourself first does not mean cutting yourself off from others or abandoning your responsibilities. It *does* mean being able to say no at times—or at the very least, "Let's discuss it." You might find this difficult at first. You may feel guilty or wonder if you're being too selfish. If you feel extremely anxious or torn, talking to a counselor might help ease your mind.

Once you decide and believe you're "number one," it will become apparent to the rest of the world, too. People will treat you with more respect because you'll respect *yourself* and it will show. If you act like you're in control, others will treat you accordingly. If you act helpless and lost, chances are you will be.

There may be someone in your life for whom your growing sense of control may be a challenge. A partner, friend, or relative may be used to you being a certain way they liked, or which may have served their needs more than yours. If this is the case and the relationship is important to you, you might try talking with this person about their fears. Together, you may be able to negotiate ways for both of you to feel more comfortable and have your individual needs met.

If anyone in your life threatens you with violence or is abusive in any way, it's time to step away from them. Take yourself and any children you have to a safe place, talk with someone you trust, and assess whether the abuser is likely to change his or her behavior. You need a positive environment and supportive people in your life. You have the power and the right to choose to be with those who respect and support you.

Many women give in to the temptation to put their children's welfare ahead of their own. It's easy to do, especially when you have a lot to think about and are stretched too thin. It's important to protect your kids, but you are as worthy of good care as your family. When you take care of yourself, you are doing something good for yourself and your kids. You are showing them that you care enough about them to make sure that you are as healthy as you can be. You're also demonstrating an important lesson every child needs to learn: how to love yourself.

Another part of putting yourself first is learning to see yourself as a person living with HIV or AIDS—not a "victim" or someone "stricken with" the virus. By the same token, you are not an "AIDS patient" unless you are in hospice or at your doctor's office or in the hospital for an AIDS-related illness. *You are a person, not a condition!* The media is quick to assign labels, and the general population is equally quick to pick up on them. Don't buy into these

---

Obviously it's hard for a woman in an abusive relationship to make demands on a partner. There's justifiable fear that it could result in an abusive episode. So we try to work on negotiating skills, coming up with a new angle. Practicing safer sex, for instance. "It's because I care about you and I care about me, and I don't want to get pregnant that I want us to use condoms"—the counselor and client both recognizing it might take a long time to get to this point, where she could even ask.

DEBORAH STEINKOPF
EXECUTIVE DIRECTOR, BEHIV—BETTER EXISTENCE WITH HIV; FORMER EXECUTIVE DIRECTOR, EVANSTON SHELTER FOR BATTERED WOMEN AND THEIR CHILDREN

Other kids are always thinking about clothes or shoes or movies or music. Yeah, I care about that stuff, but that's not my life. I care more about things like, thank God I'm alive for now. Kids don't always think, "I have to sit down and rest," or "I'm going to go out, I'd better take my coat," or "What time did I take my medicine?" I don't take life for granted. I live my life as healthy as I can.

GINA (AGE 16)

> *If I've learned anything about living with AIDS, it's this: you have to get in charge of your life. If you never have before, you've got to now or the HIV will take over. Remember, you are in control—HIV isn't. If you let your self-esteem go down, and you've given up and already decided you're gonna die—then you'll go downhill fast, believe me.*
>
> *I told my lover, "Guess what—I got a new boyfriend." He said, "What do you mean?" And I said, "My new boyfriend is <u>me</u>!" This virus forced me to make <u>me</u> the most important thing in my life, which I hadn't before. It made me realize <u>I'm</u> the number-one person here. That discovery changed my whole attitude.*
>
> — JIM
>
> *It's true, your life has changed irrevocably—but that doesn't have to be all negative. You can cast a positive light on it. Think of it like this: you now have the opportunity to take control of your life in places you've been neglecting. You now have the responsibility to <u>yourself</u> to take control.*
>
> — "GARY"

misguided attitudes—or hesitate to set others straight when they display them.

2) *Trust your own instincts.* No matter how well informed or well meaning they may be, other people cannot know what's best for you without your input. That's because they're not walking around inside your skin—*you* are. Only you know exactly how you feel, physically and mentally, at any given moment. Only you can hear that little voice in the back of your mind saying, "Go for it!" or "Don't do it!" If something is making you nervous or uneasy, even if you can't put your finger on why, there's probably a very good reason. The survival instinct is one of the oldest and most powerful known to exist. Listen to what it's telling you.

3) *Educate yourself.* It's impossible to "face reality" unless you understand exactly what that "reality" entails. The more you know about your disease, the more you'll be able to contribute to the decision-making process. Having accurate information helps you feel strong and capable. You'll have more confidence in your own input and be better equipped to resist suggestions you don't agree with. In short, "knowledge is power"—and power is what you need to fully take charge.

Don't just educate your mind; educate your spirit, too. Surround yourself with people you admire who give you energy. Find people whose talents complement your own for this fight against HIV. For instance, if you're not good at keeping up with the latest research, find an ally who is. If you're not good at relaxing or tapping into your spiritual self, make friends with people who are. If you're depressed, ask your doctor what you can do to feel better.

Finally, don't forget to train your body! Expect yourself to be strong, and make exercise a regular part of your routine. If you feel powerless and weak, surround yourself with people who are active and make you feel like challenging yourself. If you're tempted to fall into destructive habits, find a support group or talk with a professional who can help you avoid those traps.

4) *Give yourself time.* Few people are comfortable making snap judgments about important matters. Unless you're very ill and need to make treatment decisions quickly, you can afford to take time to think things through. This is not a luxury, but a necessity. When a person feels pressured or has an "every second counts" mentality, judgment often suffers. Don't allow others to rush you, and don't rush yourself with so much at stake. Get used to the idea that you *do* have time! Depending on your personal situation, you can probably take a few weeks to mull over a key decision or devise your "battle plan."

5) *Make decisions strategically.* Responsible decision making is a process, not an event. You owe it to yourself to uncover all the facts and weigh all the pros and cons before deciding on any aspect of your care. Others can help, but no one can do it for you.

The strategic approach does not have to be limited to decision making, but can enhance your life in many other ways. Take routine visits to a clinic or social service agency. To approach them strategically, you'd study the set-up there and determine how you could make it work to your advantage. This might mean getting in early so you can be first in line, having all your paperwork collected and filled out before you present it to the staff, and making friends with key people who can help you expedite things.

Your observations will lead you to many other examples—the purpose being to smooth your way to save time and energy for more important or enjoyable pursuits…which, after all, is a big part of what "being in charge" is all about.

My Suggestions for Those Diagnosed with AIDS
by Christopher D. Sherman

Well, so you have been diagnosed with AIDS! What now?? AIDS is a life-threatening illness that will take control of your life if you let it. Don't! Get angry, get mad, get enraged, but whatever you do, get control of your situation as soon as possible. You don't have to do everything at once, but take control. A lot of people will be giving you advice and telling you what you should do, what doctors you should see, where and what to get for treatment. Your job is to sort it all out.

Now for my advice: first, you must come to grips with your situation. Assess it, your life, your friends, your job; get rid of things that don't work for you. You must work on yourself, not at yourself. Don't blame yourself for your situation. Use it as an opportunity that you would not otherwise have had.

I have been lucky in some respects. I had a good job that I'm currently receiving benefits from, so I have the time to heal myself. If your situation permits, your healing should become your full-time, permanent job.

Don't cut yourself off from life, your friends or relatives. These things can be an invaluable asset when things are uncertain and you are afraid of what may happen to you. The most unfortunate tragedy of AIDS is the fear and ignorance that abound. Some people have lost their families and friends, and in some cases their jobs and homes, when others found out about their diagnosis. I was fortunate in that most of the important people in my life stuck by me, though some at a distance. If friends and relatives offer support, don't turn them away.

I've been working with handicapped, chronically and fatally ill cancer patients for over twenty years. My experience is that people with positive attitudes—those who "follow the program," whatever that is—live longer than people who are negative and bummers.

And the same is true for my AIDS patients. The ones who live longest and best learn to fight, to take an active part in their care. They get spiritual help, psychological help, medical help—whatever they need to take care of themselves. They're able to focus: what's good about today, what's important about today. What did I accomplish this <u>hour</u>, if that's all they can handle. Have a daily goal, an hourly goal. Don't just sit there thinking, "Oh, God, I'm dying!" Because when you think a week from now, a month from now, you're spoiling today.

DR. HARVEY WOLF
CLINICAL HEALTH PSYCHOLOGIST

I'm not gonna try and sugarcoat this, because it's tough. You've gotta have a lot of balls to deal with HIV. It's important for you to take control over the mayhem that's going on in your body.

When you get this disease, you become your own expert. You become the person responsible for your health. You must know what's happening in the field of research. You should subscribe to newsletters or pick them up where you can find them. You need to learn about different drugs. You have to be able to ask questions. You have to learn to tell the doctor exactly how you're feeling, and exactly what's going on if something's wrong—and that you want more treatment, or a new treatment. You'll know your own body better than most people after awhile. The doctor won't know how things are going unless you tell him.

It's important to fight for yourself, fight for your body. Look at it this way: if you don't, who will?

ADAM

When I confronted the issue of who to tell about my illness, I was scared and confused. I finally told some close friends about it, in person; others, I called; and to my family, I sent letters. The purpose of using these different methods was to retain control over each situation. Even this I did not rush out to do. I waited two or three months before I got around to telling everyone. I still haven't told everyone in my life, for it is not important, at least for me, for everyone I know to know about my illness.

You must seek treatment modalities, whether they be traditional medical interventions or holistic healing techniques, that fit within your belief system. Choose what you feel is right for you.

Remember that your doctor is a partner in your healing, and if she or he won't work with you, get another one. If your doctor won't take the time to answer your questions, get another one. Your doctor can't cure you; that is up to you.

Give yourself time to sort out your feelings and emotions. Don't panic and rush about looking for a miracle, because the only place that will come from is within yourself. Learning about your disease will give you some power over it. Don't let it control you. To the extent possible, you must control it.

There is now a lot of information available about AIDS. Use it to assist you. Check out hotlines and newsletters. Look into programs at universities, hospitals, and medical centers near your home. Be willing to take some risks in securing treatment for your condition.

My best piece of advice is to make contact with an AIDS service organization as quickly as possible. They will provide you with services and support you may otherwise not be able to get. Depending on the organizations serving your area, some benefits you could obtain include transportation for medical treatments, food, clothing, shelter, emotional support, and psychological counseling.

Lastly, don't sit around feeling sorry for yourself. This would be the worst thing you could do. Sure, you're bound to be depressed and feeling sorry for yourself at first, but GET OVER IT! Don't be afraid to assert yourself. Seek out the advice of treatment experts and apply to entitlement programs. DON'T be afraid to ask for help. Sign up with an AIDS service organization, get counseling if you feel you need it, exercise, eat right, rest, but most important, do what feels right for you. Listen to your body; it will tell you what you need. Don't be afraid to say NO!

One additional thought: for me, signing up to do volunteer work with an AIDS organization has had a very positive and healing effect. It gets me out of my own problems, and I am also doing something for someone else. Remember: there are other people out there in worse situations than you. It may not seem so, but it is true.

<u>From Surviving and Thriving with AIDS: Collected Wisdom, Volume Two</u>. ©1988, People with AIDS Coalition, Inc. Reprinted with permission.

Taking Charge as a Person of Color
by Steve Wakefield

Steve Wakefield is the former Executive Director of Chicago's Test Positive Aware Network. He has been involved with the HIV community since the early 1980s and has worked full-time with HIV issues for over ten years. As an African-American, Steve has advised agencies that serve people of color as well as those in the broader community, and has an interest in making sure that all minorities get the best HIV information and services available. His advice: "Be aggressive against HIV. Go where there's information and support, then bring it back to your home community."

As a person of color, "taking charge" of your HIV may require a special effort. This is particularly true if you live in a poor community or have few financial resources of your own. For a person of color in America, learning to live with HIV very often means learning to:

1) Accept and cope with your illness despite the denial that exists around you;

2) Seek help in places where you might not feel completely comfortable;

3) Take part in regular, organized health care; and

4) Make positive changes in your life.

Learning to Cope in a Sea of Denial

The first and most important thing for you to realize as an HIV-positive person of color is this: HIV is something you *can* live with. You've learned to live with racism, and not allowed it to stop you dead in your tracks. You've learned to take difficult situations and turn them into winning ones, and to do it without all the resources of someone who comes from a history of wealth and riches. Drawing on this experience, you can also cope successfully with HIV.

However, as a person of color, this will probably take a lot of extra determination on your part. You will find a great stigma surrounding this disease. There will be people in your community who will believe you did something wrong to get HIV. There won't be many people who will understand. The ignorance and fear will be multiplied many times over.

Since the Magic Johnson announcement, this may have eased a bit. I think many people of color now at least have the *concept* that HIV has touched them. Still, there remains a huge amount of denial, mainly because certain subjects are never, ever talked about—gay sexuality, for one. In many communities of color, there isn't a word for "homosexual," or even a slang expression. Thus people tend to say, "We don't have anyone in our community who is gay." That tends to translate into, "We don't have anyone who's at risk for HIV—let alone, anyone who actually *has* it." I think because you're not allowed to speak of it, the denial lasts a lot longer.

Denial of *any* type of sex or sexuality leads to denial of HIV. If I don't have sex with a prostitute, or if I only get a blow job and nobody knows about it, then I'm not at risk. Or if I only did it that one night when I really *had* to, because of the situation, then I'm not at risk. Or if I'm really a "nice" girl or boy, and nobody else believes otherwise, regardless of what I'm actually doing, then I'm not at risk.

Besides the denial of risk from sexual activity, there's the persistent view that HIV only affects Whites. People of color have just not had the opportunity to see themselves in the HIV picture that's been painted by the American media. Until Magic, we haven't had role models who were living with HIV. You never saw HIV-positive people of color in any stories or plays or TV specials. People with HIV were always White and lived in White communities.

So it's hard to believe that HIV is a reality in the Black or Hispanic or Asian communities. If you don't see it, you don't know it's there. If you never talk about it, then you just might decide not to do anything about it when you find it's affected you personally. And that decision could be deadly.

I think about my own family experience. I've gone to the funerals of three relatives who died of AIDS. It's never, ever mentioned that they died of AIDS. In two cases, up until the moment of death, it was denied by the mothers who were the primary caregivers for their sons and daughters. Other friends and family members were asked to help provide care, and all they were told was that the person had "cancer." If this can happen in a family where there's a member who's allegedly well-informed about HIV and AIDS, it certainly goes on in families where there's no knowledge at all.

This level of community and family denial makes it especially hard to tell other people about your HIV. Because of the oppressions and hardships you have faced, you have an urgent need to maintain those relationships that work: with your co-workers, your friends, your family, your landlord. You don't want to risk destroying these relationships by disclosing or talking about your HIV status. Worrying about how others will react can be very frightening.

You may be afraid that someone will "catch" you with HIV or AIDS literature in your home—because if you have that literature, they'll assume you must have AIDS. People won't allow the possibility that it could be just intellectual curiosity, because "the only book worth reading is the Bible." So if you've got a book on AIDS, "You must be doin' somethin' wrong, child—and if you'd been reading your Bible, you wouldn't *need* that other book." These are the negative messages the community sends out that we as people of color have to deal with.

Our churches also perpetuate this culture of judgment and silence. If HIV or AIDS is talked about in church, it's usually in a "Thou Shalt Not" context. If it's already too late, then it's "Thou Should Not Have." In the church, we don't talk about sex or sexuality unless it's in the context of making more people.

In your attempt to take charge of your HIV, you will have to go beyond this sea of denial into a place where you can accept the realities of your illness and *act* on them without fear or indecision. Most probably, this will mean keeping quiet about your HIV status as long as possible in order to avoid hassles, discrimination, and the counter-productive moralizing of people around you. And it will probably mean venturing outside your familiar environment to find the support and resources you'll need to live successfully with your disease.

Help and Comfort in "Foreign" Places

Hiding your HIV status may be necessary to your survival in the community. However, it will make you feel very isolated and alone. HIV is not something you can handle by yourself for very long. If you deny or ignore your HIV infection, it won't go away—it'll only get worse. Neglect it long enough and it may kill you.

To live with HIV, you must acknowledge two things: the virus itself within you, and your own need for support. Some of that support will come from your own inner strengths and resources. But you must also look for support outside yourself. You have to find the people, the tools, and the services to help you fight disease.

Given the denial in your own community, you probably won't find too many of these locally. Many people of color therefore have to decide that there's another community they need to start to belong to. I've heard them express it this way: "I have to find other people living with this virus who've been there and know what I'm talking about. I have to realize and accept that the resources I need to survive won't always exist in the places I want them to be."

And that's probably the hardest part of beginning to deal with HIV as a person of color: being forced to move into a new world on account of your HIV status. In most cases, this will mean creating an alliance with a gay White middle-class world, because that's where most of the services are.

So if I, as a person of color, seek services, I have two choices. I can go to the corner walk-in care clinic where they may have seen only a few people with HIV. Or I can travel into the gay White community and go to an agency or clinic where 80% of the clients are HIV-positive and most are gay White males. I have to deal with what that feels like on top of having to deal with my HIV. I have to travel farther than I might normally travel to get health care. I have to get used to surroundings that are a lot fancier and more intimidating than what I'm used to.

And though I've dealt many times in life with being the only person of color in any situation, be it a work, education, or social situation, that doesn't make things any easier or more pleasant. If I'm already dealing with a devastating illness, it's that much harder to go someplace where I have to be different one more time. Instead of being different *once*, I'm different *twice*. Or if I'm a Hispanic person of color,

I'm different three times: I'm ethnically different, I may be sexually and/or economically different, and I don't understand what these people are talking about. It's definitely not easy.

Still, if you want to survive, you've got to make the effort. You've got to be able to say, "I don't care what I have to go through or where I have to go, I'm going to get help. I'm going where I can talk about and learn the most about my HIV." There's so much stigma attached to HIV that racial barriers begin to seem unimportant. What I am anyplace else in the world is unimportant. Once I'm HIV-positive, once my life is at stake, that redefines me in such a way that I become part of a new whole, a new community.

That means if my doctor doesn't know anything about HIV, I need a new doctor. If the people at the local clinic don't know anything about HIV, I may have to go far away to a different clinic. And those are expensive choices to make, both in terms of human hardship and economics. But I have to make those choices; I have to break out of the mold so I can live with HIV a lot longer.

As communities of color gradually come to accept that HIV is in their midst, resources will begin to appear closer to home. However, it will take them a while to become fully established. So suppose I've been going to this large gay White agency, and they have this fairly nice facility, and I think I'm getting good medical care. But suddenly I hear that in my own neighborhood, there's a place that's starting to provide services.

So I go there, and they're in a rundown old building, and they're barely struggling, and I wonder if they really know what they're doing. But it feels good, because they can talk to me in a language that I'm used to talking in. Still, I question whether I'm getting the right information, because when I was at that other place, they opened a nice notebook, and they flipped through the pages and found what I needed, and were able to print a sheet out of their computer. And in my neighborhood, this woman just wrote something down on a scrap of paper and gave it to me. So how do I know which information is the best for me to have?

I would encourage you to trust the information you get in the agency where you feel most comfortable. If it's accurate and up-to-date information, it doesn't matter whether or not it's given with all the modern technology and trappings. I don't feel this puts down TPA and other organizations like it, because I think HIV has brought in a new age in terms of how we get medical information. We understand it has to come from those people who are living and dealing with the virus on a day-to-day basis. We can't wait ten years for confirmation from medical journals that a drug works. We need answers *today*.

A New Way of Thinking about Health Care

For many people of color, the emergency room doctor is the only doctor they ever see. In a survival-based community where people are transient, new, or poor, health care is not the primary issue. Finding work, staying warm, getting money, dodging bullets—*those* are the issues that matter *right now*. Protecting our children. Putting food on the table and clothes on our backs. Not preventive health care or regular check-ups.

But "crisis health care" is not enough to deal with your HIV. By the time you've been wheezing and coughing for eight weeks because you didn't do anything about it earlier, it may be too late. You may be at a life-threatening stage of your illness. Living with HIV requires a new way of thinking about your body and your health, and your interactions with medical professionals.

At first this may seem very alien, or like it's not worth the bother. That's up to you to decide. The way you make that decision is to ask yourself whether staying alive and well enough to function is worth the bother. If you decide it is, you'll need to make some changes. You'll need to make up your mind to start listening to health care workers—doctors and nurses and other people you may not trust. You might say, "I mistrust them because every time I talk to them or see them, it costs me money. Then it costs *more* money to do whatever it is they tell me to do. So I have to figure out how I can begin to trust them and do what they tell me to do in the least expensive and most creative way possible."

Sometimes, that's going to mean getting health care at a place where I pay for it with my waiting time. I may have to go to a county hospital or public health clinic and sit eight long hours because I don't have an extra $80. So how I have to think of it is, I'm paying for my health care by waiting at $10 an hour. I have more time than I have money, so I have to pay for my health care with my time. And then I can get everything I need, all the information and treatments and tests I require.

As people of color, we often lack the economic resources to pay for the latest drugs and treatments that can keep us alive and healthy. Frequently, the only way we're able to get access to experimental treatments is to join clinical trials. Whenever a doctor or a nurse says there's no proven treatment for something, always ask, "Are there any experimental treatments being tested? Is there a clinical trial I can join? If so, how do I get in?"

People of color haven't traditionally been enrolled in clinical trials in significant numbers. Primarily, this is because these trials have been mainly for people who can afford to get their medical treatment at large teaching hospitals. Trial administrators tended to favor enrolling patients who were well-educated, highly literate participants in their own health care—especially if they had good insurance.

Today, things are changing. There are community-based clinics where you can go to be in clinical trials.

But if I'm going to be in a clinical trial, I have to be willing to listen and ask questions and follow directions. I have to be willing to ask someone to read something to me if I don't understand it. I have to be willing to call back a second or third time if necessary, and ask again how to take my medicine if I'm not sure—because if I don't, I could harm myself. I have to learn that even though I feel better after the fifth day, I take all ten days' worth of medication. And though I may not like the medication, I can't tell the doctor that I took it all if I didn't. I need to tell the doctor it upset my stomach and that I stopped taking it the third day.

So I have to be honest with health care workers and realize they won't deny me services because I didn't do what I was told the first time. Maybe they can help me find a different way to get better. I have to learn to put my trust in organized medicine.

That doesn't mean I have to abandon those spiritual methods of healing that have always worked for me. On the contrary, they may enhance whatever's happening with Western medicine. Qui-gong, herbal remedies, acupuncture, massage—all kinds of things that have long been part of medicine in other cultures have become part of the way we're dealing with HIV in America today. There has been a learning process and a sharing process that is new.

Changes for the Better

I think the final thing that people of color need to recognize is that when faced with HIV, they have to start making some concrete lifestyle changes. And where do I get that list of lifestyle changes? I go back to everything Grandma told me to do. She told me to get plenty of rest. She told me to eat properly every day. She told me not to take drugs or drink too much. She told me to take all my medicine.

And everything Grandma told me to do every day is exactly what the doctor's going to tell me to do to deal with my HIV. So I need to listen to those messages even though they're now coming from an HIV professional. As if Grandma were standing there and telling me, "Honey, c'mon over here and do this." Because those are the things that will keep me alive and help me live with HIV. Paying attention to whatever will keep me healthy and well. That's the most important thing now.

See Part 1 of this book to find Resources for People of Color.

2. FINDING AND WORKING WITH A DOCTOR

As a person living with HIV or AIDS, you face an enormous challenge: keeping yourself as healthy as possible for as long as possible. To do that, you'll need to take a very active role in managing your illness. Once you've "taken charge" of the situation, you can begin to assemble a health care team that meets your personal standards for treatment and care.

You might assume the first step in this process is finding a doctor—but in reality, that's not enough. To have a real fighting chance, you'll need to find the *right* doctor for you. Your ultimate goal is to build a comfortable, ongoing relationship that will provide the foundation of your medical attack.

Coping with an Insensitive or Rejecting Doctor

You may choose to continue with your current physician or find an HIV specialist to work with your present doctor. Some physicians may resist caring for HIV-positive patients because they don't feel comfortable dealing with the complexities of the virus. This is a relatively new disease, treatments can be toxic, and recommended therapies are constantly being updated. Your physician may want you to go to a more informed and experienced colleague. (Remember, it's in your best interest to go to an M.D. with experience.)

If, however, you feel you've been denied treatment or illegally discriminated against, and you need a constructive way to channel your hurt and frustration, write a letter detailing your objection to the doctor's behavior. Send copies to the doctor, his specialty's medical society, your insurance company (if you're in an HMO or PPO), and the chief of staff at the hospital or clinic he's affiliated with. Keep a copy for yourself. You can also complain to an attorney, or contact:

The Illinois State Medical Society
20 North Michigan Avenue, Suite 700
Chicago, IL 60602
312-782-1654
312-814-4500—FAX

Then let go of your anger and move on to more important issues—namely, you and your care! There's no point in trying to force a reluctant doctor to work with you. It's a waste of time and energy, and unlikely to result in effective (or pleasant) care.

Why You Need an HIV Specialist

Even if your current doctor is extremely supportive, you'll still want to evaluate whether she or he is the best choice to help you deal with this new threat to your health. Some people with HIV go on seeing their "regular doctor" for the sniffles and such, but work with a specialist to monitor their immune system and treat HIV-related conditions as they arise. Research has shown that HIV-positive patients of

---

Doctors are learning from our lives how to deal with HIV. We're all new to this disease. More than at any previous time in history, the people with a disease are having a very active, creative part in our recovery, existence, and finding a cure. More of us have college degrees and the common sense to challenge and inform our doctors. We have the media and the Internet to connect people like never before.

"SPARKY"

doctors with more experience live longer, on average, and have a higher quality of life.

If you decide to stick with your regular doctor, you'll want to make sure that she or he knows enough to spot HIV warning signs and refer you for treatment when necessary. Don't be afraid to ask direct questions about how your doctor will stay up-to-date on new developments in AIDS care, and how she or he will pass this information on to you. Remember, you are dealing with a disease the world is just beginning to understand and have some control over. Knowledge can save or prolong your life. If you don't feel your physician will be active in learning more about HIV, see if it's possible to switch to a doctor connected with a teaching hospital or specialized HIV clinic.

Characteristics of the "Ideal" HIV Specialist

The "ideal" HIV specialist is a licensed physician who:

- is board-certified in family practice, internal medicine, infectious diseases, or a related specialty;
- has ample experience treating people living with HIV and AIDS (though it's not necessary that she or he treats these people exclusively);
- is more of a "hands-on" practitioner than a researcher;
- keeps up-to-date on the latest standard of care and encourages you to do the same;
- is open-minded, willing to listen, and follows your lead in terms of how actively you wish to be involved and how aggressively you want to fight your disease;
- is connected to a network of other specialists and willing to consult with them or refer you when necessary;
- will help you explore supplemental therapies and participate in clinical research trials, if you desire;
- encourages you to ask any question on any issue at any time, and answers in language you can understand;
- is sensitive to your particular concerns and doesn't attempt to judge or change you;
- is sensitive to any addiction/abuse history you may have, and will openly work with you on recovery-sensitive prescribing and lifestyle options;
- has a reasonable patient load so that you are not always kept waiting for appointments and don't feel rushed;
- makes sure your medical records are kept confidential;
- has a personality and "bedside manner" that make you feel comfortable and secure;
- has an optimistic attitude toward HIV infection and does not consider the disease to be inevitably fatal;
- is interested in you as a complete human being—a person, not a case or clinical problem;

- respects your wishes regarding life support and living wills; and
- is reasonably flexible about payment schedules, in case you have trouble paying your bill. If the doctor will accept delayed payment direct from your insurance company, so much the better. If you don't have insurance, you may be able to negotiate lower fees for some services. If you have Medicaid, make sure in advance the doctor accepts it.

Finding the *Right* HIV Specialist

You can get names of doctors qualified and willing to treat people with HIV and AIDS from various sources, including:

- your primary care physician (who may refer you to an HIV specialist);
- area hospitals' physician referral lines (for HIV specialists who take the kind of insurance you have);
- your health insurance company (they can tell you which specialists or HIV clinics are in their network, whether they're taking new patients, and how you can access them);
- recommendations from other people living with the disease. Support groups are an excellent place to hear the straight scoop on area doctors from people who've already screened or had experience with them.
- local health departments or HIV Care Consortia. (See the resource listings in Part 1 of this book, or call the Illinois AIDS hotline for their phone numbers.)
- local AIDS service organizations;
- your case manager; and/or
- other physician referral services.

Streamlining Your Care

You may find you need a variety of medical and non-medical services. Maybe you have children, or more than one member of your family is HIV-infected, or you have day-to-day matters you need help with. Whatever your situation, it can be tricky and exhausting trying to run all over town taking care of your business.

When deciding on a doctor or clinic, ask if other types of services are provided besides medical care. Some clinics offer a "one-stop shopping" approach, providing counseling, support groups, case management, chemical dependency treatment—a whole array of services beyond medical care. Besides saving patients valuable time and energy, staff members at these specialized facilities are more likely to be HIV experts who understand the total HIV picture and keep up-to-date in their treatment of the disease.

If child care, transportation, or other matters are obstacles for you in getting the care you need, talk with your doctor to see if the clinic you visit can offer any help.

> *Patients have a right to interview a new doctor—I found that out the hard way! But I also know if you come in belligerent and think you can psych a doctor out, it won't work. If you just go in and say you'd like to speak to him and know what his feelings are toward things, I think you get a pretty good idea.*
>
> "ELIZABETH"

Physician Referral Services

AIDS Foundation of Chicago Information Line
411 South Wells, Suite 300
Chicago, IL 60607
312-922-2322
312-922-2916—FAX
312-922-2917—Hearing-impaired TTY/TDD
• Case management coordination, information and referrals to HIV services and care.

Chicago Medical Society
515 North Dearborn Street
Chicago, IL 60610
312-670-2550
312-670-3646—FAX
312-670-3670—Tel-Med Line (24 hours)
• Confidential physician referral service for HIV/AIDS. Recorded health information to consumers through Tel-Med line. Free. English/Spanish.

DuPage County Medical Society
498 Hillside
Glen Ellyn, IL 60137
630-858-9603
630-858-9512—FAX
• Free physician referrals for DuPage County.

Gay and Lesbian Physicians of Chicago
PO Box 14864
Chicago, IL 60614
312-670-9630
• Referral service for gay- and lesbian-friendly physicians and dentists. Free.

Prologue
800-DOCTORS (362-8677)
• Hospital-sponsored physician referral service, including HIV specialists. Also has names of licensed psychotherapists, clinical social workers, chiropractors, optometrists, podiatrists, nutritionists, dentists, oral surgeons, and physical therapists in your area.

Local Hospitals and HIV Clinics

Listed below is a sampling of Illinois hospitals that have outpatient HIV clinics and HIV-related services (such as on-site alternative therapies, case management, and support groups). Call your local hospital to find out whether they offer HIV services in addition to inpatient and outpatient medical care. Call the physician referral line, or ask to speak to someone in Social Services.

Depending upon your health insurance, you may not be able to choose a hospital because it has an HIV outpatient clinic or specific HIV service. Check your options with your insurance company or health care provider.

Many health departments in Illinois also run free or low-cost HIV outpatient clinics. Call the Illinois AIDS Hotline for referrals.

Alexian Brothers Medical Center
800 Biesterfield Road
Elk Grove Village, IL 60007
888-394-9400
847-981-3580—FAX
• Infectious disease doctors experienced in treating HIV/AIDS. English/Spanish.

Chicago Department of Public Health–Englewood Clinic
641 West 63rd Street
Chicago, IL 60621
312-747-5278
312-747-0292—FAX

Lakeview Clinic
2861 North Clark
Chicago, IL 60657
312-744-2572
312-744-2573—FAX

Roseland Neighborhood Health Center
200 East 115th Street
Chicago, IL 60628
312-747-9500
312-747-2841—FAX

South Side Clinic
1306 South Michigan Avenue
Chicago, IL 60605
312-747-0120
312-747-0160—FAX

Uptown Clinic
845 West Wilson
Chicago, IL 60640
312-744-1935
312-744-5023—FAX

West Town Clinic
2418 West Division
Chicago, IL 60622
312-744-5470
312-744-5516—FAX
• HIV primary care for HIV-positive indigent persons. Also provides case management, anonymous and confidential HIV counseling and testing, and confidential STD testing and treatment. Call for services available at the nearest clinic. Free. English/Spanish.

Children's Memorial Hospital
2300 Children's Plaza
Chicago, IL 60614
773-880-3718
• Specialized outpatient and inpatient medical care, outpatient medical and OB/GYN care

for mothers of HIV-positive children, HIV counseling and testing, and clinical trials. Multidisciplinary medical team with referral to specialty clinics as needed. Public Aid accepted. Multilingual.

Children's Memorial Hospital—Hemophilia Treatment Center
2300 Children's Plaza
Chicago, IL 60614
773-880-4598
773-880-3053—FAX
• Manages children with hemophilia and other coagulopathies.

Columbia Michael Reese Hospital and Medical Center
HIV Care Program
2816 South Ellis Avenue
Chicago, IL 60616
312-791-3455
312-791-4158—FAX
• Multidisciplinary primary care services, including mental health care, case management, education, nutritional counseling, support groups, home health care, inpatient care, substance abuse treatment, pastoral care, and clinical trials. Public Aid accepted.

Cook County Hospital—HIV Primary Care Center
1835 West Harrison Street
CCSN 1268
Chicago, IL 60612
312-633-3005
312-633-3002—FAX
• Medical care, HIV counseling and testing, education, and prevention programs. Information, case management, substance abuse and mental health treatment, pastoral care, clinical trials, housing referrals, financial assistance, and food and transportation assistance. Offers legal assistance through AIDS Legal Council's on-site project. Inpatient care offered through Cook County Hospital. Free. English/Spanish.

Cook County Hospital—Women and Children's HIV Program
1835 West Harrison Street
CCSN 1200
Chicago, IL 60612
312-633-5080
312-633-4902—FAX
• Provides inpatient and outpatient care for HIV-positive adults and children, including chemical dependency counseling and clinical trials. Educational counseling, as well as psychosocial services and legal assistance. On-site child care available. English/Spanish.

Crusader Clinic
120 Tay Street
Rockford, IL 61102
815-968-0286
815-968-3881—FAX
• HIV primary care clinic, dental services, HIV case management, nutritional assessment, HIV counseling and testing, assistance with medications, financial assistance, substance abuse counseling, legal assistance, and DORS. Sliding scale fees. Public Aid accepted. English/Spanish.

Daniel Hale Williams Center
5044 South State Street
Chicago, IL 60609
773-538-6700
773-538-4325—FAX
• HIV primary care, case management, and HIV counseling and testing. English/Spanish.

Erie Family Health Center
1701 West Superior Street
Chicago, IL 60622
312-666-3488
312-666-5867—FAX
• HIV primary care, case management, and referrals. Confidential HIV counseling and testing. Public Aid accepted. English/Spanish.

Holy Family Hospital
100 North River Road
Des Plaines, IL 60016
847-297-1800
• Inpatient and home care, social workers, case managers, nutritionists, and HIV support group referrals. English, Spanish, Polish.

Howard Brown Health Center
945 West George Street
Chicago, IL 60657
773-871-5777
773-871-5843—FAX
• HIV primary care, STD and HIV counseling and testing, case management, support groups, substance abuse counseling, and referrals for legal and other assistance. Women's program offers health clinics for women, counseling, and support groups. Sliding scale fees. Public Aid accepted. English/Spanish.

Illinois Masonic Medical Center—Triad Clinic
938 West Nelson Street
Chicago, IL 60657
773-296-8400
773-296-8401—FAX
• HIV primary care clinic, and outpatient and inpatient care with special HIV/AIDS unit and hospice. On-site alternative therapies through Strong Spirit program, including massage, aerobics, and Chinese herbal medicine. English/Spanish.

Komed Health Center
501 East 43rd Street
Chicago, IL 60653
773-268-7600
773-268-9088—FAX
• Primary care facility provides HIV outpatient care, HIV counseling and testing, case management, risk reduction education, and mental health counseling. Free.

Loyola University Medical Center—HIV/AIDS Clinic
2160 South First Avenue
Maywood, IL 60153
708-216-5024
708-216-8198—FAX
• Primary medical care of adults with HIV infection, including social services, case management, nutritional assessment, and HIV counseling and testing. Referrals for dental, mental health, substance abuse, and home health services. Sliding scale fees. English/Spanish.

Lutheran General Hospital—Nesset HIV Center
1775 Ballard Street
Park Ridge, IL 60068
847-318-9320
847-318-2908—FAX
• Primary care facility of Lutheran General Hospital for persons living with HIV/AIDS in northern Cook County. Offers nutritional assessments and support group referrals. Inpatient care offered through Lutheran General Hospital. Sliding scale fees. English/Spanish.

Mt. Sinai Hospital
15th Street at California
Chicago, IL 60608
773-257-6547
773-257-6027—FAX
• Primary care facility offers HIV outpatient care and home health care services. Case management and referrals to other services. Inpatient care offered through Mt. Sinai Hospital. Affiliated with Sinai Family Health Centers on the south and west sides of Chicago.

New City Health Center
5500 South Damen Avenue
Chicago, IL 60636
773-737-5400
773-737-5567—FAX
• Primary care facility offers HIV outpatient care, HIV counseling and testing, and case management. Sliding scale fees. Public Aid accepted. English/Spanish.

Northwestern Hemophilia Treatment Center
345 East Superior Street, Suite 1407
Chicago, IL 60611
312-908-9660
312-908-1815—FAX
• Primary care, nursing care, social services, and newsletter for hemophiliacs with HIV and their partners. Also offers nutritional and psychosocial counseling, dental and genetic referrals. Public Aid accepted.

Northwestern Memorial Hospital—HIV Center
303 East Superior Street, Passavant 8E
Chicago, IL 60611
312-908-8358
312-908-9630—FAX
• Comprehensive HIV care including primary care for women and men, gynecological and prenatal care, ophthalmological care, and clinical trials. Inpatient care through Northwestern Memorial Hospital. Public Aid accepted. English/Spanish.

Oak Forest Hospital
15900 South Cicero Avenue
Oak Forest, IL 60452
708-633-3731
708-687-7979—FAX
• Inpatient care in an HIV/AIDS unit, acute care, primary care, rehabilitation services (including physical, occupational, and speech therapies), and psychological and spiritual support. Public Aid accepted. English, Spanish, Polish, French.

Open Door Clinic
164 Division Street, Suite 607
Elgin, IL 60120
847-695-1093
847-695-0501—FAX
847-695-8893—Hearing-impaired TTY/TDD
• HIV primary care clinics in Aurora and Elgin. Case management, nutritionists, and information on support groups. Free. English/Spanish.

Provident Hospital
500 East 51st Street
Chicago, IL 60615
312-572-2724
312-572-2799—FAX
• HIV primary care, inpatient care, dental services, case management, and prescription assistance. Psychological and support services on site for individuals and families. HIV support groups include women's group, co-ed group, NA meetings (12-step), and substance abuse group (for persons in recovery or current users). Public Aid accepted.

Roseland Christian Health Ministries
10248 South Vernon Street
Chicago, IL 60628
773-291-6050
773-291-6054—FAX
• Primary care, case management referrals, and low cost confidential HIV counseling and testing. Sliding scale fees or free. English/Spanish.

Roseland Community Hospital HIV Clinic
45 West 111th Street, 3rd Floor
Chicago, IL 60628
773-995-3469
773-995-3199—FAX
• Outpatient clinic for people with HIV/AIDS. On-site Family Focus support group for people with HIV and their families. Alternative therapies, dental services, and case management referrals. Inpatient care through Roseland Community Hospital. Public aid accepted.

Rush Presbyterian— St. Luke's Medical Center
600 South Paulina, Suite 143 AF
Chicago, IL 60612
312-942-5865
312-942-2184—FAX
• HIV outpatient treatment center, inpatient medical care, clinical trials, home health care, hospice services, and pastoral care.

St. Francis Hospital of Evanston
355 Ridge Avenue
Evanston, IL 60202
847-316-2775
847-316-3307—FAX
• Inpatient medical care by physicians experienced in treating HIV/AIDS.

St. Joseph Hospital
(An Affiliate of Catholic Health Partnership)
2900 North Lake Shore Drive
Chicago, IL 60657
888-712-2273—Confidential, toll-free HIV physician referral
773-665-6188—FAX
• Outpatient and inpatient medical care for adults with HIV. Multidisciplinary team includes physicians specializing in HIV treatment, access to clinical trial drugs, comprehensive social services, counseling and support groups, and HIV education/risk reduction. Offers complementary therapies through the AIDS Alternative Health Project. English, Spanish, Polish, Chinese.

Southern Illinois University School of Medicine Clinics
751 North Rutledge
Springfield, IL 62702
217-782-0181
217-782-5504—FAX
• Outpatient clinic with HIV specialists available. Comprehensive HIV services offered, including primary care, case management, social services, and nutritional assessments. Inpatient care through Memorial Medical Center.

Travelers and Immigrant Aid— Chicago Health Outreach
1015 West Lawrence
Chicago, IL 60640
773-275-2586
773-275-3689—FAX
• HIV primary health care for adults and youth, HIV counseling and testing, and referrals. Free. English/Spanish.

University of Chicago Hospitals
5841 South Maryland Street
Chicago, IL 60637
773-702-1000
• HIV testing and inpatient/outpatient medical care for persons with HIV.

University of Illinois at Chicago Hospital HIV/AIDS Project
Family Center for Immune Deficiency (FCID)
840 South Wood Street, Room Red-5
Chicago, IL 60612
312-996-8337
312-413-1421—FAX
312-413-2562—Hearing-impaired TTY/TDD
• Outpatient clinic for adults and children with HIV/AIDS in the Chicago metropolitan area. Clinical trials, adult support group, social services, and nutrition. Dental and inpatient care offered through UIC Hospital.

University of Illinois at Chicago
Community Outreach Intervention Project
4407 North Broadway
Chicago, IL 60640
773-561-3177
773-561-8813—FAX
• Primary care clinic for people with HIV. Case management, HIV counseling and testing, peer support and referrals. Free. English/Spanish.

University of Illinois at Chicago Community Health Project
4650 South Martin Luther King Drive
Chicago, IL 60653
773-536-4509
773-536-2306—FAX
• Comprehensive HIV primary care, dental services, clinical trials, case management, and HIV counseling and testing. English/Spanish.

Veterans Administration Medical Center— North Chicago
3001 Green Bay Road
North Chicago, IL 60064
847-688-1900, ext. 1551
847-578-3863—FAX
708-578-3841—Hearing-impaired TTY/TDD
• Services for eligible veterans including day and respite care, primary care clinics, long-term care, financial assistance, substance abuse treatment, housing/shelter, support services, pastoral care, and HIV counseling and testing.

Veterans Affairs Department— Edward Hines V.A. Hospital
5th Avenue at Roosevelt Road
Hines, IL 60141
708-343-7200
708-216-2410—FAX
• Services for eligible veterans including inpatient and outpatient medical care, case management, clinical trials, dental care, education programs, financial assistance, home health care, hospice, long-term care facility, mental health and emotional support, substance abuse treatment programs, pastoral care, and HIV testing for eligible veterans.

Veterans Affairs Medical Center—West Side
820 South Damen Avenue
Chicago, IL 60612
312-666-6500
312-633-2112—FAX
• Outpatient and inpatient medical care, case management, clinical trials, dental care, education programs, financial assistance, psychiatric services, substance abuse programs, pastoral care, HIV counseling and testing, and support groups.

Weiss Memorial Hospital HIV/AIDS Program
4646 North Marine Drive
Chicago, IL 60640
773-564-5333
773-564-5334—FAX
• Primary care through community-based clinic, outpatient and inpatient hospital care by HIV specialists, social work services, support groups, complementary therapies (art, massage), health education, clinical trials, financial assistance with medications, and HIV counseling and testing. Public Aid accepted. English, Spanish, Vietnamese.

Winfield Moody Community Health Center
1276 North Clybourn
Chicago, IL 60610
312-337-1073
312-337-7616—FAX
• Primary care facility offering case management, confidential HIV counseling and testing, nutritional counseling, social services, and outpatient substance abuse treatment. Sliding scale fees.

Wyler Children's Hospital of the University of Chicago
5841 South Maryland Avenue (MC 6054)
Chicago, IL 60637
773-702-3853
773-702-1196—FAX
• Services for HIV-infected children and teens include a pediatric clinic for comprehensive medical care, perinatal/women's services through the OB/GYN department, case management, clinical trials, HIV counseling and testing, mental health counseling for caregivers and patients, transportation, child care, information and referrals. Public Aid accepted.

Narrowing Down Your Options

After you've selected several good candidates for your new HIV specialist, you'll want to narrow down your list and make a choice. If you have an HMO or PPO, make certain the doctors you have in mind are on its acceptance list. You'll also want to make sure the doctor's office or clinic accepts your insurance. (In addition, it's a good idea to find out if they'll accept Medicaid, whether or not you currently have it.) If you don't have any insurance, your options may be limited to doctors affiliated with public hospitals and health clinics.

The best way to choose your new doctor is to have an initial visit with each candidate and decide from there if you want to sign on with one of them. Some doctors will charge you for this visit while others may agree to meet with you at no cost. Some insurance plans will limit your options to a finite list of care providers.

In his best-selling book *Final Exit*, author Derek Humphry offers some excellent advice on how to conduct this screening process with your "finalists":

> *Call ahead and make appointments with these doctors. Say that you would require 15 or 20 minutes of the doctor's time. You will find that most will appreciate your investigations. For the most part, doctors today are not as stuffy and formal as they used to be.*
>
> *While you are waiting to see the doctor for this selection interview, assess the appearance of the waiting room and whether the magazines are changed regularly. Are the staff pleasant and helpful? Here are clues to the level of consideration given to the patient. You do not want a doctor who is just running a business! If you are kept waiting some time, observe whether the doctor apologizes for the delay and at least hints at the reason why.*
>
> *Be quick to put the doctor at ease. You do the talking. Tell who you are, where you live, and what your health priorities will be. Be candid about why you are changing doctors….*
>
> *Don't be nervous about asking your doctor for some objective criteria. Where did qualification as a physician take place and when? At which hospital or hospitals does the doctor have privileges? Is this doctor a board-certified specialist? It is very important to ask what arrangements can be made for your medical records to be transferred from your old doctor to a new one….*
>
> *Do not sign up with any doctor on the spot. Go home and think about your research. Of course, if you have a spouse or companion, it is preferable that you make these doctor shopping visits together. When one of you is ill, it is often the companion who must communicate a great deal with the doctor. Share your thoughts about the various doctors before coming to a decision.*
>
> *When you have made your choice, find out which hospital that doctor most uses for admitting patients. This hospital may have a pre-admission procedure [which can streamline the paperwork if you enter at some point]. …If possible, get copies of your Living Will and Durable Power of Attorney for*

One of the first things I'd advise for someone who's just been diagnosed is, you'd better get a doctor who A) if you are gay, understands and accepts your homosexuality; B) is really up-to-date about this disease; and C) is not afraid to ask another doctor for advice. It's important to have a doctor who doesn't have ego problems or thinks he knows everything, because he doesn't.

Old family doctors may have brought you into this world, seen you through all the childhood diseases— but we're talking about something totally new here, a new kind of disease. And unless they are really keeping themselves current, most older doctors won't know much of anything beyond what they've read.

JIM

Health Care lodged with the hospital in advance. (You will by now have deposited them with your doctor.)…

Until tested by serious problems, you cannot make a perfect assessment of which doctor is the best for you. All you can do while "shopping around" is to check if you can communicate well with this person. But that is a big start.

From Final Exit, ©1991, The Hemlock Society. Reprinted with permission.

Working with a Doctor

Finding the right doctor is only half the battle. Once you settle on one, you'll need to learn how to work together effectively. It's important to establish a *partnership* with the doctor right up front. Make sure it's understood that you intend to take an active role in managing your illness and expect to be involved in all decisions affecting your care.

In general, be respectful but assertive. Speak as well as listen; lead as well as follow. Keep the lines of communication open at all times. Between visits, don't be timid about alerting your doctor to new developments in the field. At the same time, ask your doctor to keep you informed.

The "Baseline" Exam

Your first real appointment with your new doctor probably will involve a "baseline" examination. The purpose of this exam is to find out how well your immune system is functioning now, and to establish a point of comparison for changes that may occur later on.

If you're working with an HIV specialist, she or he will want to run tests to measure your immune function and the level of HIV in your body, order a baseline chest X-ray, give you a skin test for tuberculosis (TB), and perform a thorough physical exam. Be prepared to answer a lot of questions about yourself and your medical history. (Remember that anything you say to your physician is protected under the rules of doctor-patient confidentiality—so don't hold back. Answer the questions posed to you as honestly and completely as you can.) If you have a record of your previous vaccinations, bring it with you. If your vaccinations aren't current, now might be a good time to renew them. Bring along any medications, vitamins, or supplements you are currently taking for the doctor to review.

Female patients will need some additional tests. Women living with HIV are especially prone to recurring gynecological problems such as vaginal yeast infections and pelvic inflammatory disease. Cervical cancer is also more common in HIV-positive women. If the doctor doesn't think of it, you may want to request a Pap smear and tests for sexually transmitted diseases and cervical abnormalities at this time.

If you decide to continue working with your "regular" doctor instead of an HIV specialist, there might be some confusion as to which tests are needed or what early warning signals to watch out for. If that's the case, you and your doctor may want to do some preliminary reading, or consider a specialist for a consultation. If you don't mesh well with the specialist, tell your regular M.D. and ask for a referral to a different specialist you can check with periodically.

The first doctor I had, I think he was very good and I had nothing against him. But he was a North Shore doctor, and I think I was his only gay patient, at least that he knew of. I'm sure I was his first patient with the virus. He's probably run into it since, but in 1985, I think it shocked him as much as it did me.

I decided I should get another doctor who knew more about all this, who had a good attitude and was familiar enough with gay concerns so if you went in and told him you had done some act or something, he wouldn't say, "Well, what's <u>that</u>?!" I wanted a doctor I could be comfortable with. One man I went to was very business-like. When I mentioned this to a friend, she said, "Well, you're not going to marry him!"

But with such a serious thing as this, you have to take the whole person into account, their emotions and everything. You need a doctor who's compassionate, who isn't going to hit you over the head all the time with a sledgehammer. We're all going to have to be let down at some point; you want him to do it in the easiest way possible. You want to be able to trust him.

"PAUL"

Regular Health Monitoring: The Basics

After this baseline visit, you'll want to have regular checkups to monitor your "immune status" (meaning your ability to resist opportunistic infections). Do this even if you feel fine and have no symptoms. HIV can progress without notice, weakening your resistance without your knowing it. Keeping a close eye on your immune status will help you know when to take specific measures to prevent serious disease. You and your doctor can decide together how frequent these checkups will be. If you are ill or taking medication, you'll probably be seeing the doctor more often. Women also are advised to have more frequent gynecological exams.

At your baseline checkup and each regular visit thereafter, feel free to take notes or run a tape recorder if it will help you remember the doctor's instructions. Start a health journal in order to keep track of your symptoms and medications, and questions that come up between visits. (See the Appendices for sample forms to copy and use.) Bring this journal to your doctor's office to help you remember what you want to talk about.

At each appointment, describe as thoroughly and specifically as possible any symptoms you may have had. Learn to discuss your situation frankly. Detailed information about stressors in your life, eating, sleeping and exercise habits, sexual practices, and use of alcohol, tobacco, caffeine, and other drugs will make your doctor better able to evaluate your health and help you arrive at appropriate treatment decisions. As mentioned, anything you discuss will be kept confidential. Also, most experienced M.D.s have "heard it all." A good doctor is not likely to be shocked by anything you might choose to reveal about yourself.

You may find it difficult to assert yourself where your doctor is concerned. However, it's the only way to become a full, responsible partner in your medical care. Don't feel you have to be a "good patient" and not take up too much of the doctor's valuable time. Your time is just as valuable, and your questions and concerns need to be addressed. Also, now is not the time to worry about appearing ignorant. Don't be afraid to ask the doctor to repeat or re-explain something you didn't understand or are worried about. Doctors are not mind-readers; they won't know you still have questions or be able to answer them unless you ask.

Monitoring Immune Strength and HIV: T Cell Counts and Viral Load Testing

To fight HIV effectively, you and your doctor will want to schedule periodic tests to determine how well your immune system is standing up to the HIV onslaught, and how large that attack is at any given time. Results from T cell and viral load counts, taken in tandem, paint a clear picture of the ongoing struggle between HIV and your immune system.

To me, it seems like a lot of doctors focus in on their area of responsibility and they have blinders for the rest of your body. A foot doctor just looks at your foot. A lung doctor doesn't think of the whole picture. You need a doctor who can look at the whole person, who understands what is going on with your body and this virus that's now in it.

"LUIS"

In the past, researchers believed that after a person was infected, the virus initially was very active (sometimes causing a flu-like illness), and then lay dormant in the body for a period of time before wreaking havoc on the body's immune system. We now know that from the moment of infection the virus is active, even in those patients who have no symptoms for years. HIV takes control of the "helper" T cells (or CD4 cells) of the immune system, and uses them to create more than 10 billion copies of itself each day. Of these, 100 million are capable of "replicating," or copying, themselves.

Infected T cells die within about two days, and more are constantly being produced to replace them. If the body cannot create new cells quickly enough, the T cell count drops. When that happens, a person's resistance to disease is lowered—their immunity is down. T cell counts don't measure HIV, but the level of your body's ability to fight disease. A T cell count of 800 to 1,200 (meaning 800 to 1,200 T cells per cubic milliliter of blood) is normal for a healthy adult. Below 200 T cells, an HIV-positive person is at increased risk for Pneumocystis carinii pneumonia (PCP). The lower the T cell count, the greater the risk other types of infections will occur. Still, some people remain well (or "asymptomatic") for long periods, even after their T cell count has dropped into double digits.

Whereas T cell counts indicate the strength of a person's immune system, viral load counts measure the size of HIV's assault on the immune system. Viral load is a measure of viral particles (called "virions") that are free-floating in the bloodstream. Viral loads are measured using tests called bDNA, RNA assay, NASBA, or polymerase chain reaction (PCR).

HIV-positive patients with high viral load counts appear to be at greater risk for serious illness or death than those whose viral loads are at more moderate levels. In adults, a pattern of high viral load counts (50,000 to 100,000 copies per cubic milliliter of blood) indicates a greater likelihood that the disease will progress. Counts of 5,000 and below suggest a much lower risk of that happening.

Many things can affect your results, so it's important not to put too much weight on any single test score. What matters is how the results look over a period of time, and especially how they look in relation to one another. The best-case scenario is a high T cell count and a low viral load count.

Viral load counts in infants and children are different from those of adults. Counts can run more typically into the 100,000–200,000+ range and vary far more than in adults. Experts know very little about viral loads in children—what constitutes a high or low level and how that relates to the child's health. Many believe viral levels should be kept below 100,000 for children and toddlers.

Pregnant women with low viral load counts during childbirth are less likely to transmit HIV to their newborns. Expectant mothers will thus want to carefully consider using one of the advanced therapies to bring viral load down—not only for their own sake, but also for the health of their unborn child. However, much is still unknown about how these new drugs could affect a fetus or newborn. The decision to take them is complicated, and following through will require great commitment on your part. If you are pregnant, take your time and get as much information as you can from your doctor and other knowledgeable sources.

Patient Rights and Responsibilities

In working with any health care professional, you have certain rights and responsibilities:

1) You have a right to the best and most responsible medical treatment available without discrimination on the basis of ethnic or national origin, sex, sexual orientation, religion, ability to pay, history of drug use, or ultimate source of payment.

2) You have a right to ask questions and to have tests and procedures explained to you in language you can understand.

3) You have a right to know what medications are being prescribed to you, to have full disclosure about treatment side effects, and to a frank discussion of the pros and cons of all the different options available to you.

4) You have a right to refuse tests or treatment for any reason.

5) You have a right to a second opinion and to seek answers to your questions from outside sources.

6) You have a right to be treated like a person—not an experiment, curiosity, or teaching "visual aid."

7) You have a right to confidentiality.

8) You have a right to honesty, privacy (to the extent possible), and considerate, dignified, and respectful care and treatment from all medical professionals with whom you come in contact. You are entitled to complain to the proper authorities when these standards are not met.

9) You have a right to have whomever you want with you when you talk to your doctor.

10) You have a right to believe in your physician or in supplemental treatments as you see fit.

It's always been, the doctor is God—he knows what he's doing, and you just do what he says. You just sit there and say "yessir" and fill the prescription, and pay no attention to what it is or the dosage or what the side effects might be. It's stupid to have that mentality—it's your life, your body, your health. You're ultimately responsible for it.

CHARLIE

> *I've been to four doctors in three and a half years. My last physician, the one I'm currently seeing, I walked in with a 7-page summary of my medical history and two pages of goals and objectives I had for my physician. He laughed; but when we were done talking, I think he had a pretty good idea where I was coming from.*
>
> HOWARD
>
> *If there's anything you don't understand, always remind your doctor, "I'm not a physician—use layman's language, please. I don't understand all those fancy-dancy medical terms." Don't ever be afraid to ask, "What does this mean? What's the bottom line here?"*
>
> DR. HARVEY WOLF
> CLINICAL HEALTH PSYCHOLOGIST
>
> *I saw mistakes daily when Michael was in the hospital. Some of them were deadly mistakes. And when I go in the hospital, I'll have an advocate who'll watch out for those same mistakes. It doesn't matter which hospital it is—you cannot be confident in any one of them. I think people feel secure going into hospitals, and they shouldn't.*
>
> JOE

By the same token:

1) You have a responsibility to be honest with your doctor about supplemental treatments you may be using, risks you may be taking, sexual and other practices that could affect your health, and alcohol and other drug use.

2) You have a responsibility to take prescriptions as directed by your doctor—and to speak up if they are causing problems for you, or if you decide to discontinue taking them.

3) You have a responsibility to treat your doctor like a person, not like an oppressor or God.

4) You have a responsibility to find a doctor who will work with you on *your* terms—even if that means switching doctors more than once.

5) You have a responsibility to ask questions until you understand.

6) In Illinois and other states, you have a responsibility to help stop the spread of HIV by giving your doctor or public health authorities the names of people with whom you've had sex or shared needles. You cannot, however, be forced to name names, nor can you legally be denied treatment or other services if you decline to provide this information. In no case should your doctor judge or discriminate against you based on any information you choose to provide about how you became infected.

Anyone at risk for HIV deserves to be aware of it. If you don't want to deal with past partners face-to-face, this could be a good service for you to consider. Your past partners will be notified of their risk and offered counseling and testing without being told your name. (Of course, it's possible they will be able to guess your identity.)

These rights and responsibilities apply to any health care setting, be it a hospital, hospice, clinical trial center, or your own doctor's office.

If all goes well, you and your doctor will build an effective, trusting relationship capable of lasting for many years. If not, you may eventually decide to look for another primary care physician and/or HIV specialist. You'll probably know in your gut if things aren't working out. Don't be afraid to pursue other options at any time during the course of your illness.

Finding and Working with a Dentist

In addition to finding a doctor, you'll also want to look for a dentist who serves HIV-positive patients. It's more than simply a matter of good dental care; HIV-related infections of the mouth and gums are common and can be severe. Your current dentist may not be equipped to treat you effectively should the need arise.

Unfortunately, finding the right dentist can be more difficult than finding the right doctor. Many dental procedures are invasive and therefore viewed as "risky" to both dentist and patient. In the past, dentists often gave that as their main reason for declining to treat people with HIV and AIDS. A more likely reason was their fear of what may happen to their practice if "word gets out" they treat people with AIDS.

The Illinois Human Rights Commission has ruled that it is illegal for a dentist to refuse to treat HIV-positive patients. The American Dental Association has condemned this behavior as unethical.

That said, there *are* dentists in the Chicago area who are able and willing to treat you. You can get referrals through others living with HIV, AIDS service organizations, and by contacting the resources that follow this discussion.

In choosing the right dentist, you may decide to go through a selection process similar to that of finding the right doctor. Once you've chosen a dentist you feel comfortable with, take the same care in tracking and reporting symptoms, asking questions, and participating in treatment decisions.

Be prepared for your dentist and his staff to take the "spaceman approach" in dressing for your visit—full gloves, face masks, and eye coverings. Don't take offense; you haven't been singled out for special treatment. In fact, dental and disease control authorities now require that dentists wear those infection barriers with *all* patients.

Dental Referral Services

Chicago Dental Society
401 North Michigan Avenue, Suite 300
Chicago, IL 60611
312-836-7300
312-836-7337—FAX
• Dental referrals during normal business hours (9 a.m.-5 p.m., Mon-Fri).

Gay and Lesbian Physicians of Chicago
PO Box 14864
Chicago, IL 60614
312-670-9630
• Referral service for gay- and lesbian-friendly dentists and physicians in the Chicago metropolitan area.

Illinois AIDS Hotline
800-243-2437—Hotline staffed 8 a.m.-11 p.m., 7 days/week
800-782-0423—Hearing-impaired TTY/TDD
• Referrals to dentists and Ryan White funded dental services throughout Illinois. English/Spanish.

Illinois State Dental Society
PO Box 376
Springfield, IL 62705
217-525-1406
217-525-8872—FAX
• Referrals to dental services, including donated dental services, discounted dental programs, portable dental equipment for home use, and referral for low-cost dentures. Sliding scale fees.

3. EXPLORING THE RANGE OF TREATMENTS

Mainstream Approaches

Antiretroviral Drugs and Combination Therapies

Intensive research on antiretroviral treatments for HIV is finally starting to pay off. Just a few years ago, therapy meant only the possibility of using AZT or the handful of other drugs like it. Now several promising new treatments are available, others are in the pipeline, and there are three classes of drugs that interrupt the production of HIV. Although these medications can't "cure" you of HIV, they may reduce the amount of virus in your body, thus giving your immune system a leg up in its long-term battle.

Each of the three classes of antiviral drugs attacks HIV in a different way while the virus is replicating within a T cell. Because of this, your doctor may prescribe a "cocktail" of two or more drugs to shut down the virus to the full extent possible. This evolving approach to combination therapy has proven quite successful for some people. As we describe the three classes of antiviral drugs, keep in mind that new treatment options may have been developed since this book was printed. Check with your doctor or an AIDS group for the latest information.

Don't be scared off by how complicated these drugs may seem at first glance. You needn't be a scientist in order to benefit from these treatments! You may want to review this section quickly, or turn to this book or another resource as you need the information. On the other hand, you may decide you want to go into much more detail than is provided here. You'll be in good company; many people are surprised by how quickly they become immersed in knowledge about the various treatments. You can learn a lot by reading and talking with others who are living with HIV. (We've included resources within this chapter to help you get started.)

Either way, be sure your doctor is well-versed in the latest combination therapy protocols, that she or he is willing to take the time to help you understand your options, and that your doctor supports you but will leave the final, informed decision up to you.

As this book goes to press, there are three classes of antiretroviral drugs, as described below. All medications of this type have potential side effects, which you and your doctor can monitor and respond to. Fortunately, most of the side effects listed below are seen in only a small number of patients.

1) *Nucleoside Analogues (NRTIs or RTIs).* Nucleoside analogues, also known as nucleoside reverse transcriptase inhibitors, interfere with an enzyme that HIV uses to replicate itself. This interruption happens fairly early after HIV has infected a T cell. AZT, which was approved for use in 1986, is the oldest of the drugs in this class. (AZT is also known as ZDV, short for zidovudine, or by the brand

---

I've had full-blown AIDS, and using protease inhibitors I've gotten to undetectable levels. It's a weird thing to have AIDS and then not meet the definition anymore. I choose to believe that I have HIV, had AIDS, and am getting healthier.

"SPARKY"

name Retrovir). Others, including ddI (didanosine or Videx), ddC (zalcitabine or HIVID), D4T (stavudine or Zerit) and 3TC (lamivudine or Epivir), were first released for use during the early 1990s.

For years, AZT was the only antiviral treatment available for people with HIV. Because it can be toxic to some individuals, AZT was somewhat controversial. Taken in high doses over a long period of time, the drug may cause liver and bone marrow damage. Short-term side effects may include nausea, headaches, chills, fatigue and muscle aches, anemia (a decrease in red blood cells), and neutropenia (a decrease in white blood cells. The lower doses of AZT currently prescribed make it unlikely that patients will experience these side effects.) While some of these side effects can be managed using additional drugs, many people have found AZT difficult to take. However, when the drug was the only available treatment for HIV, deciding to *stop* taking it could be tremendously difficult.

Now there are antiviral alternatives to AZT. ddI produces a different set of side effects, which may include diarrhea, rashes, ulcers in the esophagus or mouth, chills, nausea and vomiting from inflammation of the pancreas, and tingling in the hands and feet (known as peripheral neuropathy). If you have used non-prescription drugs and alcohol heavily or have any history of neuropathy, your doctor may recommend a different RTI.

ddC can cause side effects similar to ddI. The most common side effect of d4T is neuropathy, though it can also induce fever, pancreatitis, and neutropenia. However, this drug also has been found to penetrate more deeply into the nervous system, which can be helpful for people whose brains have been affected by toxoplasmosis, dementia, or other infection. Finally, 3TC produces some of the mildest side effects: insomnia, fatigue, muscle aches, nausea, abdominal pain, and diarrhea. Children have a greater risk of inflammation of the pancreas, although the likelihood is low. Used in combination with AZT, 3TC reduces the problem of drug-resistance in some people.

2) *Non-Nucleoside Reverse Transcriptase Inhibitors (NNRTIs)*. The newest class of antiretrovirals, called non-nucleoside reverse transcriptase inhibitors, also works by interrupting the enzyme needed to create new virus. NNRTIs actually keep the enzyme from being produced. Therefore, they stop new viral material from being released into the bloodstream.

As this book goes to press, only one NNRTI has been approved for use. Nevirapine (brand name Viramune) may be a powerful tool for fighting HIV, and is most commonly used in combination with one or more of the RTIs. Use with protease inhibitors is

---

Things have changed. When I tested positive back in 1986, you couldn't get AZT, it was so experimental. And pentamidine wasn't out yet either. There really was nothing they could do for you, medically. So when my doctor said go home, take care of yourself, eat well, stop smoking, keep the alcohol to a minimum, get plenty of rest, and we'll just monitor you once in awhile—that was the standard of care back then. Today, that would be an irresponsible position.

CHARLIE

When my son goes for his infusion, that's when I get to see other mothers and kids. I met two children who were HIV-positive from birth, who are now fourteen. I think back when they didn't have a lot of the research they have now, didn't have AZT, ddI, and all those other meds. So who knows? Maybe he'll hang in there.

CHRISTINE

> *A friend of mine who had seemed to be doing well died. It was a shocker and a reminder that, although things are more hopeful because of the new drugs, we're not out of the woods yet with this disease.*
>
> WOOD

> *I'm really trying, with the medications. I've already been on and off them once. I took them for three or four days, then I had to stop because of problems from chronic hepatitis. When they took me off the medications, it just did something to me. I kind of lost faith. It was hard to start taking them again. I have a fear of them. I have to force myself to take them. I'll think, "Better take that medication. I don't really want to, because I want to be well enough to go shopping and I really want to gather some energy... but I have to anyway." That is what I'm going through. I have these medications that I fought so hard to get, and I have to get aggressive and start taking them no matter how they make me feel, no matter what the side effects are.*
>
> "SONIA"

currently being studied. Resistance to nevirapine can build up quickly, though, especially when the drug is used alone.

Most patients tolerate nevirapine fairly well. The most common side effects are skin rashes, including one called Stevens-Johnson syndrome that is potentially deadly. Other side effects can include fever, headache, nausea, and liver problems. Check with your doctor about interactions with other drugs you may be taking. Other NNRTIs are being researched (including one called delavirdine or Rescriptor) and may be available by the time you read this. Regimens for dosage and combinations are still under study. Ask your doctor or an AIDS organization about what's new or in the pipeline.

3) *Protease Inhibitors*. Is the AIDS pandemic over? Some people would have you believe so, but the story is a bit more complex than that. Protease inhibitors have been called "miracle drugs," producing amazing results in some. Scientists are studying the possibility that a few lucky users may one day be completely cured. However, for the relatively short time they've been available, protease inhibitors have shown mixed results. These drugs are extremely good news, but they're only one piece of the HIV puzzle.

How do protease inhibitors work? Once HIV has created a copy of itself inside a T cell, it assembles the new virus, packages it in a protein molecule, and releases it into the bloodstream. As their name implies, protease inhibitors prevent these final steps from taking place. They inhibit the ability of HIV to finish replicating itself.

Like RTIs and NNRTIs, protease inhibitors can cause side effects that may be severe or even intolerable. Many users have found that the first four to six weeks are the hardest and that side effects lessen as the body adapts to the drugs.

Protease inhibitors are used in combination with RTIs and sometimes an NNRTI. In some people, viral load counts have dropped to levels below what is currently detectable, while T cell counts have risen dramatically. (This does not mean that HIV is gone from the body, or that it cannot be passed on to others. It could be "hiding" in an organ or in the lymph system.) Some people have good results initially, but then "crash" as the virus develops resistance to the drugs (their viral load suddenly skyrockets while their T cells start diminishing). Others do not respond at all to the drug cocktails, or are unable to take them for a variety of medical and non-medical reasons.

Since protease inhibitors and the combination therapies in which they are used are so new, there remain a lot of unanswered questions. Researchers are still studying the best combinations of drugs, as well as optimal dosages and timetables for taking them. We don't yet know if these therapies may lead us to a way to wipe out the virus completely. We don't know what the long-term side effects will be, or how long the excellent results some people have seen ultimately will last. Finally, new therapies often work best in people who have not previously tried other medications. It's possible that when we turn the next major corner of HIV research, we will find the new protocols work best on those who have not used the current therapies.

There is currently a debate raging as to when patients should begin using protease inhibitors. Some experts believe in a "hit early, hit hard" approach, which involves using the drugs before HIV has a chance to silently do much damage. Others believe the benefits of the drugs won't last forever, so it's best to put off taking them until there are clear clinical signs that HIV is advancing. Many people with HIV see the new drugs as a chance to be around until a cure or effective long-term management regimens are developed.

One thing is certain: if you choose to try a protease inhibitor combination, it is very, very important that you think about it carefully, and that you are sure you can take the drugs exactly as you're instructed. Regimens can be quite complicated and require a rigorous commitment on the part of the user. If you miss doses or take a "holiday" from a protease inhibitor, your HIV infection has a breather during which it can mutate into a form the drugs cannot fight. Worse yet, *if you become resistant to one drug, you may actually become resistant to the whole class of protease inhibitors*. You might lose the ability to take not only the drug you've already tried, but perhaps others that are in use now or may be developed later.
A bigger public health worry is that careless or inadequate use of the drugs will lead to the development of a drug-resistant strain of HIV.

Talk honestly with your doctor about your concerns and your ability to comply with a challenging drug regimen. If you feel you are not able or ready to commit to taking the drugs on a strict schedule without a break, as well as following all other dietary and lifestyle instructions while using them, you are probably better off not trying them now. You might want to consider a different treatment approach where the stakes are not so high. No matter what anyone says, you don't have to make a decision about your treatment today or any time before you're ready.

To take your medications reliably on time, try setting an alarm on your clock or watch. Write out a schedule and hang it where you will see it. Ask your doctor or pharmacist for a schedule for taking the drugs, with boxes to be checked when you have taken your medications. Buy a special pill box if that will help. Explain your plan to your partner or spouse, and ask them to back you up with

---

I basically went to bed for about a week after I went on AZT. It was a particularly hard phase for me, starting to see the doctor and getting treatment for this. I didn't feel in any way sick— yet here I was, entering the world of sick people. Being told I was gravely ill when I had no symptoms seemed very unreal.

As time has gone on, things have been okay. I've moved away from that feeling of schizophrenia around being a sick person while still feeling healthy. I've finally come to understand for myself that being HIV-positive is kind of like having a chronic blood disorder. That's how I present it to myself in my head. And that makes everything else not seem so desperate. I'm able to rationalize taking all this medicine that way.

"RALPH"

> *It would be wonderful to feel certain that we know what the best approach is for kids, but the data is just not there yet. It's so hard to be giving multiple drugs to an infant, to be shackling a parent with the heavy responsibility that if you miss a dose two or three times a week, or if the child throws up too much or whatever, you may be doing your child irreparable harm, that they might not get a chance at the "cure." That's pretty scary pressure when you don't know for sure yet if the drugs will be effective or if you've got the right combination and dosage, what the risks are, and so on. There's still so much to learn. The absence of data makes it especially hard to ask such a difficult thing of a parent.*
>
> DANIEL JOHNSON, M.D.
> DIRECTOR, PEDIATRIC AND ADOLESCENT HIV CARE TEAM, UNIVERSITY OF CHICAGO CHILDREN'S HOSPITAL

reminders. If you miss a dose by more than three or four hours, skip it. Do not double the next dose. If you need to stop taking your medications, it's better to discontinue them altogether than taper off to a lower dose. Contact your doctor before stopping, or as soon as possible afterward. If the problem is side effects, your doctor may be able to suggest reasonable strategies for reducing them. She or he might also prescribe an alternative combination of drugs that won't make you feel so unwell.

Protease Inhibitors in Infants and Children. Studies have shown that combination therapies used during pregnancy reduce the risk that an HIV-positive woman will pass her infection on to her baby. However, there is far more uncertainty surrounding the use of protease inhibitors in infants and children. We don't fully understand the meaning of viral load markers in children, appropriate dosages, the safety of using various drugs or drug combinations in kids, or the long-term effects of using these agents on children's growing bodies.

Children are also less likely to cooperate fully with complicated drug regimens. They may hide pills or pretend to swallow them. Parents cannot always monitor if a child keeps a medication down. This can be a heavy burden, particularly when you factor in the risk of the child becoming drug-resistant and potentially missing out on the next treatment breakthrough. Still other parents are unwilling to put their youngsters through the difficult ordeal of taking the drugs. They may be tempted to skip doses if the child complains or has serious side effects. They may feel guilty, exhausted, or ambivalent about the whole process.

It's a lot to ask of parents to maintain their commitment, discipline, and vigilance in administering the drugs to children when so much is not yet known and the stakes are so high. Therefore, the decision about whether to move forward aggressively with treatments including protease inhibitors rests firmly with the parents. If you are a parent of a youngster with HIV, *you* are the one who will have to live with your child every day. You are the one whose responsibility it is to make treatment decisions in your child's best interests.

Your doctor should be willing to educate you about all your options, then let you move forward with your best idea of how you can help your child be well. Respect, knowledge, and compassion must be the cornerstones of the service your pediatrician provides for you and your child. If you are not comfortable, get another opinion before taking action, or change doctors altogether. The new therapies are nothing to take lightly. Before you use them with your child, you must be as sure as you can be that you will follow through.

Types of Protease Inhibitors. As this book goes to press, there are four protease inhibitors approved for use. The first of these is *saquinavir* (brand name Invirase). Used with RTIs, saquinavir's side effects can include mild diarrhea and abdominal discomfort or nausea. The effectiveness of saquinavir is not as great as other protease inhibitors because the drug is not easily absorbed into the body. (This can be improved through the use of other medications.) Talk to your doctor about any drugs (legal or not) that you are taking, in order to discuss side effects that may occur and make appropriate changes. One study showed that when combined with ritonavir, saquinavir was found after 20 weeks to have reduced viral load by more than 99.9 percent.

Ritonavir (Norvir) is a potent protease inhibitor. Side effects can include fatigue, nausea, vomiting, diarrhea, abdominal pain, and tingling and numbness around the mouth. In one study, this drug doubled the six-month survival rate of people with late-stage AIDS. Ritonavir has been studied in a very small number of children and was found to be safe and effective. (The bad taste of the drug can be lessened by mixing it with chocolate milk.) Ritonavir interacts negatively (at times, dangerously) with many drugs. If you use it, be sure to consult with your doctor about any and all other drugs and medications you may be taking. Be aware that alcohol and tobacco may lower ritonavir's effectiveness.

Indinavir sulfate (Crixivan) is a powerful antiretroviral. 80% of adult participants in one study whose T cells were in the 30–250 range and who were treated with AZT in combination with 3TC and indinavir showed undetectable levels of HIV after one year. Using indinavir with an RTI may decrease the chance of developing resistance to either drug. This drug is generally well tolerated, but can cause headache, nausea, kidney ailments, fever, rash, insomnia, and abdominal pain. Alcohol can increase the formation of kidney stones, which up to one-quarter of indinavir users will develop. *Drink six to eight glasses of water a day* and avoid acidic foods to decrease side effects. There are a number of other drugs indinavir should *not* be taken with—again, check with your doctor. She or he will give you full instructions as to your new regimen. As with saquinavir, indinavir drug levels in the body can be increased via the use of other medications.

Nelfinavir (Viracept) is the newest of the four protease inhibitors discussed here. This drug is safer and causes fewer side effects than other protease inhibitors, and can be used by adults or children. The most common side effects are nausea, vomiting, diarrhea, and feelings of weakness. As with all medications, check with your doctor before and during use to avoid the possibility of dangerous drug interactions.

As individualized as the effects of HIV are to each person, so are the effects of all the different treatments. It's important to do what you feel is right for you. The first time I was told to take AZT, I just did because I thought I had to. But then I freaked out and threw it away. Two years later, I was again asked to take AZT and after learning more about it, I did. But it made me sick all the time, so after a couple of months I stopped. I chose for myself to try some natural healing methods that have worked out to be the best for me.

It's been eight years since I was infected and I am still symptom-free. I'm a firm believer in the power of the mind, but that doesn't mean that I'll never take any medications. I just listen to my voice within and trust that it will lead me to what I'm supposed to do and when.

SHARI

Immunomodulators

Immunomodulators are medications designed to evoke a strengthened response from the immune system, increasing the body's ability to fight disease. These agents (of which there are about 50 in all) are not usually categorized as a group, because they include several classes of medications that target various points in the immune system. Immunomodulators include steroids, growth factors, anti-tumor agents, activated lymphocytes and other vaccines, interleukins, interferons, antibodies, immunoglobulins, gammaglobulin, and other drugs.

There's so much we don't yet know about the new drugs—the protease inhibitors, and so forth. Despite all the hype, there are still a lot of unanswered questions.

In terms of our clients, we're seeing about four different scenarios. The first is people who are on meds and doing well. I think about Bob—who had pretty much assumed he was going to die within three years of going on disability. And within three <u>months</u> of starting on the new cocktails, his viral load was undetectable and his T cells were really high. He suddenly had to start dealing with the fact that he was potentially going to be living a normal life span, maybe re-entering the job market. Even though it was a wonderful development in his living with HIV, it was really stressful. He didn't know where to start.

I remember last year, when the new treatments first came out, a whole support group session was focused around smoking cessation. There were so many people in this group who were doing so well medically, turning around their HIV situations, that all of a sudden other health aspects of their lives were a concern for them. "Oh, my God, I'd better stop smoking—I'm going to die of lung cancer before I die of AIDS!" There are all sorts of readjustments you never anticipate.

Scenario number two is people who try the new treatments, which seem to work for awhile...but then they crash. Their viral loads become detectable again and their T cells go down. For those folks, it's been a really rough ride. They've had to go through this whole process of, "Okay, I'm going to die in a couple years, better start saying goodbye to people"—to "Wow, I might live out a normal life span, I have to come back from the dead"—to "Oh, my God, the drugs aren't working! I may die prematurely after all." Which really messes with their minds.

I think some clients are still hopeful because they're hearing about new drugs in the pipeline, or their doctors are aggressive about trying different combinations. But others feel betrayed; I've heard of a few people who refuse to try the new treatments because of prior disappointments and suspicion and skepticism. But the message from the pharmaceutical industry and doctors is to hang tight, there's more stuff coming down the pike. We'll have different therapies available as soon as the FDA approves them. You can already see what's coming: they'll invent so many different drugs and combinations of drugs, no one will know what's going on. Everyone's treatments will be so individualized, it's going to be wild. It already is wild!

There are a couple of other scenarios we see around taking these new drugs—or rather, not taking them. Scenario number three involves people who try the drugs and can't handle the side effects, and so are forced to stop taking them. This is relatively rare, since combinations can be manipulated and new things tried to make treatment tolerable. Unless a patient was terribly ill—end stage—it's unlikely she or he would be unable to take any of it.

In the fourth scenario, we're dealing with clients who would like to take the drugs, but for various reasons can't access them. Some people are in a financial "catch-22"—they don't have insurance through their jobs, but they make too much money to qualify for government assistance and not enough to pay for the drugs out-of-pocket. There are clinical trials and a few other programs out there to help these people, state and drug company assistance programs, but it's still chancy. Windows close. People fall through the cracks. There's also a big concern that with Medicaid and the insurance industry moving toward managed care, coverage available for these very expensive drugs may be capped off at some point. People who once had access may be left high and dry.

Other clients can't access the drugs because their doctors won't prescribe them, often for good reason. The patients are still asymptomatic with high T cells, and have viral load counts too low to warrant the new treatment. Or they have patients where compliance is a major issue. Their lives are chaotic, or they just don't have the personal resources—the knowledge and skill level—to be able to follow very complicated sets of instructions. Some of our clients are taking up to thirty pills a day, and each pill has a different regime around it. Some pills have to be taken on an empty stomach, some after a light meal, some after a high fat meal, some at certain times of day, before or after other pills, or in the middle of the night. It's a lot to remember and organize. I had trouble taking one pill at the same time every day when I was on birth control! I can't imagine taking thirty pills a day. I'd have to hire a secretary to keep me on schedule. So the doctors have to be very cautious about whom they prescribe the new treatments to. If their patients don't take the drugs exactly as directed, totally consistently, they can crash or develop resistance.

Some people accuse the doctors of playing God; maybe some of them are. It can be a real ethical dilemma of who gets the drugs and who doesn't. With a whole class of agents that didn't even exist a few short years ago, the questions are mind-boggling and never-ending.

DEBORAH STEINKOPF
Executive Director, BEHIV—
Better Existence with HIV

Prevention and Treatment of Opportunistic Infections

The real damage HIV causes is that it weakens your body's defenses. You may become more vulnerable to a whole host of diseases that are not commonly seen in people with healthy immune systems. These problems are called "opportunistic infections," because they only have the opportunity to make you sick due to the assault of HIV on your body. Many of these conditions are on the CDC's checklist of AIDS-defining illnesses.

In addition to giving you drugs that wage a direct assault on HIV, your doctor may prescribe "prophylactic" or preventive treatments. These are medications that help prevent opportunistic infections from occurring. Ongoing medical advances make it impossible for us to outline every problem and solution, or give you all the detail you may want or need. You can obtain treatment information through newsletters, fax services, and the Internet. (See the resources in "Learning More about Drugs, Trials, and Treatments" later on in this section.)

Incidence of opportunistic infections is declining among people with AIDS. This may be the result of better preventive treatments and the positive effects of the new antiviral medications. While all the infections described below can produce serious or even life-threatening problems, the most common ones are Pneumocystis carinii pneumonia (PCP), toxoplasmosis, and mycobacterium avium complex (MAC). Your physician can tell you what prophylactic options are available to you, and help you decide whether and when to start using them.

1) *Pneumocystis carinii Pneumonia (PCP, for short)*. PCP is an infection of the lungs caused by a protozoan found in water and soil. This is the most important opportunistic infection to treat prophylactically, because without prevention it is common and deadly. Luckily, prophylactic treatments are very effective and inexpensive. Symptoms of PCP include shortness of breath, dry cough, fever, exhaustion, and unexplained weight loss. The disease can also affect the eyes, skin, liver, spleen, and heart. Preventive medication is recommended for individuals whose T cells are below 200 (even when no symptoms are present), and for anyone who has previously had a bout of PCP. Medication side effects may be minimized through a regimen of slowly increased dosages. Ask your doctor for more details about preventive treatments for PCP.

2) *Tuberculosis (TB)*. TB is caused by an airborne mycobacterium. Symptoms include coughing, fatigue, fever, and unexplained weight loss. The disease doesn't always present itself in a "typical" manner, so a regular screening test should be part of your care. Occasionally, though, even the Mantoux skin test fails to show evidence of the disease. Prophylaxis is recommended for individuals who test positive for TB or who've been in close contact with someone who has it. Drug therapy continues for at least a year, and it's important to

take your medication exactly as directed, even after symptoms disappear and you feel well again. Otherwise the disease can return, stronger than before, and future treatments may not be effective.

3) *Mycobacterium Avium Complex (MAC, MAI, Mycobacterium intracellulare)*. MAC is an infection that can attack the lungs, bone marrow, lymph nodes, or gastrointestinal tract. Symptoms can include fever, night sweats, diarrhea, fatigue, abdominal pain, unexplained weight loss, and abscesses in the skin, liver, brain, or other organs. MAC is common in people with T cell counts below 50, and can be life-threatening. Most doctors recommend prophylactic treatment for anyone with counts below 75.

4) *Cytomegalovirus (CMV)*. Caused by a virus related to herpes, CMV can produce inflammation in various parts of the body. Retinitis (decreased vision which can lead to blindness), colitis (irritation of the intestinal tract), and encephalitis (swelling of the brain) are the most common forms CMV takes. Symptoms can include blurry or altered vision, unexplained weight loss, headaches, altered consciousness, and neurological problems. Individuals who test positive for CMV and those whose T cell counts are below 50 should receive prophylactic care.

5) *Toxoplasmosis*. Toxoplasmosis is an infection of the brain and spinal column caused by a protozoan found in raw and undercooked meat, and in soil contaminated by animal feces. Symptoms can include headaches, fever, seizures, dizziness, and tingling sensations in the body. Individuals who test positive for toxoplasmosis and those whose T cell counts are below 100 should receive prophylactic care. Although the disease responds well to treatment, damage to vision can usually be slowed but not cured. Altering medications can help keep response to treatment high.

6) *Candidiasis* (thrush, esophagitis, vaginitis, diaper rash). Candidiasis is an overgrowth of a fungus called candida, which occurs naturally in the digestive tract, mouth, and vagina. It can cause pain, difficulty swallowing, a rash, itching, and a burning sensation. White, cheesy spots or discharge may be present. It's possible for your whole system to become infected, which can be life-threatening. Prophylaxis is recommended for individuals who have had candidiasis in the past.

7) *Pelvic Inflammatory Disease (PID)*. PID is an inflammation of the urinary or reproductive tract, caused by a single pathogen or a combination of pathogens (called polymicrobic infection). Sexually transmitted diseases, such as chlamydia or gonorrhea, may be underlying causes, as can other bacteria or organisms. Women with this condition may experience abdominal pain, foul-smelling vaginal discharge, fever, fatigue, and difficult menstrual periods. Treatments vary, depending on the cause of the infection.

8) *Cryptococcosis*. Cryptococcosis is an inflammation of the brain or other organs, caused by breathing a fungus found in soil contaminated by bird feces. This is the most common fungal infection found among people with AIDS, and can lead to cryptococcal meningitis. Symptoms may include headaches, coughing, shortness of breath, stiff neck, fever, nausea, seizures, altered mental states, discomfort from light, and other neurological disturbances.

9) *Cryptosporidiosis (Cryptosporidium)*. Cryptosporidiosis is an infection causing diarrhea that is unresponsive to treatment. It can also move into the biliary system of the body, causing problems such as jaundice or gallbladder attack. No preventive or prescription drug treatments have been defined. Sufferers manage the problem through fluid therapy, nutritional support, and the use of antidiarrheals. You can reduce the risk of infection by drinking bottled water, especially when traveling.

10) *Histoplasmosis*. Histoplasmosis is an infection of the lungs and blood caused by a fungus found in soil contaminated with bird feces. The fungus is transmitted by breathing or ingesting infected dust. Symptoms can include shortness of breath, fever, unexplained weight loss, lesions, anemia, and decreasing white cell counts. Individuals who live in areas with a high incidence of the disease or who have already had histoplasmosis should undergo preventive treatment.

11) *Herpes simplex (herpes)*. Herpes is a sexually transmitted disease caused by a virus. Symptoms may include itching or burning sensations, blisters, fever, body aches, abscesses, and sore throat. This is a recurring condition that may flare up many times over the course of a lifetime (although some individuals may be asymptomatic carriers). Herpes carriers focus on managing their symptoms and on avoiding unprotected sexual activity during flareups, which may pass on the disease. Many physicians recommend prophylactic treatment for individuals who have experienced many active bouts of herpes.

12) *Kaposi's sarcoma (KS)*. Kaposi's sarcoma is the most common cancer associated with AIDS. It is probably caused by a herpes virus, and can affect the lungs, lymphatic system, skin, gastrointestinal tract and other sites, creating lesions or dark patches that can be disfiguring. This disease is most common in men. Localized treatments (including surgery, laser therapy, cryotherapy, or injections) aim to decrease the size of lesions. "Systemic therapies" (in cases where one's entire system is affected) include radiotherapy or drugs. Systemic therapy aims to reduce pain, decrease tumor size, and/or reduce effects on organs.

13) *Non-Hodgkin's Lymphoma.* Non-Hodgkin's lymphoma is the second most common malignancy among adults with AIDS. Like KS, this lymphoma is associated with a herpes virus. (Epstein-Barr virus may play a role, particularly in cases affecting the central nervous system.) Standard treatments include drug therapy; ask your doctor for details.

14) *Cervical Carcinoma.* Women with HIV have higher numbers of abnormal cells (called cervical intraepithelial neoplasia, or CIN) on their cervix than do HIV-negative women. A greater number of these irregular cells go on to develop into cancers or carcinomas than is true in other women, and the mortality rate tends to be higher. Routine Pap smears and gynecological exams should be a part of health care for any woman with HIV. Treatment includes radiotherapy and surgery, used alone or together.

Clinical Drug Trials

A final treatment option is the clinical drug trial or "protocol." These corporate-, university-, or government-sponsored research studies test new medications and treatments for HIV-related conditions. People who have a certain type of illness or meet a certain set of characteristics may qualify to take part. Not everyone who applies is eligible for every trial. However, you can keep applying to different trials that interest you until you are accepted.

A clinical drug trial is not something to be entered into lightly. There are both risks and benefits to consider:

Risks
- You might be asked to discontinue treatment that has been working for you while you are in the study.
- The experimental drug may not work for you or anyone else.
- It could be unsafe—possibly making your condition worse or causing harmful side effects.
- You might be given a placebo (a "sugar pill" or shot containing no medicine) instead of the actual test drug. A placebo is used *only* in studies where there is no treatment that has been proven to be effective. You will always be told if you might be given a placebo before you sign up.

Benefits
- Many times, only trial participants have access to the drug being studied. If a new drug works, you'll be among the first to enjoy its benefits.
- The experimental medicine will be provided free. You may also receive health services (such as blood tests and checkups) free or at minimal cost. This can help cut down on your out-of-pocket and insurance costs in monitoring your health.
- The doctors and nurses running the study will be HIV experts. Expect to receive sensitive, top-quality care throughout the trial.

- Participating in a study gives many people a sense of control over their disease. They feel they're doing all they can to fight it.
- Your participation will help researchers find new ways to fight HIV, and will eventually help others living with it.
- Clinical trials are closely monitored by institutional and community review boards to make certain they are ethical and that patients are fully informed.

Special Notes
- No one can force you to join or stay in a clinical trial. You will be participating on an informed, voluntary basis. However, be aware that joining is a potentially cumbersome commitment. Get all the facts *before* signing up—and don't be afraid to ask questions along the way.
- Pregnant and nursing women are often placed in special trials where the medication's effect on the baby is better known. Contrary to rumor, women do not have to have an abortion if they become pregnant while participating in a trial. However, women are often required to use effective birth control as a condition for joining a study.
- Ask those running the study upfront what your out-of-pocket costs will be, and whether they will reimburse you for transportation or child care expenses.

If you decide the benefits outweigh the risks, ask your doctor to try and locate a study that would be right for you. Or, you can track down studies that interest you and bring them to his or her attention. Either way, your doctor will be the one to recommend you. You probably won't be able to get into a study on your own.

An increasing number of drug trials are community based, meaning patients can participate in them through their own doctors without having to travel to a test site. Before you investigate the following sources independently, ask your doctor whether she or he is aware of or already participating in any community based trials you might qualify for.

You may also hear about trials through various HIV/AIDS newsletters and from others living with the disease.

Clinical Trials Information

AIDS Clinical Trials Information Service (ACTIS)
PO Box 6421
Rockville, MD 20849
800-TRIALS-A (874-2572)
800-243-7012—Hearing-impaired TTY/TDD
301-738-6616—FAX
e-mail: actis@cdcnac.org
• Free and confidential telephone or printed information on ongoing private and federally-sponsored trials around the country. English/Spanish.

AIDS Research Alliance Chicago
2800 North Sheridan Road, Suite 108
Chicago, IL 60657
773-244-5800
773-244-0412—FAX
• Coordinates clinical trials and AIDS research through local doctors and hospitals in the Chicago area. Depending on the study, you may be able to participate and stay with your own doctor. Call for a list of doctors, current trials, and enrollment information.

CDC National AIDS Clearinghouse
800-458-5231—English/Spanish
800-243-7012—Hearing-impaired TTY/TDD
9 a.m.-7 p.m. Mon-Fri (Eastern time)
• Distributes up-to-date clinical trials publications from the American Foundation for AIDS Research. Ask for the current "AIDS Clinical Trials Handbook," which explains what it is like to be in a clinical trial. Other publications on clinical trials include "Information About the AIDS Clinical Trials Information Service" and "What Is an AIDS Clinical Trial?" (English only). English/Spanish.

Test Positive Aware Network
"Directory of Chicago HIV/AIDS Clinical Trials"
1258 West Belmont
Chicago, IL 60657
773-404-8726
773-472-7505—FAX
773-404-9716—Hearing-impaired TTY/TDD
• Updated regularly, the directory is the most complete listing of treatment trials taking place in the Chicago area. Includes a complete explanation of the clinical trials process.

Using a Computer and Modem

AIDS Clinical Trials Information Service
http://www.actis.org
• Find out what we've learned from clinical trials so far. The "AIDS Clinical Trials Results Database" gives references to the published results of HIV-related clinical trials. You can search the database by drug name, disease studied, and keywords.

Critical Path AIDS Project
http://www.critpath.org/
• Access to information on AIDS clinical trials, research, and more. Specific links for women, minorities, and youth.

The Food & Drug Administration (FDA) HIV and AIDS Page
http://www.fda.gov//oashi/aids/hiv.html
• Information on approved HIV/AIDS therapies and clinical trials. Links to other sites.

The HIV InfoWeb
http://carebase2.jri.org/infoweb/
• Provides information on HIV and AIDS treatments and clinical trials. Links to other sites.

National Library of Medicine (NLM) AIDS Information Gopher Resource
gopher://gopher.nlm.nih.gov/11/aids
• Provides access to the online databases AIDSTRIALS and AIDSDRUGS. Links to other sites.

Using a Fax Machine

NAPWA Fax
National Association of People with AIDS
202-789-2222—FAX
• Several up-to-date fax documents on national clinical trials for people with HIV/AIDS. Request the "Living with HIV" fax catalog of fax documents in English. A Spanish catalog is also available. You must be at a fax machine to use the NAPWA Fax service.

Video

"HIV/AIDS Clinical Trials: Knowing Your Options"
Mail order: CDC National AIDS Clearinghouse
800-458-5231—English/Spanish
800-243-7012—Hearing-impaired TTY/TDD

Paying for Treatment

If you're not receiving treatment free through a clinical trial, you will have to determine how you're going to pay for the medications you need. Taken regularly, antiretroviral drugs and preventive treatments may cost tens of thousands of dollars per year. Expenses can escalate quickly if you become ill.

1) *If you have insurance,* review your policy to see whether prescription drugs are covered in full or in part. If the medication is given intravenously, and/or if you need nursing or home health assistance to inject it, benefits may be spelled out under the "home care" rather than "prescription drug" section of your policy. (Coverage varies widely from policy to policy; if in doubt, contact your insurance company directly.)

   Some policies require only a small co-payment for each prescription you fill. Others require you to pay the full amount up front then submit a claim for reimbursement. If tying up cash is a problem, it may be helpful to use credit cards for your purchases. This can give you a "grace period" to get your money back from the insurance company, which you can then use to pay off the charged amount. However, many people with HIV/AIDS have gotten into financial trouble by spending their reimbursement checks instead of using them to pay off credit card debt. Credit cards, used unwisely, can be a real trap. Look for pharmacies that will provide the drugs you need up front and will work with your insurance company to do so within the allowances offered by your insurance plan.

   When trying a new medication with unknown side effects, it's a good idea to order a small amount initially. If you can't continue taking it, you haven't invested much. If it's effective, your doctor can phone in a larger order. Comparison shopping among several pharmacies can save money, too.

   Keep in mind that most insurance companies will not cover "experimental" (non-FDA approved) treatments. A few plans will cover unapproved treatments if they are considered the "standard of care" or "treatment of choice" for a particular condition by most qualified physicians. Contact your insurer if there's any doubt.

2) *If you have Medicaid,* or have met your spend-down for the month, your non-experimental HIV-related drugs will be covered in full when you purchase them at pharmacies that accept Medicaid reimbursement.

3) *If you have no insurance coverage for drugs,* but your income is too high to qualify for Medicaid, you can apply for help through the Ryan White AIDS Drug Assistance Program, administered in this state by the Illinois Department of Public Health. A number of

major medicines are provided at no cost or for a small co-payment for individuals who:

- are diagnosed as having HIV or AIDS;
- have low or no income;
- are not eligible for 80% or greater coverage of drugs through another third-party payor (such as an insurance company);
- are not eligible for medical assistance through the Illinois Department of Public Aid Medical Assistance Program on the date drugs are obtained. (Individuals with a financial/medical assistance application pending or those in spend-down unmet status may participate.)

To get into the Ryan White program, you'll need to fill out an application. Forms are available at health department HIV testing sites, public aid offices, and local AIDS service organizations. In Illinois, you can also get more information or an application by contacting:

Illinois Department of Public Health—HIV/AIDS Section
AIDS Drug Assistance Program
525 West Jefferson Street
Springfield, IL 62761
800-825-3518
217-524-8013—FAX
800-547-0466—Hearing-impaired TTY/TDD (non-hotline)
8:30 a.m.-5 p.m. Mon-Fri

You'll need to enclose documentation of your HIV or AIDS diagnosis, as well as copies of your most recent wage stubs or proof of other income or benefits with your application. You'll receive a decision within 30 days from the date your application is received. If it's approved, you must fill all covered prescriptions through the department's contracted pharmacy (they will give you all the details).

If you are turned down by the AIDS Drug Assistance Program, you have a right to appeal the decision. The denial may be reversed based upon special needs that may not have been represented when your financial information was plugged into IDPH's formula. Appeals are decided on a case-by-case basis and take into account any unusual circumstances. Your case manager can help you appeal a decision that has not gone in your favor.

In addition to this federal program, many pharmaceutical companies have programs that provide a free supply of drugs to people who don't have insurance, have low incomes, and can't qualify for other kinds of help. Drug companies call these "patient assistance programs," "payment assistance programs," or "indigent drug programs." Some have payment caps on expensive drugs—after a certain dollar amount has been spent within a given year, the program will provide the drug for free.

In almost all cases, you need to have your doctor call these numbers for an application; you will not be able to sign yourself up. However, most companies will be happy to give you eligibility information. If you're turned down, most pharmaceutical companies have an appeal system built into their drug assistance programs.

Chemical/Generic Name	Brand Name	Type	Manufacturer	Phone
Acyclovir	Zovirax	Antiviral	Glaxo Wellcome	800-722-9294
Amitriptyline	Endep	Antineuropathy	Roche Labs	800-285-4484
Atovaquone	Mepron	Antiprotozoal	Glaxo Wellcome	800-722-9294
Azithromycin	Zithromax	Antibiotic	Pfizer Inc.	800-869-9979
Blemycin sulfate	Blenoxane	Anticancer	Bristol-Myers Squibb	800-272-4878
Cefotaxime	Claforan	Antibiotic	Hoechst Marion Roussel	800-552-3656
Ceftriaxone	Rocephin	Antibiotic	Roche Labs	800-285-4484
Cefuroxime	Ceftin	Antibiotic	Glaxo Wellcome	800-722-9294
Cefuroxime	Kefurox	Antibiotic	Eli Lilly & Company	800-545-6962
Cimetidine	Tagamet	Antiulcer	SmithKline Beecham	800-546-0420
Ciprofloxacin	Cipro	Antibiotic	Bayer Corp.	800-998-9180
Clarithromycin	Biaxin	Antibiotic	Abbott Laboratories	800-688-9118
Clindamycin phosphate	Cleocin Phosphate	Antibiotic	Pharmacia & Upjohn	800-242-7014
Clofazimine	Lamprene	Antibiotic	CibaGeneva	800-257-3273
Clonazepam	Klonopin	Antiseizure	Roche Labs	800-285-4484
Clotrimazole	Lotrimin	Antifungal	Schering Corp.	800-656-9485
Clotrimazole	Mycelex	Antifungal	Bayer Corp.	800-998-9180
Cyclophosphamide	Cytoxan	Anticancer	Bristol-Myers Squibb	800-272-4878
Cyclosporine	Sandimmune	Immunomodulator	Sandoz Pharmaceuticals	888-455-6655
Delavirdine	Rescriptor	Antiviral	Pharmacia & Upjohn	800-711-0807
Dexamethasone	Decadron	Corticosteroid	Merck & Company	800-994-2111
Didanosine (ddI)	Videx	Antiviral	Bristol-Myers Squibb	800-272-4878
Doxycycline	Vibramycin	Antibiotic	Pfizer Inc.	800-646-4455
Dronabinol	Marinol	Antiwasting	Roxane Laboratories	800-274-8651
Epoetin alfa	Epogen	Immunomodulator	Amgen	800-272-9376
Epoetin alfa	Procrit	Immunomodulator	Ortho Biotech	800-553-3851
Ethambutol HCl	Myambutol	Antibiotic	Lederle	800-568-9938
Erythromycin	A/T/S	Antibiotic (topical)	Hoechst Marion Roussel	800-552-3656
Etoposide (VP 16)	VePesid	Anticancer	Bristol-Myers Squibb	800-272-4878

Famciclovir	Famvir	Antiviral	SmithKline Beecham	800-546-0420
Famotidine	Pepcid	Antiulcer	Merck & Company	800-994-2111
Fentanyl	Duragesic	Pain reliever	Janssen Pharmaceutica	800-544-2987
Filgrastim (G-CSF)	Neupogen	Immunomodulator	Amgen	800-272-9376
Fluconazole	Diflucan	Antifungal	Pfizer Inc.	800-869-9979
Flucytosine	Ancobon	Antifungal	Roche Labs	800-285-4484
Fluocinonide	Lidex	Anti-inflammatory	Medicis	800-550-5115
Foscarnet sodium	Foscavir	Antiviral	Astra U.S.A.	800-488-3247
Ganciclovir	Cytovene	Antiviral	Roche Labs	800-282-7780
Ganciclovir implants	Vitrasert	Antiviral	Chiron Vision	800-843-1137
Gentamicin sulfate	Garimycin	Antibiotic	Schering Corp.	800-656-9485
Granisetron HCl	Kytril	Antinausea	SmithKline Beecham	800-546-0420
Hydrocortisone	Cortef	Corticosteroid	Pharmacia & Upjohn	800-242-7014
Hydrocortisone	Hydrocortone	Corticosteroid	Merck & Company	800-994-2111
Hydroxyzine	Atarax	Anti-nausea/anxiety	Pfizer Inc.	800-646-4455
Hydroxyzine	Vistaril	Anti-nausea/anxiety	Pfizer Inc.	800-646-4455
Immune globulin	Gamimune	Immunomodulator	Bayer Corp.	800-246-5551
Indinavir sulfate	Crixivan	Protease inhibitor	Merck & Company	800-850-3430
Interferon alpha-2a	Roferon-A	Anti-cancer/viral	Roche Labs	800-443-6676
Interferon alpha-2b	Intron A	Anti-cancer/viral	Schering Corp.	800-656-9485
Itraconazole	Sporanox	Antifungal	Janssen Pharmaceutica	800-544-2987
Ketoconazole	Nizoral	Antifungal	Janssen Pharmaceutica	800-544-2987
Lamivudine (3TC)	Epivir	Antiviral	Glaxo Wellcome	800-722-9294
Liposomal daunorubicin	DaunoXome	Anticancer	NeXstar Pharmaceuticals	800-226-2056
Liposomal doxorubicin	Doxil	Anticancer	Sequus Pharmaceuticals	800-375-1658
Loperamide HCl	Imodium	Antidiarrheal	Janssen Pharmaceutica	800-544-2987
Loratadine	Claritin	Antihistamine	Schering Corp.	800-656-9485
Megestrol acetate	Megace	Anti-wasting/cancer	Bristol-Myers Squibb	800-272-4878
Methotrexate	Rheumatrex	Anticancer	Lederle/Immunex	800-568-9938
Methylprednisolone	Medrol	Corticosteroid	Pharmacia & Upjohn	800-242-7014
Mexiletine HCl	Mexitil	Antineuropathy	Boehringer Ingelheim	800-556-8317
Morphine sulfate	Roxanol	Pain reliever	Roxane Laboratories	800-247-8651
Nelfinavir	Viracept	Protease inhibitor	Agouron Pharmaceuticals	888-777-6637
Nevirapine	Viramune	Antiviral	Roxane Labs	800-274-8651
Nimodipine	Nimotop	Antineuropathy	Bayer Corp.	800-998-9180
Nizatidine	Axid	Antiulcer	Eli Lilly & Company	800-545-6962
Nystatin	Mycostatin	Antifungal	Bristol-Myers Squibb	800-272-4878
Octreotide acetate/Sandoz	Sandostatin	Antidiarrheal	Sandoz Pharmaceuticals	888-455-6655

Paclitaxel	Taxol	Anticancer	Bristol-Myers Squibb	800-272-4878
Pentamidine	NebuPent	Antiprotozoal	Fujisawa U.S.A.	800-888-7704
Pentoxifylline	Trental	Blood thinner	Hoechst Marion Roussel	800-552-3656
Phenytoin	Dilantin	Antiseizure	Parke-Davis	800-223-0432
Prednisone	Deltasone	Corticosteroid	Pharmacia & Upjohn	800-242-7014
Prochlorperazine	Compazine	Antinausea	SmithKline Beecham	800-546-0420
Pyrazinamide	Pyrazinamide USP	Antibiotic	Lederle	800-568-9938
Pyrimethamine	Daraprim	Antiparasitic	Glaxo Wellcome	800-722-9294
Pyrimethamine	Fansidar	Antiprotozoal	Roche Labs	800-285-4484
Ranitidine HCl	Zantac	Antiulcer	Glaxo Wellcome	800-722-9294
Rifabutin	Mycobutin	Antibiotic	Pharmacia & Upjohn	800-242-7014
Rifampin USP	Rimactane	Antibiotic	CibaGeneva	800-257-3273
Ritonavir	Norvir	Protease inhibitor	Abbott Laboratories	800-659-9050
Saquinavir	Invirase	Protease inhibitor	Roche Labs	800-282-7780
Sargramostim (GM-CSF)	Leukine	Immunomodulator	Immunex Corp.	800-334-6273
Sargramostim (GM-CSF)	Prokine	Immunomodulator	Immunex Corp.	800-334-6273
Scopolamine	Transderm Scop	Antinausea	CibaGeneva	800-257-3273
Somatrem	Protropin	Antiwasting	Genentech	800-879-4747
Somatropin	Humatrope	Antiwasting	Eli Lilly & Company	800-545-6962
Somatropin (hGH)	Nutropin	Antiwasting	Genentech	800-879-4747
Stavudine (d4T)	Zerit	Antiviral	Bristol-Myers Squibb	800-272-4878
Streptomycin sulfate	Streptomycin USP	Antibiotic	Pfizer Inc.	800-646-4455
Sucralfate	Carafate	Antiulcer	Hoechst Marion Roussel	800-552-3656
Terfenadine	Seldane	Antihistamine	Hoechst Marion Roussel	800-552-3656
Testosterone	Testoderm	Hormone	Alra Pharmaceuticals	800-321-3130
TMP/SMX	Bactrim	Antibiotic	Roche Labs	800-285-4484
TMP/SMX	Septra	Antibiotic	Glaxo Wellcome	800-722-9294
Trimetrexate glucuronate	Neutrexin	Antiprotozoal	U.S. Bioscience, Inc.	800-887-2467
Valacyclovir HCl	Valtrex	Antiviral	Glaxo Wellcome	800-722-9294
Vinblastine	Velban	Anticancer	Eli Lilly & Company	800-545-6962
Vincristine sulfate	Oncovin	Anticancer	Eli Lilly & Company	800-545-6962
Zalcitabine (ddC)	Hivid	Antiviral	Roche Labs	800-285-4484
Zidovudine (AZT)	Retrovir	Antiviral	Glaxo Wellcome	800-722-9294

Adapted and updated from Pharmaceutical Company Patient Assistance Programs, National Association of People with AIDS (NAPWA FAX), and The Access Project patient assistance program listings.

Patient Assistance Program Resources

For the most complete, up-to-date listings of patient assistance programs, use both of the following resources. Each offers some listings not included by the other.

NAPWA Fax
National Association of People with AIDS
202-789-2222—FAX
- Fax documents on pharmaceutical company patient assistance programs. Request the "Living with HIV" fax catalog of fax documents in English. A Spanish catalog is also available. You must be at a fax machine to use the NAPWA Fax service.

Access Project: Patient Assistance Programs
800-734-7104
http://www.aidsnyc.org/network/access/pa.html
- Easy to use listing of pharmaceutical company patient assistance programs, including eligibility criteria and toll-free company numbers.

"Chicago Area HIV/AIDS Services Directory"
Bejlovec, Rick, Editor
Test Positive Aware Network, 1997
Mail order: Test Positive Aware Network, 773-404-8726, or 773-404-9716—Hearing-impaired TTY/TDD
- Includes a listing of national pharmaceutical assistance programs. Free. English/Spanish.

4) *If you want to purchase "experimental" drugs* without participating in a clinical trial, or wish to locate approved drugs at a discount, there are buyers' clubs operating in several U.S. cities. These "underground" organizations offer domestic and imported prescription and non-prescription drugs for use by individuals under a doctor's care.

Your doctor may be opposed to your taking medicines that have not yet received FDA approval. If you're committed to pursuing this kind of treatment, you may have to switch doctors. *It is extremely important that you keep your doctor informed about all drugs and medications you are taking,* regardless of their source or legal status.

Pharmacies and Buyers' Clubs

You can often get up-to-date information about pharmacies, mail order pharmacies, and buyers' clubs from your health care provider, case manager, or local AIDS service organization. State and national AIDS hotlines may also have this information. Some national AIDS organizations have their own buyers' club (such as the People with AIDS Coalition, 800-828-3280) or pharmacy (such as the National Association of People with AIDS, 800-808-8060). These organizations can give you names of others around the country.

> *Another thing that's keeping my spirits up is the alternative treatment I'm going through. I believe—no, I don't "believe" in acupuncture. I do acupuncture three times a week. But I believe that trying something, actively doing something for my health, is good for me. I don't even know if it will add a day to my life, but I feel better while I'm alive attempting something.*
>
> JOE

> *Early on, I tried to do the least intrusive, most supportive things possible—not to attack the virus but to support my immune system. I didn't want to take experimental drugs so I took herbs. I've recently gotten back to doing herbs because I really think I shouldn't have stopped, I think they were doing me some good. But I just got bored with it after awhile.*
>
> CHARLIE

> *Meditation has helped. It lets you forget for thirty minutes you've got this virus in your body.*
>
> "MARIE"

> *I'm a believer in Western medicine, as opposed to alternative or holistic kinds of medicines. But for others, I say do what's best for them.*
>
> JIM

AIDS Treatment News
800-873-2812
http://www.aidsnews.org
• Annually publishes the most comprehensive listing of buyers' clubs in their newsletter. Call to request a back issue. Or find it easily on their Web site by searching for "buyers' clubs" in their newsletter archives.

NAPWA Fax
National Association of People with AIDS
202-789-2222—FAX
• Fax information on buyers' clubs. Request the "Living with HIV" fax catalog of fax documents in English. A Spanish catalog is also available. You must be at a fax machine to use the NAPWA Fax service.

Statscript Pharmacy
912 West Belmont Avenue
Chicago, Il 60657
773-665-8900
773-665-9766-FAX
• Pharmacy service with an emphasis on counseling to HIV-impacted persons.

Stadtlanders Pharmacy
600 Penn Center Boulevard
Pittsburgh, PA 15235
800-238-7828
800-426-9613—FAX
800-336-8675—Hearing-impaired TTY/TDD
• Confidential pharmacy service with no membership fee. Provides over-the-counter medications and durable medical equipment, and operates a free medication counseling hotline covering the gamut from emotional to financial concerns. Publishes the Magazine "Lifetimes 2."

"Complementary" or "Holistic" Approaches

Dovetailing with the Mainstream

Some treatment approaches are different from mainstream medical care in that they may address not only your physical needs, but also your spiritual, psychological, and social needs. These are known as "complementary" or "holistic" therapies. Among the most popular are meditation, yoga, massage, acupuncture, herbal remedies, macrobiotic or other special diets, visualization, chiropractics, stress reduction and relaxation techniques, vitamin therapy, homeopathy, and tai chi.

You will sometimes hear these types of approaches referred to as "alternative medicine." However, while one or more of them may help you feel more relaxed and better able to cope with your illness, it's best to view them as things you can try to *supplement* your doctor's recommendations. Reputable holistic therapists will urge you to discuss complementary treatments with your doctor before pursuing them.

Complementary therapies have shown only limited results in strengthening the immune system. However, the benefits they can provide in such areas as pain management and stress reduction should not be overlooked in creating a strategy for living with HIV. These therapies can also help you cope with troubling conditions resulting from HIV or the prescriptions you are taking, such as nausea, diarrhea, dry skin, or muscle aches.

Before trying any non-medical approach, it's extremely important to consult your doctor. If not properly administered, special diets and other interventions can jeopardize your health, as well as limit the effectiveness of prescribed drugs you may be taking. Any change in your treatment program should be closely monitored by a licensed physician.

Doctors have different opinions on the subject of complementary therapies. Some consider them helpful to the extent that they enhance a patient's sense of empowerment and well-being. Others consider them potentially dangerous. If you're not sure how your own doctor feels, ask. A good way to get into the topic is to pose questions: "Is this therapy accepted by the medical profession? Why or why not? Could it benefit me in addition to my conventional treatment? Is there any possibility it could harm me or be counterproductive to what we're trying to accomplish? How vigorously should I pursue it?"

Notice that by broaching the subject this way, you enlist the doctor's advice. You haven't attacked the doctor's form of healing or questioned his or her competence. Instead, you've invited the doctor into a dialogue as your partner in the care of your health.

Keep in mind that *not all complementary approaches are equal.* You'll have to employ your intuition and common sense to separate "snake oil" products from truly helpful folk medicine and alternative techniques. If you find yourself watching desperately for magic remedies, enlist a trusted friend or call a fraud hotline to help you sort through your options.

AIDS Fraud Is Dangerous!

When people are confronted with a serious illness like AIDS, they're often willing to try almost anything that promises to help. Some of these alternative treatments may be helpful or at least harmless, but others can be dangerous, even deadly. For example, immune system "booster" capsules were promoted as a remedy, but were found to contain heavy metals such as lead and chromium that can cause anemia, central-nervous system damage, and kidney failure. Another product being brought into the U.S. from the Caribbean turned out to be contaminated with HIV and the hepatitis B virus.

If you're looking for treatment for AIDS or HIV infection, protect yourself! Question any treatment that:

Early on, I did a lot of reading of the medical studies in terms of how to be healthy, how to deal with an illness. I got very much into ayervedic medicine. It's the foundation for Greek medicine, which is the foundation for the Western medical model. But it originated in India, and a lot of the traditions of it are being revived. It's tied in with transcendental meditation and diet.

I've been trying to find a balance between Western medicine and some other forms of medicine, which was a new experience for me because I've never been into meditating or anything like that. I still haven't started meditating, but I think that period of exploration of alternatives was an important stage for me to go through. The ayervedic approach touched me personally and fit into my way of thinking about things. It was simple and doable and not too far out. I'm really not into far-out philosophical schools.

"RALPH"

- claims to prevent or cure AIDS or HIV infection. Right now, there is no cure.
- is promoted as "miraculous," "foolproof," "revolutionary," "painless," or makes other fantastic claims.
- sounds too good to be true. (It probably is.)
- claims to have been discovered by a "foreign doctor" or is advertised as "tested in another country."
- is an experimental drug or treatment that you have to pay for. (Patients are rarely charged for experimental treatments or drugs.)
- uses personal success stories to sell the product. Endorsements are not proof that a product or treatment works.
- is sold as a "cure" for other illnesses, such as cancer or arthritis, in addition to AIDS.
- uses big, scientific-sounding words or other medical jargon in its advertisements. While it may sound sophisticated, it could be untrue.
- claims to enhance your immune system.

From "What You Need to Know about AIDS Fraud," by the Illinois HIV Health Fraud Information Network. For more information, contact the Network at: PO Box 804678, Chicago, IL 60680. Reprinted with permission.

Complementary Treatment Resources

AIDS Alternative Health Project
4753 North Broadway, Suite 1110
Chicago, IL 60640
773-561-2800
773-561-8225—FAX
• Complementary therapies, including chiropractic, massage therapy, acupuncture, psychological services, nutritional counseling, and energy work, provided in a cooperative environment with on-site medical physicians.

Center for Natural and Traditional Medicines
PO Box 21735
Washington, DC 20009
202-234-9632—Voice/FAX (same line)
• Information and resource center on the use of natural and traditional healing methods from various cultures worldwide. Provides telephone information, materials by mail, and referrals nationwide.

Coach House Drop-In Center—Woodlawn Organization
1445 East 65th Street
Chicago, IL 60637
773-288-4088
773-288-5871—FAX
• Provides acupuncture, massage, and herbal therapy for people with HIV/AIDS. Also offers case management, counseling, recreational activities, emergency care, testing, and other programs with a holistic approach. Free.

Cook County Department of Public Health
1010 Lake Street, Suite 300
Oak Park, IL 60301
708-445-2530
708-445-2130—FAX
708-445-2406—Hearing-impaired TTY/TDD
• Offers massage therapy off-site at locations throughout suburban Cook County for suburban residents with HIV/AIDS. Free. English/Spanish.

Cook County HIV Primary Care Center
1835 West Harrison Street
CCSN 1268
Chicago, IL 60612
312-633-3005
312-633-3002—FAX
• Massage therapy and acupuncture for patients who receive primary care at the center. Free. English/Spanish.

Illinois HIV Health Fraud Information Network
PO Box 804678
Chicago, IL 60680-4108
312-744-9400—Report fraudulent HIV/AIDS treatment claims in the Chicago area
312-353-4423—Federal Trade Commission, report fraudulent claims outside Chicago
• Write for a free brochure on how to identify HIV/AIDS fraud. (The phone numbers listed above are for fraudulent claims only, not ordering publications.)

Illinois Masonic Medical Center–Triad Clinic, "Strong Spirit" Program
938 West Nelson Street
Chicago, IL 60657
773-296-8400
773-296-8401—FAX
• HIV primary care clinic, outpatient and inpatient care with special HIV/AIDS unit and hospice. On-site alternative therapies through "Strong Spirit" program, including massage, aerobics, and Chinese herbal medicine. Public Aid accepted. English/Spanish.

Project VIDA
2659 South Kedvale Avenue
Chicago, IL 60623
773-522-4570
773-522-4573—FAX
• Alternative therapies for people with HIV. English/Spanish.

Roseland Community Hospital HIV Clinic
45 West 111th Street, 3rd Floor
Chicago, IL 60628
773-995-3469
773-995-3199—FAX
• Outpatient clinic for people with HIV/AIDS, including alternative therapies. Public aid accepted.

St. Joseph Hospital
2900 North Lake Shore Drive
Chicago, IL 60657
888-712-CARE—Confidential, toll-free HIV physician referral
773-665-6188—FAX
• Outpatient and inpatient medical care for adults with HIV. Multidisciplinary services include complementary therapies offered through the AIDS Alternative Health Project. St. Joseph Hospital is an Affiliate of Catholic Health Partnership. English, Spanish, Polish, Chinese.

VIDA/SIDA
2703 West Division Street
Chicago, IL 60622
773-278-6737
773-278-6753—FAX
• Alternative health clinic and STD/HIV prevention project. Acupuncture, massage, and chiropractic services. Resource library. Public Aid accepted. English/Spanish.

Weiss Memorial Hospital HIV/AIDS Program
4646 North Marine Drive
Chicago, IL 60640
773-564-5333
773-564-5334—FAX
• Primary care through community-based clinic. Outpatient and inpatient hospital care by HIV specialists. Complementary therapies include art and massage. Public Aid accepted. English, Spanish, Vietnamese.

On the Web

Critical Path AIDS Project
http://www.critpath.org/
• Access to information on mainstream and complementary treatments, clinical trials, research, and more. Specific links for women, minorities, and youth.

Test Positive Aware Network
http://www.tpan.com/alternat/index.htm
• Alternative Health Center at this site offers information from the TPA newsletter "Positively Aware" on acupuncture, Chinese medicine, ayurveda, homeopathy, biofeedback, massage, reflexology, and other complementary therapies. Includes a list of dangerous therapies to avoid.

Books and Publications

"Chinese Medicine and HIV"
Mail order: Impact AIDS, 505-995-0722
• Brochure explaining how Chinese medicine, including acupuncture and herbal medicine, may enhance the immune system and reduce or prevent certain HIV-related symptoms. Discusses how to combine Chinese and traditional Western medicines. English only.

A Holistic Protocol for the Immune System, (Sixth Edition)
Gregory, Scott J., O.M.D.
Palm Springs, CA: Tree Life Publications, 1995
Mail Order: Impact AIDS, 505-995-0722, or
Amazon.com Books:
http://www.amazon.com
• The book describes a range of natural treatments, including homeopathy, therapeutic massage, holistic medicine, and others.

The Honest Herbal: A Sensible Guide to the Use of Herbs and Related Remedies
Tyler, Varro
The Hayworth Press, 1993

Immune Power: A Comprehensive Treatment Program for HIV
Kaiser, Jon
St. Martin's Press, 1993
Mail Order: Impact AIDS, 505-995-0722
• Outlines a treatment program including nutritional support, psychological care, and standard medical therapies.

Reader's Guide to Alternative Health Methods
Zivicky, J.F.
Milwaukee, Wisconsin: American Medical Association, 1993

Treating AIDS with Chinese Medicine
Ryan, Mary Kay and Arthur Shattuck
Pacific View Press
Mail order: Lambda Rising Books, 800-621-6969
• Comprehensive guide for practitioners of Chinese medicine. Identifies the acupuncture and herbal strategies most effective in maintaining well-being, reducing drug side effects, and minimizing the impact of opportunistic infections. Addresses the concerns of Western medicine, explaining what Chinese medicine can offer.

Video

"Sun Chi: Techniques of Relaxation and Positive Imagery"
Mail order: Lambda Rising Books, 800-621-6969
• Self-care video for people with HIV and other illnesses. Teaches the basic principles of tai chi, positive thinking, and relaxation.

Learning More about Drugs, Trials, and Treatments

Your own doctor will be a key source of advice in deciding whether you should try one or a combination of medically approved drugs and complementary therapies, or participate in a clinical research trial. Your local AIDS service organization and the various AIDS hotlines can also help you learn as much as possible about the treatment issues surrounding HIV.

If you really want to get immersed in the treatment area, there are a number of excellent newsletters and magazines available from sources around the country. Staff members at AIDS service organizations can advise you on which ones deal exclusively with treatment issues and are easiest for non-professionals to read.

Some of these publications will reduce or waive their subscription fees if you can't afford them; be sure to ask when you call. In addition, your doctor, clinic, and/or AIDS service organization may subscribe to one or more of these publications and have current and back issues available for you to browse through, free of charge. Check with university and medical school libraries, too.

Treatment Newsletters and Magazines

"AIDS/HIV Treatment Directory"
• The most comprehensive source of information about approved and experimental treatments available for people with HIV or AIDS. Published twice per year by the American Foundation for AIDS Research. To subscribe, call 800-392-6327. You can get a free copy of the current issue from the CDC National AIDS Clearinghouse, by calling 800-458-5231.

"AIDS Treatment News"
• Published twice per month. Summarizes the latest developments in research, experimental therapies, and available treatment options. John S. James, PO Box 411256, San Francisco, CA 94141. Subscription fee on sliding scale. 800-873-2812.

"BETA" (Bulletin of Experimental Treatments for AIDS)
• Quarterly treatment publication of the San Francisco AIDS Foundation, available in English and Spanish. Fairly easy to read. Subscriptions: San Francisco AIDS Foundation, 1250 45th Street, Suite 200, Emoryville, CA 94608. Call 800-959-1059 (subscription office). Scholarship subscriptions available for those unable to pay. For scholarship requests, write to: Subscriber Services, SFAF, PO Box 426182, San Francisco, CA 94142.

"Body Positive"
• Monthly newsletter specifically for people with HIV. A Spanish newsletter is published quarterly. Distributes the 1996 book, Positive Options. 19 Fulton Street, Suite 308B, New York, NY 10038. 212-566-7333. Reduced or free subscriptions available for people with HIV.

"Critical Path AIDS Project"
• Published quarterly, the newsletter includes current news on approved drugs, alternative therapies, clinical trials, drug assistance programs, and medical alerts about drug interactions. 2062 Lombard Street, Philadelphia, PA 19146. 215-545-2212. Free to HIV-positive persons who cannot afford it.

"Notes from the Underground"
• Current information on therapies and treatment strategies, concentrating on "underground" AIDS treatment access. Published by the PWA Health Group. Also offers a buyers' club and fact sheets in English and Spanish. 150 West 26th Street, Suite 201, New York, NY 10001. 212-255-0520.

"Positively Aware"
• Provides comprehensive HIV/AIDS news, treatment updates, and other articles of interest to people affected by HIV. Published bimonthly by Test Positive Aware Network, 1258 West Belmont, Chicago, IL 60657, 773-404-8726 (or 773-404-9716—hearing-impaired TTY/TDD). Free to TPA members and persons with HIV who cannot contribute. Recent issues are posted on their Web site <http://www.tpan.com> English/Spanish.

"POZ"
• Monthly national, glossy magazine for anyone affected by HIV/AIDS. Subscriptions: PO Box 417, Mt. Morris, IL 61054. 800-973-2376.

"PI Perspective"
• Published quarterly by Project Inform; other information is sent out in a confidential treatment information packet. Project Inform, 1965 Market Street, Suite 220, San Francisco, CA 94103. 800-822-7422. Or visit them at <http://www.projinf.org>. Donations for subscriptions are appreciated.

"PWA Coalition Newsline"
• Monthly newsletter covering all aspects of HIV/AIDS. Reports on alternative and experimental and community-based research programs. Written primarily by people living with the disease and their friends from around the world. PWA Coalition also offers a buyers' club. 50 West 17th Street, 8th Floor, New York, NY 10001. 212-647-1415. Free to people with HIV.

"TAG"
• Half English/half Spanish publication on AIDS research and policies by New York's Treatment Action Group. 212-260-0300.

"Treatment Issues"
• The Gay Men's Health Crisis Newsletter of Experimental AIDS Therapies is the world's largest monthly community-based newsletter devoted to HIV treatment and medical information. Provides information on drug research, how to access special "compassionate use" programs, and other timely news. The groups' "AIDS Medical Glossary" is a good summary of terms in plain English. Call or write for a free sample issue. GMHC, 129 West 20th Street, New York, NY 10011. 212-337-1950.

"Treatment Review"
• Newsletter of the AIDS Treatment Data Network (ATDN), published at least eight times per year. ATDN also offers a treatment guide and an excellent set of simple fact sheets on treatments, conditions, and common lab tests. English/Spanish. 800-734-7104.

Book

HIV Drug Book, (Second Edition)
Petrow, Steven
Pocket Books, 1997.
• A comprehensive, user-friendly guide to all the drugs most used by people with HIV and AIDS. Produced by Project Inform. Formatted for quick reference and written in nontechnical language, the handbook features an extensive master index (from AZT to Zantac). In most bookstores.

Using a Computer and Modem

AIDS Research Information Center (ARIC)
http://www.critpath.org/aric/aricinc.htm
• ARIC is a private, nonprofit AIDS medical information service committed to making complex medical information understandable to the average person. Issues of ARIC's newsletters and excerpts from other publications are accessible through this site.

AIDS Treatment News
http://www.aidsnews.org
• Contains issues of their newsletter "AIDS Treatment News." Information about approved treatments and experimental therapies available in English, Spanish, Italian, French, German, and other languages.

The AIDS Treatment Data Network
http://www.aidsnyc.org/network/index.html
• Good information source on treatments and clinical trials. Contains glossaries of drugs and opportunistic infections, issues of their newsletter "Treatment Review," and more.

The Body: A Multimedia AIDS and HIV Resource
http://www.thebody.com/cgi-bin/body.cgi
• An excellent site offering HIV/AIDS treatment information. Topics include Information on Treatments, Antiviral Medications, Infections/Complications, Research, Experimental Drugs, and Alternative Medicine. Links to other sites.

The Food & Drug Administration (FDA) HIV and AIDS Page
http://www.fda.gov//oashi/aids/hiv.html
• Information on approved HIV/AIDS therapies, clinical trials, articles and brochures. Links to other sites.

The HIV/AIDS Treatment Information Service (ATIS)
http://www.hivatis.org/
• This Public Health Service site provides information about federally approved treatment guidelines for HIV and AIDS. English/Spanish. Links to other sites.

The HIV InfoWeb
http://carebase2.jri.org/infoweb/
• Provides information on treatments and clinical trials. Includes a search engine and links to other sites.

The Journal of the American Medical Association (JAMA) HIV/AIDS Site
http://www.ama-assn.org/special/hiv/hivhome.htm
• An interactive collection of useful and high-quality resources for physicians, other health professionals, and the public. Includes information for patients, support group information, a glossary, and more. Links to other sites.

National AIDS Treatment Information Project
http://www.kff.org
• Provides very up-to-date most since 1996) fact sheets on treatments and the meaning of many medical tests. Sponsored by the Kaiser Family Foundation with Beth Israel Hospital.

National Library of Medicine (NLM) AIDS Information Gopher Resource
gopher://gopher.nlm.nih/gov/11/aids
• Provides access to the online database AIDSDRUGS. Links to other sites.

Using a Fax Machine

NAPWA Fax
National Association of People with AIDS
202-789-2222—FAX
• Provides many fax documents on mainstream and alternative treatment options. Request the "Living with HIV" fax catalog of fax documents in English. A Spanish catalog is also available. You must be at a fax machine to use the NAPWA Fax service.

National AIDS Treatment Information Project
800-399-AIDS—FAX
• Very current, easy-to-understand information available toll-free. Fact sheets can help people with HIV understand medical conditions and the latest treatments. To order the entire set, enter #1156. The voice instructions for using this fax service are in English or Spanish, but the faxes come through in English only.

4. TELLING OTHERS

One of the most urgent questions people face after their diagnosis is whom to tell. This is an intensely personal matter and one of the most important decisions you'll make. It is usually not a good idea to make a decision to disclose your HIV status immediately after receiving your diagnosis or when you are in a time of crisis. Wait until you've had time to talk to trusted friends or qualified professionals about your decision.

Whether to Tell

In your "public" life, you will want to think carefully before telling many people about your HIV status. The lay public is still very ignorant and fearful about the virus and how it is transmitted. People may form negative opinions about you based on your having it. Many HIV-positive men, women, and children have faced ugly and damaging discrimination from schools, landlords, neighbors, employers, classmates, co-workers, insurance companies, even health care workers. Much of this discrimination is illegal and you do have recourse if it occurs. You might want to protect yourself from negative encounters, however, by choosing to keep your health information confidential. This is especially true if you have just learned you are HIV-positive. Do yourself the favor of waiting to share this information with anyone except a physician until you've had a chance to get over the shock.

In your personal life, be aware that by telling friends and family members you have this disease, you will forever change the way you relate to one another. This may be a bad thing or a good thing. Some people living with the virus have had friends abandon them and relatives disinherit them. Others say sharing the news has led to warmer, deeper relationships than they ever dreamed possible. It's almost impossible to predict how others will take the news. Even if you think you know people very, very well, their reactions may surprise you—pleasantly or otherwise. You'll want to take great care in choosing your confidants so you won't create more problems than you solve. You will also want to consider if they will respect your need for confidentiality.

When to Tell

It *may* be a good idea to tell someone about your HIV if any of the following apply to you:

- you are very clear in your own mind about why you want to tell that particular person at that particular time.
- you feel comfortable enough with your condition to present the news effectively to others.
- they're a past, current, or potential sexual partner who may be at risk personally, or has the potential to transmit the virus to others unknowingly.
- they're providing you with medical, dental, or psychological care related to your illness.

In 1989, my best friend died of AIDS. I took a week off work, going back and forth to Detroit helping out with funeral arrangements. I told my boss all this, straight out, because I figured this was my chance to sort of begin to open up the question at work.

When I got back from Detroit, I found out that everyone thought there had been a death in my family, of cancer. My boss had "translated it for my benefit," and other people were, in effect, covering for me. I actually was kinda pissed, because I had told them about the AIDS on purpose to establish okay, there's some way little indirect connection between Charlie and AIDS. I wanted that to get out there because I knew that down the road, it would have to come out. It didn't fly that time; but later on, when I did tell my boss, it didn't come as such a shock.

CHARLIE

- you're fairly certain they're going to guess or find out anyway, and you want to have control over when and how they're told.
- you're already ill and you need them to help take care of you.
- you're feeling fine, but want to prepare them in case you get sick in the future.
- it will help you make the most of your life right now.
- it will help you make important future plans for things like custody of your children, living wills, and administration of your estate.
- your child is having emotional or other problems as a result of HIV in your family, and telling a key person outside your family could help your child.
- you need help finding, paying for, or getting resources.
- you need emotional support.
- you don't go in with any preconceived notions of how that person will take the news.
- you're ready to open up and share other issues in your life, such as sexuality or drug use, that may be related to your HIV.
- you are prepared for the flood of emotions that will come from both of you, and are ready to help that person come to grips with your news, however long and difficult that process might be.
- you are prepared for the possibility of a disappointing, negative, or violent reaction, and for the possibility that the person could walk out of your life temporarily or permanently.
- you are prepared for the possibility of having your status disclosed to others without your knowledge or approval.
- you have "rehearsed" the best way to break the news, either alone or with a trusted friend, relative, or therapist.
- you do not feel forced into the disclosure by circumstances beyond your control (such as being in the hospital). If possible, it's best to tell while you're feeling well, are in a comfortable and private setting, and are strong enough to handle the repercussions.

Remember, you are under no obligation to tell another living soul, as long as your behavior does not put anyone at risk of infection. If someone else reveals your HIV-positive status against your wishes, you may have grounds for legal action. Still, there probably will be people in your life you'll want to inform, out of a sense of responsibility or to help you cope in some way. Just be certain their "right to know" doesn't interfere with your needs in living with the disease.

As you disclose the facts of your illness, you may find yourself being forced into the role of HIV educator and "support center." People naturally gravitate to and lean on those who know more than they do. This can be very flattering and empowering—but it can also be very frustrating, coming at a time when you need support yourself. It may help to keep a few copies of a favorite HIV/AIDS brochure on hand to give people, to take off some of the pressure. HIV/AIDS educational materials are available from many of the resources listed at the end of the first chapter. You can usually obtain a few free of charge by asking.

You might also refer a person who wants or needs to learn more to a counselor at an HIV service agency. Often, it is helpful to have the realities of living with HIV and AIDS explained by a caring, knowledgeable person who is not emotionally involved in your particular situation.

How to Tell

There's really no easy way to tell someone close to you that you have a life-threatening illness. Test Positive Aware Network suggests the following approach for breaking the news to the "significant others" in your life:

1) *Assess the reasons you want to tell your friends or family.* What do you expect from them? What do you *hope* their reaction will be? What do you expect it to be? What's the worst possible reaction they could have?

2) *Prepare yourself.* Gather clear, simple, educational brochures, hotline numbers, pamphlets, and articles on the disease. Take these with you to leave after your discussion.

3) *Set the stage.* Call or write and explain clearly that you have to meet with them to discuss something extremely important. This is a once-in-a-lifetime experience for all of you—don't treat it in an offhand or rushed manner.

4) *Enlist help.* Ask a close friend or family member who knows the situation to come along or write a letter to your folks asking them to try to understand and reminding them that their acceptance and support are vital. Ask your physician or therapist to write a letter to your folks as well. This can be most effective—many parents will believe or listen to a stranger before listening to their own child.

5) *Be optimistic.* Accept the possibility that your parents are caring and rational adults. Likewise, you need to be as caring and rational; having a chip on your shoulder or selling your parents short is not going to help win the support you need.

6) *Let the emotion come through.* You are not asking to borrow the family car. The prospects to be considered are as frightening for them as they are for you. Now is not the time to assume false fronts or joke away the more serious implications.

7) *Let them know you are in good hands.* Explain how you are taking care of yourself, that your physician knows what to do, that a support network exists for you. The single thing you are asking of them is love.

8) *Let them accept or deny it in their own fashion.* Do not try to change their position right there. Leave them the material and put an end to the discussion if things go very badly. Try not to revisit past discussions about lifestyle.

9) *Give them some time* to digest the information and adjust to the news. After a reasonable period, call them back to assess their reaction.

10) *ACCEPT* their reaction and move on from there.

Attempt to keep the lines of communication open. Approach the process of telling with the best expectations. Still, with all the preparation possible, there may be surprises. Be willing to pull out, pull back, and give them some room. If you're prepared for the worst, the best will be a blessing.

Adapted from an article by Chris Clason in "Positively Aware" (formerly "TPA News"), July, 1990. Reprinted with permission.

Telling Your Employer

Deciding if and when to tell your employer about your HIV status is an extremely critical decision. Timing is everything. If you haven't had any HIV-related symptoms or illnesses and are not on medication that is affecting your job performance, there's probably no need to open up that particular can of worms.

If, on the other hand, your illness is interfering with your work such that your job might be in jeopardy, it may be time to reveal your situation to your boss. Federal, state, and local laws prohibit employers from discriminating against people with HIV or AIDS. If you wish to discuss your HIV status with your employer, it is a good idea to consult first with an attorney. While there are good anti-discrimination laws on the books, they do not guarantee that your employer will treat you in a fair or rational manner.

Once you decide to disclose your HIV status, it is best to do it in writing. Bring a letter from your doctor explaining the current state of your condition and how it might affect your ability to perform your job. (Make a copy for your own records.) Let your boss know you want to continue to do your job to the best of your ability, but that because of the effects of your illness or medication, there are times when your schedule or workload may have to be adjusted. Make specific requests for accommodations of your disability, if needed. Because the law regards a person with HIV or AIDS as a disabled person, your employer is required to reasonably accommodate your needs if you are otherwise qualified to perform the essential duties of the job.

Ask your boss to keep your condition confidential, only notifying those people in the company who absolutely have to know. Illinois law requires this of anyone you tell, but many people (employers included) are not aware of their legal obligation. For your own protection, you may want to decide on a noncombative way to make the people you tell aware of this. For example, if you live in Illinois, you can mention the requirements of the state's AIDS Confidentiality Act in your letter. (You can get the particulars from your case manager, a local library or HIV/AIDS service organization, AIDS Legal Council of Chicago, or a private attorney, to name a few sources.) Again, it's always a good idea to have a few pamphlets or hotline numbers available to help your employer understand your illness and locate resources. The Centers for Disease Control in Atlanta can provide training materials, sample policies, and training referrals to help ensure that an employer provides a friendly atmosphere for the HIV-positive worker. For more information, call:

CDC Business and Labor Resource Service
800-458-5231

Once you present the facts of your condition to your employer in this manner, you may be protected from job discrimination under the federal Americans with Disabilities Act (ADA), the Illinois Human Rights Act, and local ordinances.

As long as you are able to do the essential functions of your job, your employer cannot legally fire you, demote you, refuse to promote you, or force you to work separately from others on account of your condition. It is illegal for your employer to discriminate against you in any way or treat you differently than other employees, except to help you accomplish your work. Also, the Americans with Disabilities Act may prohibit your employer or insurance company from terminating, limiting, or "capping" your medical benefits or life insurance coverage.

For your own protection, carefully document any communication with your employer or questionable incidents on the job for future reference. Keep notes of conversations or incidents, and keep copies of any documents you give to or receive from your employer regarding your health condition. (See the Appendices for a form to copy and use in documenting conversations with your employer and others.)

In certain circumstances, if you are qualified as disabled, your employer is required to take reasonable steps to help you stay on the job. These accommodations might include purchasing special equipment, making changes in your work schedule, restructuring jobs, and more.

It is important for employers to be proactive about HIV. They should have an informed staff and policies related to disabilities in place, whether or not they are aware of any employees who are HIV-positive. The Centers for Disease Control in Atlanta can provide training materials, sample policies, and training referrals to help ensure that an employer provides a friendly atmosphere for the HIV-positive worker. If your employer doesn't measure up, consider making an anonymous suggestion to your human resources department about CDC and other materials that are available.

If you're applying for a job, be aware that under the ADA, prospective employers do not have the right to make inquiries about your health or the existence of a disability prior to a conditional job offer. However, they may inquire if you are aware of any physical limitation that would interfere with your ability to perform the essential job functions.

If you are asked on an employment application or in an interview whether you have HIV, any symptoms of AIDS, or even whether you are associated with anyone else who does, it's best to tell the truth or decline to answer. Although the employer has violated the ADA, you do not want to raise the matter at this time. An employer may not legally refuse to hire you based on your perceived or actual HIV status; thus, most will come up with some other reason if questioned. Still, if you do not get the job, you may have an easier time proving discrimination if the employer had concrete knowledge of your status. You would also be better protected from on-the-job discrimination if hired.

Employers can request a medical examination only after a conditional offer of employment has been made, and when two other conditions apply: the request can be shown to be job-related, and the same examination is required of all other entering employees of the same classification. All medical information obtained by the employer must be kept confidential.

Keep in mind that you cannot be forced to take an HIV test as a condition for getting or keeping a job. However, many HIV-positive people are also active users of illegal drugs. While the ADA protects you from discrimination based on your HIV status, it does not protect you from discrimination based on drug use. Pre-employment screening for illegal drugs is permitted in some states (including Illinois), and an employer or prospective employer may terminate or refuse to hire you based on drug test results.

After July 26, 1994, all employers with 15 or more employees were subject to the provisions of the ADA. If you feel you have been discriminated against in any employment situation, consult an attorney to determine whether the ADA or any of several anti-discrimination laws apply to your situation.

Working with Your Child's School

You may have heard "horror stories" about children who were taunted, discriminated against, or encouraged not to attend school when their HIV status became known. You may also have heard stories about families with HIV-positive children who enjoy an excellent, cooperative relationship with their schools. Telling others about your child's HIV infection is a highly personal decision that must be carefully planned and considered. In most cases, it is in your child's best interest to notify certain school professionals.

In Illinois, physicians must report to local health departments the name, if known, of any person ages 5–21 who tests positive for HIV.

By law, the health department must then notify the child's school principal of the student's identity. The law allows the principal to notify others in the school, specified as the school nurse and classroom teacher, of the child's identity on a "need to know" basis.

Many Illinois principals have proceeded to notify the entire staff or school community that there is an unnamed HIV-positive student in the school. Although public health officials do not advise this practice, it is legal for schools to do this—with or without parental consent—so long as the child's identity is not publicly shared.

Your first step as parent or guardian of a school-aged child with HIV is to schedule a meeting with the school's principal. The purpose of this meeting is to establish a good working relationship between you and the school, enlist their cooperation to ensure that an HIV policy is in place and being observed at the school, and reassure yourself that training has been provided for school personnel. At this meeting, work with the principal to determine which school professionals need to know your child's HIV status to provide safe care. Some parents have found it helpful to invite their child's physician or someone from the local health department to advise the school on handling the situation.

After this initial meeting, request that the principal schedule a follow-up meeting with the principal, yourself, the school nurse, and your child's classroom teacher (as well as anyone else mutually agreed upon as having a "need to know" about your child's HIV status). The purpose of the second meeting is to review your child's health and educational needs and to discuss how all involved, working as a team, can best meet these needs. Remind those you meet with at both meetings that your child's HIV infection is confidential information protected by law. Ask what steps will be taken to ensure your child's right to confidentiality. Also, ask for a written copy of the school's HIV policy and review it with those present.

At this second meeting, you will want to request information on what inservice training on HIV is provided to students, staff, and parents. By educating on HIV and reducing anxiety, training can create an atmosphere at the school that will help HIV-positive children feel welcome. It can also help protect their health and that of their classmates and teachers. Information for children should be designed by educators using age-appropriate vocabulary, concepts, and teaching techniques. Where possible, discussion of HIV and how it is (and is not) spread should be presented as a part of the school's health information, without mention of whether there is an HIV-positive child currently enrolled.

Many local and national AIDS service organizations and other public and private agencies can provide educational and training materials for school personnel and students. A source to consider:

Kids with AIDS should be treated the same as any other kid! We all need love.

KARISSA (AGE 10)

CDC National AIDS Clearinghouse
800-458-5231—English/Spanish
800-243-7012—Hearing-impaired TTY/TDD
9 a.m.-7 p.m. Mon-Fri (Eastern time)
• Questions answered and publications mailed confidentially, free or low-cost. Reference specialists do free database searches on any aspect of HIV/AIDS, including effective training and educational resources for school staff and students.

Most Illinois school policies require periodic meetings of the parent or guardian, child's physician, and selected school staff to assess the child's health and educational needs on an ongoing basis. Because your child's needs may change, this team should meet regularly.

In consultation with your child's doctor, the school nurse can help monitor your child's health by checking for any changes, and by reporting outbreaks of infectious diseases in the school. The school nurse can act as a liaison between you, the school, and your child's health care provider. The nurse can also function as the support and resource person for your child's teacher.

An informed teacher can reinforce educational and developmental goals established for your child, and observe and report to you any educational, physical, or emotional changes she sees in your child. Children who are unable to attend school because of a health condition are eligible to receive a "homebound teacher" who will come to your home five days a week for one hour each day.

As this book goes to press, the Chicago Board of Education policy states that a student with HIV may be given a temporary exclusion from school if there is a risk of transmission of HIV. That policy is currently being revised. For current information on exclusion policies that may affect your child, contact your local board of education (or have an attorney do so, if you wish to protect your privacy).

In consultation with your child's principal, your child may be advised to remain out of school for his or her own protection due to an outbreak in the school of an infectious disease. Measles, chicken pox, and mumps can be dangerous to a child with a compromised immune system. Your child's doctor should be notified of outbreaks in the school.

Personal Perspectives on Telling

It may also be helpful to know how HIV professionals and men and women who are living with the disease have dealt with telling others. Following are some of their perspectives.

As far as telling people goes, that's an individual decision. I personally think your doctor needs to know. If she or he can't handle the diagnosis, then go to a doctor who can.

You should only tell people whom you really know, who'll be on your side and be supportive, not judgmental. But realize there's only so much they can handle. They may be wonderful and loving and caring and open—but they're still going to be flipped out. If you know the news is going to give someone a heart attack, don't tell them.

In terms of how to tell, just be direct. People know when you have something bad to tell them. The minute you say, "Let's talk"—they'll hear it in your voice. It can be a double coming out for a lot of people. I also think it's important to let the person you're telling know how you're handling it. That will give them some clue of how to deal with it.

There's no easy way to tell someone, and there's no such thing as breaking the news gently—because once the point comes across, it hits them like a hammer anyway. If you have to tell someone, just tell them you're HIV-positive, then ask if they have any questions. Then you can just answer yes or no, open up a discussion. That can make it a little easier on you because you don't have to reveal everything all at once. You can just answer questions a little bit at a time.

In the hospital, you can call in a professional to talk with the family and give them the straight story. Reassure them that even though you're sick, you are getting good care and will follow doctor's orders. A lot of people tell their families they have cancer, but the families always figure it out after a while. Lying about this won't help anyone learn to face it any faster.

DR. HARVEY WOLF
Clinical Health Psychologist

If someone brings up telling their parents, I always say you'd better plan on supporting them first. They know less about this than you do. It violates the law of nature—kids don't die before their parents. That's what they'll be thinking, and you've just turned their world upside-down. You'd better be able to help them deal with it before you can expect to get any support back.

You'd also better be prepared to answer a lot of questions. I was suddenly faced with the fact that I was going to have to tell my family about my gayness. Suddenly it's out of your hands—you're "outed." The only control you've got left is when to tell, and how.

People at work have noticed the weight loss and they ask what's going on. I work among a relatively sophisticated, progressive group of people. I'm not afraid for the most part that they would go, "Eww! I can't work with this guy." But there are some people in the company who could react that way. I guess what I'm more concerned about is people treating me weird or talking about me, because as soon as people find out you're positive, they start to speculate: "Is he a junkie or is he gay? He certainly ain't Haitian! Transfusion? Hemophiliac?" I don't want all that hassle and mess. Most people won't pry, but some don't know when to stop.

If someone is being really nosy or prying, the temptation is to just lie and say no. But in most cases, my strategy has been to sidestep. I learned early on, the instant you start lying about things, it gets really complicated and awful. Now you've got to remember your lies, and back them up and embellish them. It's easier just to say, "It's none of your business."

With certain people you can be a little more subtle, because they have a better understanding of things like privacy. If someone were to ask me point blank, "What's the matter, Charlie—do you have AIDS?" I guess at this stage I'd have to say yes. Four years ago, I probably would've said, "What a question!" trying to deflect and make them feel ashamed for asking. Now, depending on who it is, if it's somebody I work with closely, I might say, "Well, sometime we'll talk about that, but it's really not appropriate right now." That's basically a "yes," but it's a "yes" that discourages further discussion then and there. Let them seek me out privately later.

CHARLIE

After my "stoic" period, there was a period of feeling very isolated. It made me want to be around my friends and talk about this a whole lot. At times, I wanted to tell <u>everyone</u> I was HIV-positive—just go to the top of the building and scream it.

Finding out any news like this that is health-related and mortality-related accentuates a lot of what you don't like or what irritates you about your partner. It also accentuates and brings to light a lot of what you don't like about yourself. All the old behaviors, fears, anxieties—attitudes you've been able to keep under control or channel in a slightly different way—that all comes gushing out and there's a lot of garbage that gets dumped on the dinner table. Sometimes, you almost feel like you're starting from scratch. Issues in the relationship you thought were resolved are triggered all over again in a slightly different configuration.

"RALPH"

Many people are still treated poorly by employers, pushed into disability before they need to be. My own case went badly. At 11:00, I told my employer I had AIDS. At 12:00, the senior managers met over lunch. At 1:00, a senior officer from my firm, along with an attorney, were ready to meet with me. They notified me they wanted me out on disability— now. I cautioned them about the legal issues around disclosure and protecting my privacy. Then I excused myself and called the Minnesota AIDS Project. In the next week I was able to clarify my legal position.

I was shocked at how ill-prepared my supervisors were. All of a sudden, I didn't have a job because my boss had no compassion. All this happened within an organization that employs 600 people. My advice is, don't expect your company to be up to date, even on information that's now "common knowledge." Also, don't think that you can turn to the employee relations office, human resources, or your shop foreman and tell them about your HIV status and expect them to keep that confidential. They work for the company, after all. And learn what your benefits are—not just in the public sector, because corporations have disability policies, too.

WOOD

Re-entering the work force, interviewing for jobs after you've been on disability—that's tricky. Chances are, you'll be asked about any lengthy gaps in your employment. It's a strategic decision, how you respond to that. I'd recommend being very brief and vague…saying you took time off for personal reasons. You took a sabbatical to study privately on your own. You don't need to volunteer that you're now an expert on HIV disease!

Before you start interviewing, I'd say talk to a lawyer or someone from AIDS Legal Council. They can give advice from a legal perspective, in terms of what questions are inappropriate in an interview setting and what you're absolutely obligated to respond to.

DEBORAH STEINKOPF
Executive Director, BEHIV—
Better Existence with HIV

I feel obligated to tell anyone who's interested in me that I'm HIV-positive before they get too interested. If they're going to get real interested in me, it's almost like betting on a three-legged horse. They're not gonna win in the way they might like. They can't have children with me; I'm not going to keep them company in their "golden years." I'm gonna be checkin' out long before then. I just feel like I have to let them know what they're getting into.

"MARIE"

There are certain people in my life who I'm terrified to tell. I've had some real bad experiences. People who found out I had AIDS wouldn't let their kids play with mine or even come in the house. Many people have a very poor understanding of how the virus is spread. I figure, the fewer people I have to tell, the less I have to deal with.

Before I decide whether to tell somebody, I try to figure out <u>why</u> I am telling them. What is my <u>reason</u>. Once in a while, it's to get someone to feel sorry for me. Mostly it's to share it with them, or because they're close to me and kind of have a right to know.

People do treat me different once they know. Sometimes they're nicer to me. Not always. It kind of goes from one extreme to the other. Some people will totally stay away from you. They're out of your life for good. Others will try to be very supportive. There aren't too many people in the middle—it's one or the other. I haven't really had anyone come out and try to hurt me or be mean because I have it.

I know it's impossible, but I wish people could kind of disconnect me from my illness. Look at me, and if they want to judge me, fine—but don't keep bringing AIDS into it. Since most people can't separate the two, I really don't volunteer it much. I don't feel it's necessary for everyone to know about my illness.

GEORGE

You can't tell what the response to your child will be. I talk to the teacher and principal, and based on their response to our situation, I get a pretty good idea. It's a gut feeling. With all the problems for families in dealing with HIV, school shouldn't be one more.

Legally, you are accepted at your neighborhood school. So you have to decide whether to stand your ground or not. It really depends on the experience that your child is having. If your child is enjoying school and has good friends and gets along with the teacher and is doing the work well, then if you have to put up with something, put up with it. But if a child is not having a good time, if they are discriminating and the child is feeling it, you have to consider challenging it. If you have to fight a little and it's your fight and not the child's fight, then okay. But it if is going to be an all-around unhappy, miserable experience for everybody, then it isn't really worth fighting for.

TERRY RUCKER
Foster Parent

You may think that telling would be too stressful, but in truth, the fear of people finding out will haunt you and the secrecy will cause you stress—stress that right now, you don't need in your life. For me, to tell was to be set free.

SHARI

For those who are incarcerated, I would say tell your doctor so that in jail you can receive medical care and have your condition monitored. If you became infected because you've been abused, don't tell anybody other than the doctor. I would tell the doctor an abuse situation happened and identify the abuser. I wouldn't give permission to reveal my name, out of fear that in retaliation I'd lose my life. If telling would mean your life, don't tell.

HIV can spread like wildfire in jails. We need to have access to condoms in jails, because there is sex happening. We need bleach, too, because there also are drugs in jail.

ANNIE MARTIN
Clinical Nurse Specialist,
Women and Children's HIV Program, Cook County Hospital

I was at a TPA meeting a few years back about who, when, and how to tell. The speaker and some other people were advocating that you should tell your parents, and some parents were there advocating that they had a right to know. As far as I'm concerned, <u>nobody</u> has a right to know anything about me that I don't want to tell them. I couldn't understand why everybody was so tied up in saying they had to tell their parents they were gay, or HIV-positive, or anything else. That is up to you. You don't have to tell anybody <u>anything</u>!

STEVEN

At first I thought a lot about, "What are my friends going to say? What is my family going to say?" Now I just don't care. I know my family and they are with me. If others are my friends, they will stay. If not, they will go.

GAIL

I still have a lot of fears and resentment about how people would feel about me, how they'd look at me if they knew. I work, and every day I go to work I am fearful: "What if somebody says or finds out something, and they all shun me?" When my daughter found out quite by accident that my partner was positive, she told her boyfriend. He said to her, "Don't you ever take the kids over to your mother's again!" That was even before they knew about me. So the rejection is the biggest fear. But truthfully, most of the close friends I've told have accepted me.

"ELIZABETH"

In deciding who to tell, consider whether the person is able to keep your confidentiality, is mature, cares about you, is knowledgeable, honest, and open. Helping people learn more is important to me. I feel I was meant to have this disease, to educate people. My husband and I are interracial, and I think we were meant to be that way, too. God has given me this to tackle. We're all here for a purpose, to help each other.

EVIE

I haven't told the neighbors in my apartment complex yet, because you never know how they'd take it, or how management would take it. It could be like their swimming pool, a big sign: "THIS DAY FOR ADAM ONLY." You never know, so you don't especially want to tell them.

If a stranger came up to me and asked if I had AIDS, I'd say it's none of their business. I'm not going to run around town waving a sign, "I've got AIDS!" It's a private, medical thing. You don't tell just anyone, but you tell the people you're close to.

Telling potential girlfriends is a big ordeal. The third date is about the right time to do it. You start out with the term "hemophilia," then work your way from that to "HIV." You have to start there because the word "AIDS" will send people diving out of third-story windows. You explain that it's a virus that may or may not kill you. You have to say "may or may not," because if you say it's definitely going to kill you, she won't stick around.

It's like the Paris Peace Talks; it's horrible. I dread that whole conversation. How do you say it in a nice way—in a way that will make her not run away? It makes dating a nightmare, because who wants to date if it's never going to lead anywhere? It's a shitty set of circumstances.

ADAM

Some people have this image that the people they tell will get really hysterical and freak out and stuff, but what is more common is <u>denial.</u> All of a sudden, nobody talks about it. You can't get them to ask how you are. I go two months with no problems and my lover will go, "Are you sure you're sick? Do you think about it often?" And I'll say, "Every five hours, when I take a pill."

JIM

I wish I'd had something to help me decide whether to start telling people right away. That was my biggest thing. Right away you feel alone, scared, and then you wonder, "Should I tell my mother and father, should I tell my friends—and what friends <u>shouldn't</u> I tell?" You're afraid to tell your neighbors because they might burn your house down or something. I was very worried about my kids and how they might be teased at school, so I didn't tell them. I didn't tell my neighbors, either, but I figured maybe I should tell my immediate family.

I asked my doctor what she thought I should do. Should I just lie and say I have lung cancer, or should I come right out and tell everybody it's AIDS? She said I had to be the one to make that decision.

I still to this day don't think it's a great idea to run out and tell everyone. You want to share it with people, but then later, some of the aftereffects may not be worth it. I had an incident where my sister told a friend of hers who lives in Wisconsin, and the friend has a brother who lives in Las Vegas, and within a day or so they both knew. The brother happened to be in town at a garage sale and he blurts out real loud to someone who knew me, "What's this I hear about Sam having AIDS?" It was supposed to be confidential. I had asked my sister to keep it within the family. Taught me a good lesson, I guess.

"SAM"

Talking with Your Children

A difficult decision you face as a parent is when, if, and how to tell your child about your own or their HIV infection. Children have varying abilities to cope depending on their age and situation. A lot of people will be eager to offer you advice, but don't be pressured. It's your family, and you know your child best.

For the most part, children under the age of five or six understand and care about only what immediately affects them. Most parents choose to offer basic explanations when questions come up, and stop there. Because kids often forget things or listen selectively, it's best to use the simple approach. However, even young children have done well with more information when the parent follows the child's cue.

To protect your family's privacy, you may want to be careful how you talk about HIV around your child until you feel sure she or he can

---

As far as my relationship with my kids goes, the time that we spend together— it's much more meaningful. What we say to each other is real significant. It cuts out a lot of the having to test each other. I think it has brought us closer together. From that perspective, I can see a positive in having this disease.

SANDI

Usually I try to talk to my mom every day, but sometimes I can't. I don't talk about AIDS much with her, because I don't want her to feel bad that she has it or that I'm worrying about her too much.

JENNY (AGE 10)

keep a secret. Also, it is important to teach young children to get help if someone is bleeding, and not to touch other people's blood or let anyone touch theirs without gloves.

Some parents talk to their school-age children frankly, shielding them only from the tougher realities of HIV. If you choose this route, pay close attention to the signals your kids send. A child may react differently at various points in time. Sometimes children will deny that they or someone in their family is infected, even when they've heard the facts directly. You and your child might be more comfortable talking about specific health problems you are facing, or about the fact that you have more health problems than most people do.

Children can be terribly afraid of death or illness. Parents and family are a child's whole world; the idea of losing that can be impossible for them to imagine. Many times children can't emotionally afford to talk, they may want to avoid hurting you, or they magically believe HIV will just go away. They may become overly protective of you. Don't force your kids to "face facts" in order to make yourself feel better. Indicate your willingness to talk, and open up opportunities for communication. Always respond as openly as possible to their questions and statements about their feelings. Talk about your own feelings, mistakes, or fears so they know it's okay to do the same. Children can have many of the same anxieties about HIV that you face, but they're not yet fully equipped to process these feelings. That's where *you* come in. Now is the time to let your kids know you love them, and that there's nothing you can't talk to each other about. Explain that you, not they, are responsible for taking care of your health.

Young people may also respond to HIV by acting out or doing poorly at school, lying, creating a fantasy world, or reverting to bed wetting or other behaviors they had outgrown. They may become sullen or aggressive toward other children, or withdraw into escapes such as computer games, television, friends, or drugs. Intervene if your child's escapes have become destructive in any way. But remember that, like denial, escaping behaviors can serve as a useful buffer against matters that are too difficult or painful to face. Although you may be irritated by your child's behavior, be patient and try to understand the changes she or he is going through. These changes are signs that your child needs more support and reassurance.

Some parents choose not to discuss HIV with school-age children because they sense their child does not want to talk or couldn't handle the news. However, kids are intelligent and sensitive little human beings. They can pick up on very subtle cues, and may be more aware of the situation than you think. Your silence could be sending them messages you don't intend: that HIV is something to be ashamed of, that you don't trust them, or that you're not in control.

Without open communication, your child may develop scary misconceptions about HIV. They might believe you could die at any

---

I think a good time to tell my son about my HIV would be when I got sick and knew I only had a few years left. He's 9; he couldn't handle it now. He's the type of kid that during the Iraqi War, he was just waiting for Iraq to bomb us. So when he worries about something, he worries and worries and worries and worries and worries. He already worries about me; he's always asking how I'm feeling. Maybe that's because his father already died. And we're real close. I think telling him would affect his schoolwork. I don't think I'd want to tell him alone, either.

"MARIE"

Telling my 8-year-old boy I was HIV-positive was pretty simple, because we already knew a lot of people who had AIDS. My best friend had died of it. Also, he pays attention, even when you think he's not, so he knows stuff.

He's negative, thank God. It took me awhile to get him tested, because I knew it was possible he might be infected, and I was afraid. That had to be the hardest thing I've ever done. I never told him what I was having him tested for.

WENDY

moment, that a minor illness like a cold or rash could kill you, that if they aren't "good" you will die, or that they in some other way have control over your health. If you sense this kind of stress is overtaking your family, let your children know they can come to you or someone else to talk—even if only to acknowledge what is going on.

Some parents don't talk to their children because they can't bear the thought of it. Maybe inside, you feel that if you don't talk about HIV, it won't be real. Maybe you have feelings of guilt or sadness you'd rather not think about.

If you're trying to get a handle on your own feelings or on what path to take with your child, discuss your situation with your case manager, a relative, or a trusted friend. A social worker or psychologist who works with young people can help you assess your children's needs and find effective ways to help them be healthy and happy. Try to create situations where your child can communicate freely by talking, painting, acting, or playing. A trained therapist can help you direct and learn from these sessions.

A Note to Teens

If you're a teenager who's just learned you're HIV-positive, you may face some stress that adults and children don't have. You aren't little anymore, but you're not quite an adult yet either. You may just be getting comfortable with your body, your family, your friends, or your sexuality. There can be a lot of pressure, both from within yourself and from the world around you. It can be hard to relate to people you've just met, and to those who've known you a long time but aren't quite sure how to approach you now.

The news that you're HIV-positive can feel like one big thing too many on your plate. It's very common for young people who learn they are infected to try and make the news "go away" by ignoring it. It can be good not to let something get to you when you need to be busy living your life. Unfortunately, ignoring HIV can leave you feeling lonely and depressed. It can also keep you from getting medical attention that can help you live longer. Remember, *you're* the one whose job it is to take care of yourself—but you can't do it by yourself. Be sure you have the best medical care possible. Take steps to keep yourself healthy and well.

A key thing to remember is, *you are not alone!* There are many other people your age who are going through the same thing. Telling a friend who will respect your privacy can be a big relief. If you're not ready to tell anyone you know personally, try talking anonymously to someone at a hotline or HIV service agency. There also are support groups strictly for teens or people in their 20s. They're a great place to get information, vent strong emotions, and make new friends.

You may be reluctant to talk to adults because you feel there's no way they can relate to your concerns. However, there are many adults

---

Sometimes parents don't want to tell their kids that they, the children, are infected. We have to follow the parents' wishes and not disclose to the kids if they don't want us to. Still, kids wonder why they're coming to the clinic all the time and seeing people get sick. They can't go to camps or special outings for HIV-affected families because the parents are afraid they'll find out. They miss out on a lot if the parents won't let them know or talk about it.

ANNIE MARTIN
CLINICAL NURSE SPECIALIST,
WOMEN AND CHILDREN'S
HIV PROGRAM,
COOK COUNTY HOSPITAL

My son's only 3. He knows he gets infusions and medications, but I don't think he's old enough to know what all that means. I'm sure he's not old enough to use discretion. I don't want him walking down the street saying, "Look, I'm HIV."

I'm not sure when I'll tell him he's infected. It just depends on when I think he'll understand. Or maybe it'll be when he really bleeds for the first time. Maybe I'll say, "See how you're bleeding here? Don't let anyone touch you except Mommy or Daddy, or someone with gloves."

CHRISTINE

who can be a great resource for you. An older person can be your advocate, or help you solve practical problems by lending you money, giving you a place to stay, helping you find services, or just being there.

If it's not you but a relative or friend who has HIV, hook up with people who can support you. You are not responsible for the illness your loved one is facing, but you *are* responsible for taking care of yourself. You deserve to have the love and attention of your family and friends, and you deserve to have your feelings taken seriously. Take time to get away and enjoy your life. Seek out other kids who are in situations like yours. You may be surprised at how good it feels to talk to someone who knows what you're going through.

Surviving the Company Blood Drive

To avoid passing the virus along to others, HIV-infected people must *never* allow their blood to be used for transfusion purposes. You'll see this expressed in warnings such as, "Do not donate blood or blood products."

In reality, there are times when you may find yourself pressured to give blood. Church- and company-sponsored blood drives are a prime example. *Even if your viral load is currently below measurable levels, you can still pass on HIV.* It is vital that you do whatever it takes to avoid donating blood. In addition to the risk of passing on HIV, you would also be putting unneeded stress on your body.

To gracefully get out of donating while still protecting your confidentiality, it may be necessary to tell a "white lie." You could say that you faint when you give blood, that you are anemic, that you are not feeling well that day, are on antibiotics, or have just gotten over the flu. If all else fails, consider calling in sick on the day of the blood drive.

If you're not comfortable with these options and feel you have to go through the motions, go ahead and fill out the screening questionnaire, but check the "NO" box in answer to the question about whether you believe your blood is safe to use. You can also tell the blood-service personnel that you don't feel like giving blood, that you feel ill today, or that you are feeling pressured to donate but don't think it's a good idea. These personnel are trained to be very discreet, and will excuse you without any questions.

If you fail to let the blood collection service know of your blood's unsafe status, they will test it for HIV anyway, just as they now test all donated blood and blood products. If your test comes out positive, your name will go into a computerized donor deferral registry. While only blood banks are supposed to have access to these records, you *don't* want to have your name placed on file in connection with a blood disorder if you can possibly avoid it.

Don't rush into telling a lot of people. You need to find someone you trust who will have your best interests in mind. Think about the people in your life. Who can provide care and affection? Who has been there for you in the past? It should be someone you feel comfortable being with and talking to. You don't want to exclude your friends, but think about how they treat you. Do they call you names or treat you badly in any way? Then they are not someone you'll want to tell.

FELICIA RODRIGUEZ
DIRECTOR OF ADOLESCENT EDUCATION, WOMEN AND CHILDREN'S HIV PROGRAM, COOK COUNTY HOSPITAL

Adults probably understand more than teens do. For teens, it's harder to learn about stuff. That's one reason I haven't told nobody about my HIV. My mom has told some of the family, but that's about it. She told me it's important to keep it quiet.

"AL" (AGE 13)

Blood Donation or HIV Test?

Some people who aren't sure of their HIV status, but are unwilling or afraid to be tested, wonder if giving blood might be a way to find out if they have the virus.

This is a bad idea for several reasons. Namely:

- The test used to screen donations may not detect antibodies to the virus early in the infection. If the donated material does contain HIV, the person or persons receiving it could become infected. If you think there's any possibility you have HIV, do not donate blood, plasma, sperm, body tissue, or organs.
- Attempting to learn your HIV status by giving blood means you will not be provided with follow-up testing to confirm your diagnosis. The EIA (or ELISA) test used to screen blood for HIV is overly sensitive, producing many false-positive results. This helps make the blood supply safer (since the test tends to err on the side of caution). However, you could be informed that you are HIV-positive when you're not. In normal HIV testing procedures, any positive EIA result is double-checked with a second, more accurate test called the Western Blot. This test weeds out the false-positives from those samples that really are infected with HIV. You owe it to yourself to get accurate results, and not put yourself through any needless trauma.
- Being tested through proper channels also ensures you'll receive valuable counseling both before and after you are tested. Trained counselors can help you cope with your results and begin to formulate a game plan. Blood donors who turn out to be infected are not automatically provided with help or guidance.

Two additional facts. First, you *cannot* get HIV from giving blood. New, sterile equipment is used on each person, and each needle is discarded properly after use. Second, HIV can be spread through the transplanting of organs (such as heart, liver, etc.) from an infected person. Potential organ donors are screened for HIV, bringing the risk of infection to near zero. Donated blood products and organs are desperately needed to save lives. Encourage your non-infected friends and loved ones to continue donating blood and plasma regularly and to register to be organ donors.

Home Testing for HIV

There are also mail-in kits that allow you to test for HIV infection at home. Home kits, such as Confide or Home Access, cost from $35 and $50 and can be purchased by phone or at a pharmacy. You place a sample of your blood from a fingerprick onto filter paper and mail it to a laboratory for testing. Later, you call the company that produces the kits, give them a code number, and they confidentially inform you of your results. Often, a recording is used to give negative results, while a "live" person comes on the line to inform you if your test is positive.

Our company has very aggressive blood drives. The woman who used to run them, after about the third year of my refusing them, came by and said, "Should I even bother asking you this year?" I told her, "No, there's no point in asking me, ever. I'd love to, but I can't." Finally, I just explained that I'd had hepatitis several years before and couldn't ever donate. But hepatitis is already kind of pushing it, because most people don't get hepatitis in this country. Here, it's primarily homosexuals and IV drug users. You've got to be careful what you say, because you can tip your hand either way.

CHARLIE

Home testing kits may be a helpful resource for individuals who would not otherwise seek out testing. Many people do not have access to a public testing site where they feel confident their anonymity will be protected. Others are uncomfortable with the prospect of talking with a counselor, even anonymously, about intimate matters such as sexual history or drug use. Still others may not be uncomfortable discussing these matters but value home testing as the most private and convenient way to confirm their HIV status.

There are several reasons why home tests may *not* be the best choice. First, there are many testing sites throughout the country where you can receive the same information at no cost. Second, privacy is an issue. Your materials may not arrive in the mail confidentially, and/or you may be concerned that others will see your testing kit. Finally, the counseling that comes with home tests may not be adequate or sensitive.

Free public health clinics offer you the physical presence of a human being with whom to discuss your test results. Those who test positive can really be helped by the information and face-to-face emotional support only a "live" person can offer. Those who test negative can receive counseling about the limitations of the test (such as the fact that if you were infected in the last few months, you might not be showing up as positive yet but could still infect others with HIV). A person who is tested in these settings can ask questions, talk about what they're feeling, and discuss what they can do to protect themselves and others.

A person retrieving test results from a recording might hang up before listening to the full message, or they might not understand parts of the message or get all of his or her questions answered. Someone who calls in and is connected to a live voice may hang up without talking, because they believe the live voice means their test came back positive. If they do speak to the counselor, they may hang up before the discussion is over or before they're given a contact number for support services in their area. They may be too numb to listen or to write down information. Without human contact, they may be more likely to make rash and harmful decisions. The counselor, meanwhile, misses the chance to read the caller's body language, calm down the caller in person, or intervene if they seem to be in real trouble. Finally, while the companies that manufacture the tests may be prepared to refer callers to organizations in their home city for counseling and follow-up care, testing sites in one's own immediate area will tend to have better knowledge of local resources.

The practical issues surrounding the use of home tests are currently being evaluated by the CDC. If you know someone who is considering using a home test, encourage them to call a hotline, such as 800-AID-AIDS (800-243-2437). Your local health department or Red Cross chapter can also answer questions about home tests, as well as identify area clinics that do free confidential or anonymous HIV testing.

Needle-Free HIV Testing

For those who dislike needles, there is now an alternative way to test for HIV. Orasure, developed by Epitope, uses no needles. Instead, a cotton pad is placed between a person's cheek and gum and held there for about two minutes. The pad absorbs HIV antibodies, if they are present, direct from capillaries in the mouth. The pad is then placed in a vial with preservative solution and sent to a lab for testing. The test is more than 99% accurate. (For the record, this does not mean that HIV can be spread through saliva. The test measures antibodies, not HIV.)

To learn more, call the National AIDS Hotline (800-342-2437), or SmithKline Beecham toll-free at 888-672-7873. Visit the company's Web site at www.orasure.com.

PART 4

Learning to *Live* with HIV

- Nutrition
  Nutrition Assistance
- Food Safety
  Food Safety Resources
- Exercise
  Exercise Resources
- Rest and Relaxation
- Emotional Support
  Support Groups and Mental Health Services
- Spiritual Support
  Spiritual Support Resources
- Sex
  Safer Sex Resources
- HIV in Newborns and Children
- Having Children
- Alcohol and Other Drug Use
  Syringe Exchange Programs
  Finding Chemical Dependency Treatment and Support
- HIV and Homelessness
- HIV in Prison
  Prisoner Resources
- Hygiene
- Pets

Throughout this book, we've used the phrase "living with HIV." Not just "surviving," not merely "existing"—but *living*, in the fullest sense of that word. As you gradually get used to the facts of your illness and take steps to get it under control, you may notice a rather remarkable thing happening: your life returning to normal.

True, certain things have changed forever. You now have a different set of physical and life-expectancy potentials. You'll be facing big decisions about work, relationships, family, and the future. You'll be immersing yourself in a whole new area of knowledge. Where the virus is concerned, there's no going back.

And yet, despite all the upheaval you're going through and the challenges up ahead…life *will* go on. You can choose to let it pass you by or jump on and be a part of it. But then, that's the same choice you've always had. Having this virus has changed everything and nothing, all at the same time. A paradox? You bet. Just like life.

On a day-to-day basis, there *are* things you can do to improve and safeguard your health. For the most part they're "common sense" measures you've been doing or hearing about for years: eat right. Get plenty of rest. Exercise. Reduce stress. Don't abuse alcohol, tobacco, caffeine, and other drugs. Practice good hygiene and safer sex. Avoid too much sun.

Nothing magical here—but in the face of HIV, the choices you make to follow or ignore these measures can greatly impact your immune system. HIV slowly drains a person's strength and stamina. By pursuing a more healthful lifestyle, you may be able to retard or reverse this process. You'll be giving your immune system every possible advantage.

The following guidelines can help you determine which health-related areas you might want to make changes in, and what the nature of those changes might be. As with every other aspect of your care, the decision to do anything or nothing is completely in your hands. It's probably best not to try and become an overnight paragon of health, as most people who attempt this fail. However, you may find that moving in the "right" direction in a few select areas makes you feel so good, you'll want to experiment with others.

The thing that upsets me sometimes in reading the literature is the notion that treatment is somehow just buying time. That no matter what I do, I'll still eventually progress to AIDS. It upsets me, because it interferes with the way I've constructed my illness for myself, in my mind. I'm not interested in thinking about treatments that will buy me time in six-month intervals. My first interval is five years. I don't harbor any fantasies about a magic bullet, in terms of a cure anytime in the near future. What I do think is that research may continue to uncover treatments and more new information that can sort of keep me at the same place I am now. So that I can move ahead and live my life in the way I choose to live it.

"RALPH"

I know it sounds unbelievable, but a lot of good things can happen from HIV if you take charge of it. It can be a launching-off point in terms of personal growth, emotional growth, spiritual growth. People become more health-conscious; they begin exercising, eating better. They start taking care of themselves—sometimes, for the first time.

"GARY"

I think if I regret anything about the way I've handled my HIV, it's not having understood nutrition better. I actually paid a lot of attention to it but went about it in the wrong way. When you talk to one of these private "New Age" practitioners, what you get is really detailed biochemical advice that's so superweird and technical and complicated and confusing, you eventually feel—why bother?

But if I had understood something as basic as my calorie intake a year ago, I might not be as wasted as I am now. Turns out, I was only taking in two-thirds of the calories I needed as a healthy, non-infected person. I've been trying to retrain myself to have three square meals a day. The mere fact that your body has been invaded by something means it needs more energy. I wish someone had explained that to me when I first learned I was positive.

CHARLIE

Nutrition

As human beings, we need energy from food in the form of carbohydrates, proteins, and fats. Vitamins and minerals are also required to function effectively and stay healthy. When there is physical trauma or illness, the body needs more energy than it normally would. It's important for people with HIV to get enough of the right kind of fuel to meet the demands of living with their disease.

People with advanced HIV and AIDS often lose a lot of weight. In extreme cases, this can be life-threatening. You may find you need to take in more calories than you did before you became infected to avoid this "wasting" effect. However, that doesn't mean simply eating more pizzas and candy bars; you must eat nutritionally-balanced foods to meet all your body's energy needs, maintain an appropriate body weight, and support your immune system.

Your ideal body weight is determined by your height, physical build, sex, and age. The amount of fuel required to maintain that weight depends on how active you are, and on any special problems you may be experiencing. In general, someone with HIV will require about 16–18 calories per pound of body weight each day to maintain weight.

The carbohydrates, proteins, and fats we eat all supply energy, but they each impact the body very differently. For instance, carbohydrates satisfy the brain's need for glucose (sugar) and regulate the appetite. Protein helps the body build cells and repair tissue. Eating too much fat can interfere with the delivery of these nutrients. That's why it's vital to take in a balanced diet: typically, 2 to 3 servings from the milk or dairy group, 2 to 3 from the meat or protein group, 3 to 4 fat servings, 5 or more servings of fruits and vegetables, and 6 to 11 servings from the grain or bread group, every day.

Vitamin and mineral needs for people with HIV are currently being studied, with some results suggesting new reasons for hope. If a person isn't absorbing food properly or has a nutrient-poor diet, a vitamin and mineral supplement containing 100% of the RDA is recommended. If a doctor suggests them, more potent supplements may be taken. Avoid megadoses of vitamins and minerals, however—excesses can cause problems and impair the immune system. Ask your doctor or local HIV/AIDS organization for more information on what current vitamin research is underway, and be sure to discuss with your doctor any dietary supplements you are taking. This is especially important if you are pregnant, as some types of vitamins can build to toxic levels in your body, leading to birth defects and other problems.

Since individual needs can vary even more when you are ill, you may want to ask your doctor to put you in touch with a registered dietitian (R.D.) who is experienced in working with people with HIV. If your doctor doesn't work with an R.D., get the names of those in your area from the American Dietetic Association. Your case manager and/or the staff at a local HIV organization may also be able to recommend someone. The R.D. can plan your meals and make selections from foods you need and like. Custom diet plans are important because medications can sometimes require strict meal schedules, and HIV-related symptoms can greatly affect your individual nutritional needs.

Kids with HIV need the help of an R.D. as early as possible after their diagnosis. Children have lower stores of fat and muscle than adults, and nutritional deficiencies can lead more quickly to serious problems. The weight loss that often accompanies AIDS can impact negatively on a child's development. In working with children, dietitians watch for potential problems and give valuable advice on enticing children to eat, battling nausea and diarrhea, and addressing food-related behavioral or emotional problems.

Any problems with eating, digestion, or food absorption can put a person at risk for malnourishment—a potentially dangerous situation with HIV. Some people can digest food better and feel more comfortable if they eat small, frequent meals rather than two or three large meals each day. Drinking enough fluids is also important—at least eight 8-ounce glasses of water each day in addition to other beverages.

The following table can help you manage some common nutrition-related problems:

All of us wish we could do things we cannot, like live forever—but the fact that we cannot do that just proves that we are not our bodies. We are more. The body follows the mind and is not equivalent to our selves. I believe that food can help us be well and be present in our bodies and health. Koreans use food like Americans use pills, for medicinal purposes: to heal, correct, soothe, or strengthen you. We can help ourselves be well, even if we are all mortal.

BO GYUNG, CHEF
AMITABUL RESTAURANT, CHICAGO

My health is a big topic of conversation around our house. My wife is always asking, did I take my medicine? Did I eat today, and how much do I weigh? She's being a nurse. She's constantly monitoring me, health-wise. It gets to be a little much, after awhile. At times, it kinda bugs me. She makes these high-calorie milkshakes—if I don't have three a day, I'm in trouble! She's gonna carry on, we're gonna have words. She's going to make it real uneasy for me.

GEORGE

Problem	Possible Solutions
Weight loss	Eat high protein foods: milkshakes, peanut butter, cheese, meats; nutritional supplements designed for weight gain; and snacks between meals.
Anorexia (loss of appetite)	Consume small, frequent meals of high calorie/high protein foods like cheese, yogurt, and peanut butter and jelly sandwiches.
	Drink milkshakes or commercial nutritional supplements.
	Eat with friends or family and have favorite foods.
	Exercise before meals. A short walk can increase your appetite.
	If condition persists, ask your doctor about medications.
Chewing/swallowing problems	Eat soft, tender foods. Avoid foods that are too spicy or hard. Experiment with food texture to find what is best for you.
	Cold food may be easier to tolerate than hot.
	Rinse your mouth often and keep it clean and fresh. Use a straw or tilt your head forward or backward to ease swallowing.
	Drink non-acidic juices such as nectars, grape or apple juice.
	If the mouth is dry or sore, eat soft, moist foods and take fluids often. Hard candy and gum may help.
Taste changes	Add flavor by marinating food for a few hours in salad dressing, wine, soy sauce, or fruit juice.
	Experiment with different spices and seasonings.
	Try changing food temperature.
	If meat is not appealing, take protein in the form of eggs, cheese, dried beans, peas, peanut butter, nuts, or tofu.
	Suck on hard candy or chew gum to keep the mouth fresh.
Diarrhea	Continue to eat, and drink lots of fluid.
	Limit foods high in fiber, like bran, dried beans and peas, nuts and seeds, whole grains and fruits, and vegetables with skins and seeds. Don't eat prunes or raisins.
	If dairy products make it worse, choose low lactose foods such as yogurt, reduced-lactose milk and soy milk, and commercial lactose-free nutritional supplements. Pills containing an enzyme (lactase) that breaks down milk sugar (lactose) are also available.
	Persistent diarrhea should be brought to your doctor's attention.
Gas and bloating	Consume small, frequent meals.
	Avoid gas-forming foods, such as broccoli, cabbage, cauliflower, onions, or cucumbers. Try Beano, a product that contains an enzyme that helps in digestion.
	Restrict your use of chewing gum, caffeine, and carbonated beverages.

Nausea and vomiting	Eat slowly. Consume small, frequent meals.
	Try soft, bland foods. Saltine crackers, pretzels, and dry toast or cereal can decrease nausea.
	Avoid cooking odors.
	Eat foods cold or at room temperature.
	Avoid highly seasoned or spiced foods. Limit excessively sweet or fatty foods.
	Avoid liquids at meal times. Drink beverages 30–60 minutes before or after meals.
	Juice, soda, or hot tea may be soothing.
Fatigue	Eat at regular intervals during the day.
	Accept help from family or friends with buying and preparing food.
	Freeze leftovers in single-serving portions for later use.
	Keep easy-to-prepare food items on hand.
	Use restaurant take-out foods and foods from the deli or salad bar at grocery stores.
	Participate in home-delivered meal programs.
Constipation	Drink enough fluids. Have at least eight 8-ounce glasses of water daily in addition to other fluids.
	Exercise regularly and include a daily walk.
	Develop a regular meal pattern.
	Speak to your doctor about using fiber products available over-the-counter.

For people who cannot take food by mouth, nutrients can be supplied through the intestine (enteral nutrition, EN) or intravenously (parenteral nutrition, PN). EN may involve feeding tubes. The content of the food supplied is usually chosen by physicians and dietitians. There should be fully-informed consent before any artificial feeding takes place. There are risks as well as benefits with tube feedings.

Nutrition Assistance

Many hospitals and AIDS service organizations offer nutritional counseling and related services. For a referral to a Registered Dietitian, ask your doctor or contact:

American Dietetic Association Consumer Hotline
800-366-1655
9 a.m.-4 p.m. Mon-Fri (Central time).
• Names of Registered Dietitians (R.D.s) in your area.

Books and Publications

The AIDS Caregiver's Handbook
Eidson, Ted, Editor
New York: St. Martin's Press, 1988
• See the chapter on "Nutrition and the Immune System." Includes bibliography.

"HIV Nutrition Guidelines: Practical Steps for a Healthier Life"
Wong, Gustavo, R.D.
1992
Mail order: Stadtlanders Pharmacy, 800-238-1548
• Free booklet, available in Spanish only.

Howard Brown Health Center
945 West George Street
Chicago, IL 60657
773-871-5777
773-871-5843—FAX
• Request their free pamphlets, "Eating Well," "Problem Solving," and "Nutritional Supplements."

"Living Well with HIV/AIDS: A Guide to Healthy Eating"
Davis, Margaret, Cade Fields Newman and
Sharon B. Salomon
Mail order: American Dietetic Association, 312-899-0040
• Booklet covering all aspects of nutrition and the role it plays in HIV disease. English/Spanish.

Nutrition and HIV: A New Model for Treatment
Romeyn, Mary, M.D.
Mail order: Lambda Rising Books, 800-621-6969
• Shows how HIV-positive men and women can treat and prevent the causes of HIV-related wasting. Offers advice on using vitamins, increasing appetite, and dealing with malabsorption, depression, and anxiety.

Positive Cooking
Mail order: Avery Publishing Group, 516-741-2155
• Terrific source of calorie-dense recipes. Symptoms charts indicate which dishes can help relieve various ailments.

Surviving with AIDS: A Comprehensive Program of Nutritional Co-Therapy
Calloway, C. Wayne, M.D., with Catherine Whitney
Boston: Little, Brown, and Company, 1991
• Includes a low fat/high calorie regimen as well as a cookbook and information on drug/nutrient interactions.

Videos

"HIV+ Survival Guide: Diet for Living in the Age of AIDS"
Mail order: Lambda Rising Books, 800-621-6969
• A complete nutritional guide for rebuilding, strengthening, and maintaining a healthy immune system.

"Nutrition and HIV"
Available for viewing at:
Test Positive Aware Network (TPAN or TPA)
1258 West Belmont
Chicago, IL 60657
773-404-8726
773-472-7505—FAX
773-404-9716—Hearing-impaired TTY/TDD
• A short video stressing the important role nutrition plays in managing HIV.

Using a Computer and Modem

ACT UP: Real Treatments for Real People
http://www.aidsnyc.org/rtrp/index.html
• Web site providing nutritional information, including a guide to micronutrients, vitamins, and contact numbers.

The Body: A Multimedia AIDS and HIV Resource
http://www.thebody.com/cgi-bin/body.cgi
• Offers HIV/AIDS information on topics including Diet & Nutrition. Links to other sites.

NOAH: New York Online Access to Health AIDS Information Page
http://www.noah.cuny.edu/aids/aids.html—English
http://www.noah.cuny.edu/spaids/spaids.html—Spanish
• Extensive information on nutrition. Includes a search engine and links to other sites.

Using a Fax Machine

NAPWA Fax
National Association of People with AIDS
202-789-2222—FAX
• Several nutrition publications available by fax, including nutritional considerations for women. Request the "Living with HIV" fax catalog of fax documents in English. A Spanish catalog is also available. You must be at a fax machine to use the NAPWA Fax service.

Food Safety

HIV-infected people must be on guard against harmful bacteria, parasites, and other micro-organisms found in certain foods. The same germs that can cause an upset stomach or mild case of food poisoning in a healthy person can cause serious or fatal illness in someone with a damaged immune system. If your body is in a weakened condition to start with, you may be more vulnerable to food poisoning. The main symptoms of food contamination are diarrhea and vomiting, but they may also include fever, abdominal cramps, nausea, and gas.

Contamination typically occurs because of improper food handling. All cooking utensils, cutting boards, bowls, and so on in contact with raw meat or chicken and uncooked eggs should be thoroughly washed with soap and rinsed with hot water before being reused. Don't use cutting boards that cannot be sanitized. Stone or hard plastic is preferable to wood or soft plastic. Scratched surfaces may house bacteria. Wash your hands thoroughly and often while preparing food, as well as before and after eating.

In general:

1) Buy pasteurized milk and cheese and intact eggs only. Pasteurized egg products (such as Egg Beaters) are safe. Store eggs in cartons on the refrigerator racks and not in the refrigerator door where they may not stay cold enough. Soft cooked, poached, or "runny" fried or scrambled eggs may not be safe. Foods containing raw egg—even a little—should be avoided. Store products labeled "Keep Refrigerated" appropriately. Also pay close attention to "sell by" and "use by" dates.

2) Do not eat raw or undercooked poultry, meat, shellfish, or other seafood. Raw or rare ground meat can be especially risky. Thoroughly reheat frozen or refrigerated processed meat and poultry products before eating them.

3) Scrub all fresh produce to remove visible dirt. Be aware that organically grown fruit or vegetables may have been produced with substances (like manure) that can cause serious illness. If you use them, make sure they're cooked or peeled. Avoid organic lettuce altogether.

4) Drinking untreated contaminated water can also be dangerous. Be very cautious when traveling in foreign countries. Drink bottled water whenever possible.

5) Keep foods below 40° F or above 140° F. Never let food sit at room temperature. Wrap and cover foods in the refrigerator; use airtight containers whenever possible.

6) Never thaw frozen food by letting it sit at room temperature. Thaw in the refrigerator or under very cold running water, and use at once.

7) Reheat leftovers to an internal temperature of 165° F. Don't keep leftovers for more than three days. When in doubt, throw it out.

8) Don't buy or keep rusted, dented, or bulging cans or jars.

9) Avoid mayonnaise-based potato, egg, chicken, and macaroni salads unless you know the conditions under which they were prepared and stored.

Food Safety Resources

CDC National AIDS Clearinghouse
800-458-5231—English/Spanish
800-243-7012—Hearing-impaired TTY/TDD
9 a.m.-7 p.m. Mon-Fri (Eastern time).
• Request the brochure or video, "Eating Defensively: Food Safety for Persons with AIDS."

NAPWA Fax
National Association of People with AIDS
202-789-2222—FAX
• Food and water safety publications available by fax, including the "Eating Defensively" brochure listed above. Request the "Living with HIV" fax catalog of fax documents in English. A Spanish catalog is also available. You must be at a fax machine to use the NAPWA Fax service.

Exercise

Many people with HIV manage their lives by trying to pursue a healthier lifestyle. Exercise can be an important part of the positive changes you decide to make now. The more physically fit you are, the better able you will be to fight off opportunistic infections. Research suggests that regular aerobic exercise can boost your T cells. Some of the side effects of AZT can be lessened by exercising. Regular exercise may also help you maintain or improve muscle mass, strength, flexibility, and endurance. Finally, physical exertion can be a great mood enhancer on days when you're down or frustrated.

It's very important to exercise at an intensity, frequency, and duration that will improve your fitness level but not overdo your capacity. Develop an enjoyable cross-training program that includes aerobic exercise (dancing, bicycling, swimming, running), strength training (lifting free weights or using resistance machines), and stretching. All three types of exercise will produce beneficial results to people living with HIV. Yoga and tai chi are other ways to replenish the mind and body.

If you're already exercising, keep it up! If you were exercising but have stopped because of problems associated with HIV, consult your doctor or a physical therapist. Ask what, if any, exercise would be the most therapeutic for you. If you have never been physically active, you may need guidance and support from a knowledgeable friend or a trainer to get started on the right foot. Check around—special exercise classes for HIV-positive individuals may be available in your community.

Exercise Resources

Test Positive Aware Network
773-404-8726
773-404-9716—Hearing-impaired TTY/TDD
• Ask about TPA's exercise and stress reduction programs designed especially for persons living with HIV/AIDS.

Take-A-Hike
3525 North Broadway
Chicago, IL 60657
708-366-5713
• Offers indoor and outdoor nature activities year-round for people with HIV/AIDS on Chicago's north side. Families welcome. Includes transportation and lunch. Free.

Rest and Relaxation

Rest and relaxation are something few people get enough of. Now that you're battling a serious illness, you may want to rethink some of your priorities. You may decide that preserving your physical and mental health is more important than running yourself ragged.

Try to get a good night's sleep as often as possible. Take short naps to refresh yourself during the day. If you're having trouble sleeping, talk to your doctor.

"R & R" during your waking hours may be a little harder to achieve. We live in a very go-go, stressful society. You may feel overloaded with responsibilities at work or at home. Now is a good time to take some of the pressure off yourself. There are many excellent techniques available to help you do this.

For help in finding the right stress-relievers for you, talk to the people at your local AIDS service organization. Your doctor or case manager may know of other resources.

Emotional Support

It's been said that HIV is as much an emotional virus as it is a physical one. You may have experienced an intense array of feelings when you first learned you were infected—or you may have felt nothing at all. This "numb" response is every bit as common and valid as the immense sadness, anger, panic, or depression that may also be triggered by the news.

You may feel you "should have known better," or have let down those who love you. You may have friends or family members who are actually angry with you. Or perhaps you feel a sense of relief that "it's finally happened." You can finally let yourself off the hook for remaining well while you stood by and watched friends and loved ones grow sick and die of AIDS.

There's this thing called stress that will destroy you if you let it—and HIV just loves it. A stress-weakened immune system lets the virus happily replicate. Stress, worry, anxiety—that's exactly what you don't need.

JIM

You have to remember to get the proper rest, the proper nutrition—but don't forget to have fun! I think that's real important in eliminating stress—having a good time. Going out for a walk, being able to look at the sky. Just appreciating all the things that are going on around you.

"ELIZABETH"

I think it's important not to depend too much on your doctor. You need to seek other medical people and alternative healing practices. That means time. You've got to take time. You can't work twelve hours a day and then deal with this. I'm not working that hard anymore. I'm putting in 40-hour weeks now. I've been lucky; my boss is very supportive. A lot of bosses aren't, and I don't have any answers for that.

JOE

> *For me, it was really hard to even fathom going to an HIV support group. I have yet to do that. Because I can deal with—that there is some one person who understands how I feel. A group of people who can understand, I have a difficult time with. But there again, as I get more solid in recovery and use my recovery experience to support things that are available to the HIV community, it may be more helpful to me at some point.*
>
> SANDI

Sound outrageous? Not if it's how you feel. Remember, there is no right or wrong way to feel, and there is nothing to be ashamed about admitting how you feel. You don't need anyone's "permission" but your own! In time, and with support from others, you will most likely feel better. Your view of yourself and your HIV status will change and become more life-affirming.

If you're HIV-positive, it's important to find someone else who's in the same situation as you…someone nonjudgmental, who can be really sad or mad or scared with you. Someone who will try to help you make some kind of meaning out of this. At the same time, allow for the possibility that you will *never* find that meaning. You may never experience the "silver lining" that many people with HIV find.

You may not go through a predictable list of stages with your disease. Still, certain people may try to force you along an emotional continuum—saying things like, "get over it" or "move on" before you're ready. If you're not ready to travel that path, don't let them push you. It's valid to feel what you need to as long as you need to, with whatever intensity naturally occurs.

If you are pregnant, or were infected by a partner you had assumed was not infected, you may have feelings of rage, guilt, or fear. Not only your life, but your family and your relationship may be in danger. Your ability to trust, your whole sense of what life is about, may be lying in pieces around you. Still, no matter how you may feel now, try to remember: *knowledge is power*. Educate yourself all you can about HIV. This process will allow you to take back control of your own life and health, and prepare you to help your loved ones when they need you most.

Many HIV-positive parents feel more angry, sad, or afraid for their children than they do for themselves. Some find themselves obsessing about their children's health and being overprotective in day-to-day situations. Others react by lavishing gifts and treats on their kids, in an attempt to lessen feelings of guilt and panic. Other parents "space out," and are hardly able to interact with their families. Some lash out at those around them with violent words or actions.

If these feelings and reactions persist and cause problems for you and your family, or threaten to cause you to harm yourself or others, seek outside counsel from someone who cares and is trained to help. There are hotlines you can call 24 hours a day, 7 days a week.

There is no single approach to dealing with the emotions surrounding HIV. You may choose to consult an individual therapist or join a support group. Or, you may decide to deal with this on your own, or with the help of a trusted friend or loved one. You may also decide not to do anything at all for a time while you let your feelings settle down, and that's okay too. The important thing is to make a conscious decision to do whatever feels right, then follow through and do it.

Some of your options include:

1) *Individual Therapy.* If you decide to seek help from a professional therapist, you'll want to make sure that person has the right education and experience. Equally important, the therapist you choose should be well-versed in HIV-related immune disorders and chronic illness. A background of working with substance abusers, teens, people of color, or gay and lesbian clients can also be very helpful, depending on your own personal issues.

   Whether you decide to see a psychiatrist, psychologist, social worker, or clergyperson, it's important for you to confirm that they are licensed to practice psychotherapy by the state. Besides assuring yourself of the highest quality care, licensed clinicians (like M.D.s) are the only professionals who can accept third-party insurance and Medicare payments. (If your insurance does cover psychotherapy, check your policy to see how many visits are covered, what percentage of the bill will be paid, and whether there are any restrictions on the type of therapist or therapeutic setting.)

   Finding an individual psychotherapist is much like finding a doctor. You can get referrals by word-of-mouth, from AIDS service organizations and hospitals, via classified ads, or through physician referral services. Once you have a few names, you can schedule some initial "get acquainted" visits to see which therapist you feel most comfortable with. (Many will be happy to talk with you for a short time at no charge.)

2) *Group Therapy.* Instead of an individual therapist, you may decide to try a support group. You can find one by calling major hospital centers in your area and asking for the department of social services or pastoral care office.

   Independent support groups may come and go; they often disband without warning. Your support group choices will be much greater in the city than in the suburbs or rural areas. Through the various AIDS service organizations there, you'll find sessions for substance abusers, gays and lesbians, people of color, women, teens, hemophiliacs, and many other special interest groups as well as those open to all.

   If you don't have a car or are too sick to get to the group by yourself, call the facilitator (group leader) and ask what arrangements can be made to assist you.

   Support groups may or may not be led by a trained or professional facilitator. Many groups are "peer-led," meaning the group leader is a volunteer member of the organization sponsoring the session, and may be living with HIV.

One of my first questions was, "Where do I turn?" I was told to go to Howard Brown, and I went, and they were perfect. For me, if I walk into a room with strangers to talk about this, I would prefer that they be gay strangers. My experiences at Howard Brown and in the gay community have been very comfortable.

"PAUL"

It's easy to isolate yourself, living in the city. I imagine it's even easier living thirty miles outside the city. I'll never forget my first TPA meeting—it was just, a body blow! I realized, I am not the only being on this planet who's going through this. It was astounding.

JIM

> *A lot of times, all the attention goes to the sick child. Uninfected children face a lot of loss, too: the possible loss of a sibling or parent, the loss of their parents' attention, the loss of their carefree childhood. They really need to have positive outlets and positive attention in order to have a quality life. Pay attention to them, and get them involved in after-school programs, camps, or other things so they have some space of their own. Healthy kids should not always have to accommodate a sick sibling or parent.*
>
> ELIZABETH MONK
> AIDS PROJECT DIRECTOR, DCFS AIDS PROJECT

> *A few months ago I sprained my ankle, and didn't go anywhere for three days except to the bathroom. My son refused to go to school and he wouldn't sleep in his bedroom. I figured we'd better talk to a psychologist.*
>
> *It turns out my son was really scared that I was going to die then. He was afraid of losing me. He had to sleep with me, to hear me breathe. I don't know how or when he got through it. I think it was when my ankle got better.*
>
> WENDY

In any group setting, it's best not to ask others to reveal too much personal information about themselves. They'll disclose the details of their lives as they feel comfortable. Likewise, your own privacy will be respected until you feel ready or willing to talk about yourself. No one can force you to answer questions about your lifestyle or your illness, nor can anyone make you join or continue with a group against your wishes. Many ongoing groups are set up to accommodate drop-ins, who may come to a group only when they have specific questions or issues they need to talk about.

Many people believe that only "mentally ill" people go to psychotherapists or join support groups. These days, that's simply not true. Therapists and groups offer advice and support to people from every walk of life. Reaching out for help is not a sign that you are crazy or weak or out of control. Rather, it means that you could use some time with an objective, compassionate individual or group of individuals who understand what you're going through and want to help you face this new reality.

3) *Interventions for Families and Children.* Although not every family member may be infected with HIV, each can be *impacted* by the virus in many ways—emotionally, socially, financially, and more. Your ways of interacting may shift wildly, or you may revert to earlier patterns you thought you'd left behind. Those who aren't ill can get "lost in the shuffle" when the spotlight is turned to a family member who is battling AIDS.

A serious illness can deepen your relationships by forcing you to consider what is most important in life. HIV can make us mindful that life is to be treasured, and that it's most meaningful when we celebrate the people we love. Good relationships build a sense of hope and positively affect our physical and mental well-being. Try to find ways every day to appreciate and have fun with those you care most about.

If you have children, or are the primary caregiver of someone with AIDS, try to give yourself some private time now and then to avoid burnout. There are agencies that provide child care and respite services for HIV-impacted families. Some will even bring a care provider to your home so you can go out.

Children and teenagers with HIV face many of the same psychological pressures that adults do. However, they are often less able than adults to talk about their feelings or beliefs. You might be shocked to learn that your little one believes you may die if he doesn't stay near you, or stay awake, or keep praying—or any of a hundred other things. No parent should abandon a child to his or her fears, rational or irrational, during a difficult time like this.

In addition to talk therapy, trained professionals may use play groups or techniques using dolls, art, music, movement, or play-acting to access the inner world of children. Much of the child's emotional "work" may be accomplished through non-verbal means. Interventions like these can help kids feel safer and less lonely, sad, or afraid. As Nina Beaty, art therapist at the HIV Primary Care Center at Cook County Hospital, points out:

The old saying, "A picture's worth a thousand words," really is true. The feelings surrounding HIV can be overwhelming—too big or too scary for words. Art therapy is a safe and powerful way of expressing things that may be too hurtful to speak about. Art is more basic than words, and every member of a family can do it. It's a direct communication from your mind and spirit, and it can be a direct path to learning about yourself and healing.

Don't forget, *you* can have a tremendous impact on your children's emotional well-being. Pay close attention to what they're telling you, verbally and non-verbally. Remember that kids, too, need a break from illness. Even if your child seems well and your home is calm, be sure to create "safe" places and/or activities where kids can be themselves and have fun. If you're unable to protect your children adequately or give them a healthy environment, consider asking a relative or trusted friend to serve as an "alternate parent" during difficult times.

There are as many ways of coping with HIV as there are people affected by the disease. Following are firsthand accounts of some of the many ways people experience living with HIV.

As a hemophiliac, I probably had less and more to deal with emotionally than people who got HIV in other ways. Less, because I already know what it's like to live with a chronic disease that's basically a pain in the ass. More, because I kinda felt like I'd paid my dues by having this damn hemophilia and didn't deserve to get anything else.

I think anyone who gets this disease—even though it sounds so "Dear Abby-like"—should probably go and talk with a professional counselor, at least in the beginning. You can find cheap ones who work at clinics with a sliding fee scale who are great. You have so many things to work out, and you've got to talk about it. You go through a million different feelings and emotions—depression, rage, anxiety—you name it. One person might say go see a shrink, another person might say take a pill, a third might say talk to a friend or go to a group—but you do what you gotta do.

I wish my mom was well. I hate the hospital. I don't want to go there. I want her to come home.

When I take my medicine, I just try to take it really fast, like, "Gulp!" and then go on and play with my friends and stuff. Sometimes when I'm mad at my mom or something, I am bad. I only pretend to take my medicine, or say "NO WAY!" She gets really mad then. Usually we have a fight and I get in trouble.

"CARMEN" (AGE 8)

> *I don't think immediately, initially, that you are ready for a support group. I think you have to be ready to turn to support.*
>
> GAIL

> *I never thought of myself as the "support group type." But I realized it was real important for me to connect up with people. When I walked into TPA the first night, I had no idea what to expect; but after the first meeting, I thought, "This is neat! They're talking about some real stuff here. It's not like a bunch of people sitting around going, 'Well, I'm gonna die pretty soon, and God, it's so unfair.'" There just wasn't any of that stuff, which a lot of people expect from these groups. There are some groups like that, but you don't have to stay in them.*
>
> CHARLIE

I personally don't believe in support groups. I tried a couple in the beginning, but I didn't get much out of them. I've got a couple of friends I can talk to about anything at any time. If I'm really bummed out, I can call one of them up and go on for hours on the phone, express my emotions, my fears, my thoughts. Maybe support groups are for people who don't have friends like that to talk to.

ADAM

The things I do to cope with this are things I wouldn't recommend to <u>anybody</u> else, but they work for me. The day I go to find out my T cell results, I medicate myself; I take a Valium. I've started smoking, too. Sometimes I'll get these days when I'm thinking about things a real lot, and I just can't stand another minute—and I take a Valium and get into bed.

I've been to two counselors since being diagnosed and I think there has been something lacking in both of them, probably because I'm their only HIV patient. The sympathy and compassion may be there, but if they've never worked with HIV people, they don't really know the issues or questions.

I have two friends who are also HIV-positive. They don't go to support groups either, because none of us feel we have that much in common with the other women there. Most of those women don't know where they got it, so they don't have anyone to hate—like we do. We know exactly who the assholes are who gave this to us. And I find that every once in awhile, I like kicking back and thinking, "That son of a bitch!" And so do these friends. So the three of us found we had a lot in common, and we stay in touch. We call ourselves "The HIVster sisters." That's where I kind of get my support. I guess it's one way of dealing with my anger.

"MARIE"

It was hard at first, because some of the kids around here started talking about Mom, and making fun of her and stuff. I didn't know much about AIDS then, so I didn't know what to do. Then I talked to Mom and got prayer cards from her and advice—like it didn't matter what other people said as long as I took care of myself. As long as she takes care of <u>herself</u>, that's all we can do.

PATRICK (age 11)

HIV is kind of like incest in that it's an unwelcome invasion that brings a sense of powerlessness—there is nothing you can do to fix it or change it. And your options are to totally deny it or deal with it. Being a good addict, I worked very hard to deny it, but it just creeps out everywhere and I am forced to deal with it. I think it also really ties into that whole less-than-human kind of thing—"What is wrong with me? Why me?" It's another thing that happened without my permission. No one goes out and says, "I think I'll go get AIDS," just like nobody says, "I hope I grow up in a family where someone will molest me all the time." When it happens, you just think, "It's done now, and I have to deal with the wreckage."

Incest is a pain that is inside of you all the time, just as the virus is there all the time. Even though sometimes you can't see its effects, they're there. One of my main incest issues was that the people who were supposed to take care of me didn't do so, and actually hurt me. Now my body, which is supposed to take care of me, isn't—and is actually hurting me. Where do you go when you can't rely on yourself or your caretakers? Where do you <u>go</u>? That is where my recovery is so important. It's the only place I have to go right now.

SANDI

I'm not around many people who have HIV, and I think that makes it hard—like double jeopardy. It's almost like I feel I belong to a different population now, and I haven't found it. I haven't found my tribe.

I talked to two women who were HIV-positive, but they both had really bad attitudes. When I got off the phone I just wanted to cry. I thought—am I going to get so ill that I would get like that? One of them acted embarrassed to be positive, and the other one was just <u>mean</u>. That depressed me. Since then, I have learned that I have to be careful of who I socialize with right now, because they could have a good impact on me or a bad impact on me.

"SONIA"

The list of burnout symptoms for caregivers is pretty long, and pretty obvious. You're losing your patience, you're angry, you're raising your voice—or becoming physically abusive to the person you're caring for. Changes in your own daily functioning, changes in sleep and eating patterns are all signs you're stressed out and not coping well. If you're feeling the need to use substances as a way to cope—drugs, smoking, drinking—that's certainly a strong indicator that stress may be getting out of control.

Last week for the first time, I went to a support group. It was really helpful for me because I was sort of at my limit. I needed to be with people who had the same condition that I have. And I felt I needed to take some of the pressure off Fred in terms of my wanting certain things emotionally from him that are hard to articulate, and him not being able to understand or give them to me.

I was really terrified about going. I didn't know if it was going to be a roomful of sick people, or what. It wasn't. Just a very mixed bag of gay men who are at different points in dealing with this. Basically, people talking and answering questions and giving information to each other. It was just what I needed—finding out that some of the issues I'm experiencing with Fred are the same issues other people experience in their relationships.

"RALPH"

And depression. A lot of caregivers get depressed because the work is exhausting and endless and stressful. They know it won't end until their loved one dies. There's a lot of guilt associated with that. I've talked to many caregivers who have a really difficult time acknowledging their relief, once it's all over. They have a lot of mixed feelings as they watch someone die. To deal with that on their own, without support, is a really difficult journey.

A lot of caregivers don't ask for support because they don't realize they <u>need</u> it. Because all the focus is on the sick person. But asking for help is not a selfish act. You have to keep the well person well to continue to care for the sick person. It's important to seek out support before it all really starts to get to you.

DEBORAH STEINKOPF
Executive Director, BEHIV—
Better Existence with HIV

Because of my mom's illness, I attend a group at my school for kids with problems. It's a bunch of teenagers, people I know, and we all talk about little problems that we have. The social worker and psychiatrist are really cool. Before, I didn't talk about it with anybody. I didn't want to go to a group, I didn't want to speak about it, and I didn't want to hear about it. I didn't want nothing! I knew my mom was sick and that was all I wanted to know.

I think I understand HIV more than I did before. I think I am coping with things better. Now, me and my mom have talks about it; I go to groups, I talk to a few of my close friends, and I talk to my father about it. It's more open, family-wise.

Kids like me, who have a parent with HIV, should spend as much time with their loved one as they can. Because if they don't, they'll regret it. I know that when my mom goes I want to remember, "Oh, me and my mom had fun." I don't want to think that I didn't talk to her, no negative things. So be close to them; be their friend.

ALYNA (age 17)

In the first years following my HIV diagnosis, I became more and more depressed. My parents still didn't acknowledge my illness, and my husband and I had a relationship only to the point that we were both Shane's parents. The two doctors I saw only depressed me further by telling me there was nothing they could do. They told me I had two years left if I was lucky. A few months of living and some painful times in a hospital were to be my future. It was made worse by a comment from one of the nurses that, "It's too bad for people like you." People like me, I thought? Who exactly are "people like me"?

The depression overcame me. I was sick all the time. I was sure I was dying; I could feel it inside. The fear haunted me all through the day and endlessly through the night. I was afraid of everything. I developed phobias of all kinds. I was afraid to leave the house. I was afraid to drive. I was afraid to talk to anyone. I was afraid of myself. I was terrified that someone was going to find out I had this disease and of what would happen if they did.

I isolated myself from the world. I was frightened, lonely, and lost. I would lock myself in my room and cry until there were no tears left. I sat trying to will myself to death, until one night I thought—this doesn't make sense! Here I was so depressed that I wanted to die? But how could I <u>live</u>?! If there was a way through, I decided then and there I wanted to find it.

SHARI

Support Groups and Mental Health Services

(Note: For crisis intervention and emergency mental health services, refer to the hotlines listed in Part 1 of this book.)

AIDS Care Network
221 North Longwood, Suite 105
Rockford, IL 61107
815-968-5181
815-968-3315—FAX
• Support groups for HIV-positive individuals, their families and friends.

AIDS Support Coalition
PO Box 1548
Crystal Lake, IL 60039
815-459-1985
• Support groups and services for HIV-positive individuals, their families and friends in McHenry County.

Ascension Respite Care Center
1133 North LaSalle Street
Chicago, IL 60610
312-751-8887
312-751-3904—FAX
• Individual counseling for family members of people with HIV. Mothers' support group.

Better Existence with HIV (BEHIV)
PO Box 5171
Evanston, IL 60204
847-475-2115
847-475-2820—FAX
• Individual and group counseling for those with HIV/AIDS and their partners and families. Serves northern Chicago and north/northwest suburbs. Free. English/Spanish.

Brother to Brother—Mt. Sinai Family Health Centers
5401 South Wentworth Avenue
Chicago, IL 60609
773-288-6900
• Support groups and referrals for African-Americans, primarily gay men.

Center for New Beginnings
10300 West 131st Street
Palos Park, IL 60464
708-923-1116
708-923-6524—FAX
• Individual and group support for bereavement and for persons affected by HIV/AIDS. Serves the Chicago metropolitan area.

Chicago Women's AIDS Project
5249 North Kenmore Avenue
Chicago, IL 60640
773-271-2242
773-271-2618—FAX
• Support groups for women. Individual counseling for children and teens of parents living with HIV/AIDS.

Circle of Hope
PO Box 1152
Woodstock, IL 60098
815-334-9116—Voice/FAX (same line)
• Support, networking and peer counseling to persons impacted by HIV/AIDS. Call for support group locations in northern Illinois.

Community Response
225 Harrison Street
Oak Park, IL 60304
708-386-3383
708-386-3551—FAX
• Comprehensive support services for people with HIV/AIDS and their loved ones, including peer-led support groups, mental health counseling (off-site), volunteer services, and companions. Free. English/Spanish.

Comprension y Apoyo a Latinos en Oposicion al Retrovirus (CALOR)
2015 West Division Street
Chicago, IL 60622
773-235-3161
773-772-0484—FAX
• Support groups for Spanish-speaking persons with HIV. Free. English/Spanish.

Cook County HIV Primary Care Center
1835 West Harrison Street
CCSN 1268
Chicago, IL 60612
312-633-3005
312-633-3002—FAX
• Offers mental health services and several on-site support groups, including groups for men, women, people in recovery, Latinos, and others. Other support services available through the Cook County Hospital Women and Children's HIV Program. Free. English/Spanish.

DuPage County Health Department AIDS Program
111 North County Farm Road
Wheaton, IL 60187
630-682-7979, ext. 7310
630-462-9439—FAX
• Support groups for HIV-positive persons, including a group for those in recovery. Monthly event night for people with HIV and their loved ones.

El Rincon Community Clinic
1874 North Milwaukee Avenue
Chicago, IL 60647
773-276-0200
773-276-4226—FAX
• Support groups, including groups for Spanish-speaking persons with HIV. English/Spanish.

Family Service and Mental Health Center
120 South Marion Street
Oak Park, IL 60302
708-383-7500
708-383-7780—FAX
• Mental health counseling for people living with HIV/AIDS in Oak Park and River Forest.

Fox River Valley Center for Independent Living
730 West Chicago Street
Elgin, IL 60123
847-695-5818
847-695-5892—FAX
847-695-5818—Hearing-impaired TTY/TDD
• Independent living skills counseling, peer counseling and support. English/Spanish.

The HIV Coalition (HIVCO)
1471 Business Center Drive
Suite 500
Mount Prospect, IL 60056
847-391-9803
847-391-9826—FAX
• Referrals to HIV support groups in Chicago's suburbs, including Cook, DuPage, Lake, McHenry, Will, and Kane Counties. English/Spanish.

Horizons Community Services
961 West Montana
Chicago, IL 60614
773-472-6469
773-472-6643—FAX
773-929-4357—Lesbian/gay Helpline, 6-10 p.m. daily
773-871-8873—24-hour Anti-violence Crisis Hotline
773-327-4357—Hearing-impaired TTY/TDD hotline
• Offers individual and group psychotherapy services. Provides short-term counseling for PWAs, their lovers, or the couple together. Group support sessions are peer-led. Offers services for lesbian and gay youth, and youth with questions and concerns about HIV/AIDS. Sliding scale fee for psychotherapy. Offers short-term professional help for individuals who cannot afford a private practitioner or use insurance. English/Spanish.

Horizon Hospice
833 West Chicago Avenue
Chicago, IL 60622
312-733-8900
312-733-8952—FAX
• Provides support services to terminally ill people, including persons with HIV/AIDS and their families and caregivers. Bereavement support group.

Howard Brown Health Center
945 West George Street
Chicago, IL 60657
773-871-5777
773-871-5843—FAX
• HIV support groups, including groups for current substance users and persons in recovery. Alcohol/drug abuse counseling and referrals. Women's program offers counseling and groups. English/Spanish.

Illinois AIDS Hotline
800-243-2437—Hotline staffed 8 a.m.-11 p.m., 7 days/week
800-782-0423—Hearing-impaired TTY/TDD
• Referrals to HIV support groups and mental health services throughout Illinois. English/Spanish.

Lake County Health Department
2400 Belvidere Road
Waukegan, IL 60085
847-360-6891
847-360-9274—FAX
• HIV support groups; referrals to mental health and support services in Lake County. English/Spanish.

Lutheran Social Services of Illinois—Second Family Program
1144 West Lake Street
Oak Park, IL 60301
708-445-8341
708-445-8351—FAX
• Support group for parents affected by HIV, including gay and lesbian parents. Free. English/Spanish.

Minority Outreach Intervention Project (MOIP)
1579 North Milwaukee Avenue, Suite 314
Chicago, IL 60622
773-276-5990
773-276-3002—FAX
• Peer support groups and prevention education for HIV-positive gay and bisexual men of color. Free. English/Spanish.

Northwest Community Hospital
Joshua Ministries Support Group/Positive Approach To Health (PATH)
800 West Central Road
Arlington Heights, IL 60005
847-618-4255
847-618-7739—FAX
• Support groups for HIV-positive persons, their families, friends, and caregivers. Bereavement group for persons who have lost loved ones to AIDS.

Parental Stress Services
600 South Federal Street, Suite 205
Chicago, IL 60605
312-427-1161
312-427-3038—FAX
312-427-1102—Enrollment in groups/classes
10 a.m.-2 p.m. Mon-Fri (Central time)
312-3PARENT (372-7368)— 24-hour Parental Stress Hotline
312-427-1102—Hearing-impaired TTY/TDD
• 24-hour hotline offers support, problem-solving, and referrals. Parent education classes, parent support and children's groups. HIV-affected families welcome. English/Spanish.

Test Positive Aware Network (TPAN or TPA)
1258 West Belmont
Chicago, IL 60657
773-404-8726
773-472-7505—FAX
773-404-9716—Hearing-impaired TTY/TDD
• Self-help support and information groups, including meetings for people under 30 years of age, gay/lesbian couples, straights, women, African-Americans, Latinos, substance abusers, people in recovery, those experiencing grief and loss, HIV-positive clergy, and those recently diagnosed with HIV/AIDS. English/Spanish.

Trinity United Church of Christ
HIV/AIDS Support Ministry
400 West 95th Street
Chicago, IL 60628
312-409-AIDS (409-2437)
• Support groups and spiritual support for individuals impacted by AIDS.

Using a Computer and Modem

America Online (AOL) AIDS and HIV Resource Center
• Accessible if you have AOL via keyword "AIDS" or "HIV" (without the quotation marks). This area provides connections to "The Positive Living Forum," Web sites featuring HIV/AIDS information, and more. For a live chat room and support area, go to the "Positive Living Room" within "The Positive Living Forum."

The Body: A Multimedia AIDS and HIV Resource
http://www.thebody.com/cgi-bin/body.cgi
• Offers HIV/AIDS mental health information and support resources. Get online support and post messages to others in "Connecting to Others." Links to other sites.

POZ Magazine
http://www.POZ.com
• HIV-positive people from all over the country post messages to each other in the forum offered by this national magazine.

Test Positive Aware Network
http://www.tpan.com
• Site includes full listings from the "Chicago Area HIV/AIDS Services Directory," including dozens of mental health and emotional support programs. Up-to-date meeting times and listings for TPA support groups. National resources and state hotlines for persons outside Illinois.

Spiritual Support

At times of crisis or unexpected change, people often feel the need to get in touch with or strengthen their spiritual beliefs. "Spiritual" can be a hard word to deal with. It might mean something very specific to those who've been raised in a particular religious tradition. On the other hand, it might be a very fuzzy word that doesn't mean much at all to those raised in a non-religious home. "Spiritual" can also have negative connotations for people who have walked away from or been rejected by their church, or who dismiss organized religion as illusory. For many, the idea that "spirituality" and "religion" are always interrelated can present a significant obstacle to spiritual growth and discovery.

Whatever your beliefs, you will probably find yourself grappling with some very difficult and deeply personal life issues. What does life mean? Why am I here? What will happen to me when I die? How am I connected to the earth, the solar system, the universe—and God (if I happen to believe in God)?

HIV makes us very aware that life has a definite end. It can be a frightening thing to contemplate, especially if you've never thought that much about your death. Oftentimes, people with HIV feel a lot of guilt around their illness. You may find yourself wondering if this is God's way of "punishing" you because of things you've done or failed to do.

John Fortunato, a pastoral psychotherapist and Executive Director of the North Suburban Counseling Center in Skokie, has this to say in response:

> *Right here and now, I want to help you question some of those standard guilt-tripping things that people sometimes think and say about those who get infected with HIV. Things like, "They deserved it—they're homosexual (or drug users)."*
>
> *First of all, if you believe in God and you believe God is Love, then no God who is all love and mercy could be so hateful as to make His own creatures suffer for being who they are, and who He made them. That God would have no mercy.*
>
> *Second, it isn't logical to say that AIDS is God's punishment on people because of their sinfulness in being gay or a drug user. Think about it. Lots of gay people (even some who have had a lot of sex) don't get AIDS. So does God punish some people because they're gay and not others? What about the fact that lesbians are the lowest risk group for HIV in the whole U.S. population? Does that mean God has a special love for lesbians?*
>
> *By the same token, some IV drug users just happen never to meet the virus and never get AIDS—while others do. What does that mean for the babies and little kids and wives or husbands of those unfortunate*

enough to bring HIV home by accident? What did they do to "merit" God's punishment?

You see, it doesn't make sense. So blow off all of that terrible, blaming moralizing if anyone tries to lay it on you. It's as simple as this: HIV is a virus. Speaking from a believer's vantage point, I don't know why God let this virus come into existence on the earth. I don't have any clearer idea why God allows the viruses that cause meningitis or yellow fever or polio on the earth, either. Are they God's punishment on the people who get those diseases? Of course not. It's no different for HIV.

Just as you will seek out doctors and counselors for your physical and emotional care, you will also want to find ways to care for yourself spiritually. If you belong to a church, synagogue, or other religious community you feel nourished by, talk to a clergyperson there. Together you can explore worship, prayer, or meditation practices from your tradition that will help you find at least hints of answers to the enormous questions you're dealing with.

If you're not a member of an organized religious group, or feel your own clergy wouldn't understand what you're going through, find spiritual support and guidance outside the church. Seek out someone wise, calm, and centered in their life. It might be a neighbor, a co-worker, a companion in a recovery group, or an older relative. It might also be a therapist who is comfortable giving you space to explore and doesn't feel the need to "fix" anything in you. Explain to this person that you would value their spending some regular time with you as you try to work through the meaning of this disease in your life.

Personal Perspectives on Spirituality and HIV

What I think the Lord has shown me, through my HIV, is that no matter what happens, He'll be there to carry me through. I think that's real important—knowing that Jesus is there always, and that He knows what's best for you, and if you just ask Him, He will help you. Whether it's God or Jesus or Allah or whomever—He is there for you. You are not alone. Even if you don't have a single friend here, you always have one friend you can trust. And you can turn to Him and He will love you no matter what, with no questions.

In the beginning, I was so afraid of dying. But I think I've become a lot stronger as a result of faith and prayer and meditation. The belief that God is forgiving, that He's not doing this to punish me. That He has a reason for everything He does. And now, whenever the time comes, I'm not afraid to die. I'm not looking to have excruciating pain—but I'm not afraid to die.

Besides, I now know that AIDS doesn't have to be the end; I may not even die of it. I may live to a ripe old age! No one knows what He has in store. Sometimes, I look at this and say, "I'm grateful." If it hadn't been for HIV, I probably would've just gone along and done the things I was doing, and never really felt the closeness with Jesus I do now. When things are going bad I just say, "Lord, I've had enough." And it's like, He kind of wakes me up.

"ELIZABETH"

My ex-husband was Catholic; my parents were Jewish and never practiced. So I was kind of in limbo; I didn't have a church. But I met this priest through AA, and he's helped me a lot—not with the "Why me?" part, but with the "What's gonna happen?" part. When you find out you're going to die pretty young, you want the security of at least trying to believe it's not gonna be the end, at least for your soul. I really needed that. I just couldn't handle things without it. It's been real comforting. My outlook was so drastically changed after HIV, religion kind of modified it. Believing in something higher, a higher power, has helped. So I took out of Catholicism what I needed from it, their teachings on the spiritual afterlife, and left the rest.

"MARIE"

I've given a lot of thought to the afterlife. I really don't believe there is one. To me, it's patently absurd. It doesn't disturb me; I think if I believed in an afterlife, I'd be much more concerned about death.

I have gotten somewhat more in touch with my spiritual life since HIV. I'm attracted to stuff that's influenced by Buddhism. Not the religious aspects, but the stuff about the relationship between the individual and the universe, and between the individual and other people. It's almost like a mental health thing—how do you work with the world and come to terms with it? I've gotten some comfort and insights through those ideas, though I don't really see them as "religious" ideas. It's not a God-system.

CHARLIE

I just pray to God and the Holy Spirit to shine on me. I lean on my faith. Not long ago, I had to go into the hospital for a few days because I was very ill. They did a spinal tap, and I never imagined I would have the strength to sit there and have somebody poke me with a needle in my back, you know? Basically humor got me through that one, but then I started to cry and I just leaned on my faith. Without that, I would have done something stupid by now. I would've started getting high or resorted to destructive-type behavior—but I haven't gone back to anything like that. People who have faith are going to weather this better.

"SONIA"

We are each given a set of circumstances, and it is our job to live in them, to be ourselves fully. There is a reason we are here now. We can't look to the future or to the past without causing ourselves pain, but we can create ourselves and our universe now. We can choose whether we want our lives to be heaven or hell, and we can create heaven or hell in our lives. Things may seem overwhelming, but if we take one thing at a time and do what we can today, then we will create a heaven for today. When we do that, the future takes care of itself and there is no room for regret.

BO GYUNG, CHEF
Amitabul Restaurant, Chicago

I'm not a religious person, though I do believe in God. I thank God every morning, first thing, for helping me make it through another day and night—and let's go for another one. I think that's helped me tremendously.

JIM

I have something no one can help me with: the guilt that you feel as a mother knowing your child is sick because of you. Friends try to say it's not my fault, but you know what? It is.

One guy helped me, when he told me that Buddhists believe babies pick their parents. He said, "How do you know that Phillip didn't see you and Louie on the streets and think your life was worth saving, and pick you? Maybe that's why he's here, to save you." That helped a lot, to think of it that way.

CHRISTINE

Spiritual Support Resources

AIDS Ministry of Illinois
68 North Chicago Street,
Suite 240
Joliet, IL 60432-4380
815-723-1548
815-740-5910—FAX
• Provides comprehensive support services to people with HIV.

AIDS Pastoral Care Network/ Equipo de Cuidado Pastoral Contra el SIDA
4753 North Broadway, Suite 800
Chicago, IL 60640
773-334-5333
773-334-3293—FAX
• Direct spiritual support services include pastoral care and counseling, support groups, bereavement support, and pastoral support in hospital and other institutions. Offers faith-based domestic assistance to clients through the "Communities of Care" program. Outreach and education efforts include education for clergy and congregation of all faiths with specialized services in African-American and Latino communities. Quarterly newsletter, "The Spirit." English/Spanish.

Bethany Ministries
Deerfield & Wilmot Roads
Deerfield, IL 60015
847-945-1678
847-945-9511—FAX
• Non-denominational support group for families and friends of those with HIV/AIDS.

Bishop's Task Force on AIDS of the Greek Orthodox Diocese of Chicago
40 East Burton Place
Chicago, IL 60610
312-337-4130
312-337-9391—FAX
• Medical and pastoral education for priests and laity surrounding HIV/AIDS issues. Pastoral support for HIV/AIDS-impacted Orthodox faithful. Grief and loss counseling. Free.

Catholic Charities
126 North Desplaines Street
Chicago, IL 60661
312-655-7715
312-263-4290—FAX
• Services include professional family, bereavement, and in-home counseling. Referrals.

Catholic Charities— Lake County
671 South Lewis Avenue
Waukegan, IL 60085
847-249-3500
847-623-6750—FAX
• Professional and volunteer support services for people with HIV. English/Spanish.

Circle Family Care
4909 West Division Street,
3rd Floor
Chicago, IL 60651
773-921-8100
773-921-4428—FAX
• Provides services from a Christian perspective, including case management, confidential HIV counseling and testing, primary health care, and women's support group.

Jewish AIDS Network Chicago, U.A.H.C.
4753 North Broadway, Suite 800
Chicago, IL 60640
773-463-7251
773-334-3293—FAX
• Rabbis, social workers, and volunteers offer support and counseling for individuals affected by HIV/AIDS and their families and loved ones. Affiliated with the AIDS Pastoral Care Network.

Lawndale Christian Health Center
3860 West Ogden Avenue
Chicago, IL 60632
773-521-5006
773-521-2742—FAX
• Support groups, including a group for persons in recovery, and pastoral care. Primary outpatient care, case management, HIV counseling and testing, transportation, and referrals. Sliding scale fees. English/Spanish.

Love & Action Midwest, Inc.
107 South Hi Lusi
Mount Prospect, IL 60056
708-392-3123
• Interdenominational Christian ministry for those with HIV/AIDS and their loved ones. Spiritual, emotional, and physical support; volunteer training.

The Night Ministry
1218 West Addison Street
Chicago, IL 60613
773-935-8300
773-935-6199—FAX
• Nighttime street outreach and ministry service for youth and young adults. Free.

Pastoral Counseling Center of Lutheran General Hospital
1610 Luther Lane
Park Ridge, IL 60068
847-518-1800
847-823-9222—FAX
• Pastoral counseling on a sliding scale. English/Spanish.

Trinity United Church of Christ
HIV/AIDS Support Ministry
400 West 95th Street
Chicago, IL 60628
312-409-AIDS (409-2437)
• Provides spiritual support and support groups for individuals impacted by AIDS.

Books and Publications

AIDS and the Healer Within
Bamforth, Nick
Amethyst Books, 1993
• Focuses on emotional and spiritual energies that can be used to combat living with HIV/AIDS.

AIDS, God and Faith: Continuing the Dialogue on Constructing Gay Theology
Long, Ronald and J. Michael Clark
Publishers Associate
• Insight into the issues of AIDS and religious faith. Supplement to the "Gay Men's Issues in Religious Studies" series.

I Know the Time Is Now: A Journey Living with AIDS
Kavanaugh, W. J.
Alamo Square
• A man comes to terms with AIDS in a spiritual way.

In the Lap of the Buddha
Harrison, Gavin
Random House
• A teacher of insight meditation speaks openly about his own struggles with memories of childhood sexual abuse and with being HIV-positive. He reveals how the teachings of the Buddha and the practice of meditation offer support.

Video

"Positive Faith"
Mail order: Lambda Rising Books, 800-621-6969
• A film about being Christian and HIV-positive.

Sex

You know that unprotected sex is one of the main ways you can transmit HIV to others. What you may not know is that unsafe sex remains extremely risky for you, too. You might believe that once you have the virus there's nothing more to worry about. You can't catch it again, right?

Wrong. The virus can have slightly different characteristics from one person to another (or even in different tissues within the same person). If you're HIV-positive and have unprotected sex with a person who is also positive, you could be reinfected with a new, potentially more deadly strain of HIV. This could speed up the damage that HIV does to your immune system and make it easier for you to get sick. If you've thought it's okay to have unsafe sex with another person with HIV, think again.

Besides being reinfected with the virus, having unsafe sex can also put you at risk for catching other sexually transmitted diseases (STDs). Syphilis, herpes, genital warts, chlamydia—all these and more can cause problems that are especially dangerous for you now. They're also much tougher to control or cure with HIV in the picture. Having a sexually transmitted disease increases the risk of passing along HIV to a partner through unprotected sex.

Some people on antiretroviral drugs find their viral loads dropping to levels so low the HIV in their system can no longer be measured. This does *not* mean they're no longer infected with the virus. They are, and are still capable of passing it on to others. Don't assume, if you or a partner experience success with these drugs, that you no longer need to practice safer sex. You do.

The only completely "safe" sex is no sex. Obviously, lifetime celibacy is not a realistic option for most people. Still, doing your best to cut back on sexual risk for yourself and your partners is highly advisable.

Many "safer" sex practices are not 100% guaranteed safe, but they are known to be less risky than no protection at all. According to the San Francisco AIDS Foundation and other sources, safe sexual activities include:

- masturbating alone.
- masturbating others with healthy skin (especially while wearing thin rubber gloves, like doctors' examination gloves, or "finger cots"—like a little condom for your finger. Do not share or reuse these.)
- massage, back rubs, hugging, body rubbing.
- social (dry) kissing.
- sex talk, phone sex.
- role playing, fantasy, dressing up, showing off.
- watching others, live or on video.
- sex toys or dildoes that are clean and not shared.
- light S&M (without bleeding or bruising).

I just found out my former boyfriend gave me HIV. He knew he had it! This man committed murder!

I don't know how I didn't go insane. No one should pass this on to anyone. If you know you have AIDS, you are responsible to take care not to hurt anyone like that!

"SONIA"

Recently, I've started seeing somebody. It's like, we date, but we don't make love. Every once in awhile we get kind of sexual. We don't get anywhere near intercourse; we cuddle, do some touching. Once we got a little bit heavy, almost to an intense sexual experience between us—but we both started laughing real hard. I think that was a defense. I'm sure he's afraid. In a way, it's fine, but it's kind of weird and frustrating, too. I don't know if it's ever gonna turn into anything more.

"MARIE"

My 8-year-old son finds it really surprising that people don't use condoms, don't protect themselves. He asks, "Are they stupid or don't they care?" I told him, not everyone cares about themselves or others.

WENDY

My wife and I are careful. Sexually, there are "do's" and "don'ts." There are things we never do. Like, we never, <u>ever</u> have any kind of penetration without a condom. Before I'll put it on, we'll put some kind of cream with nonoxynol-9 in the condom—I call it "glue." We'll also put it on me, she'll even put it into her with this syringe thing she has. At times that's a pain in the ass, but at other times it's kind of fun. It's become part of our lovemaking—it's like a ritual, we've got to get ready. It's crazy, but it's okay. She can put the "glue" in, and she can put it on for me, or I can put it in her—we experiment with different little things like that.

Keeping all that as a rule, we've kept her HIV-negative. Up until now, that's done the trick. Our sex life's been very active.

GEORGE

Activities with some risk (a gray area):
- wet or "French" kissing, because people may have bleeding gums.
- oral sex on a man using a condom, or on a woman using a "dental dam" (a latex condom cut lengthwise, used as a barrier. You can also get dental dams through a dentist. Plastic wrap may not provide an adequate barrier. <u>Note</u>: While spermicides found on some condoms may numb your tongue, they are non-toxic.) Besides HIV, syphilis, chlamydia, gonorrhea, and herpes may be transmitted orally.
- water sports without swallowing.
- anal or vaginal intercourse using a condom with a water-based lubricant entails some risk because condoms can break and must be put on and removed correctly every time.

Activities with more risk (a gray area):
- anal or vaginal intercourse using a condom alone.
- oral sex without a condom or dental dam, without cumming in the mouth. (Risk is increased when there are cuts or sores in the mouth or on the lips, or bleeding gums.)
- masturbating others unprotected with open or broken skin.
- fisting with a latex glove.

Activities known to be dangerous:
- anal or vaginal intercourse without a condom.
- unprotected oral sex on a man to climax, or on a woman who is menstruating or has open sores, or where blood is present.
- rimming (licking the anal area) or fisting without a latex glove (dangerous because of other infections and damage to delicate tissue).
- sharing IV needles, syringes, cookers, or works.
- sharing enema equipment, sex toys, or dildoes.
- semen in the mouth, vagina, anus, or open skin area.

In addition:
- Using alcohol, poppers, or other drugs can weaken your resolve to practice safer sex. As a rule, "sober is safer."
- It's best to lay the ground rules and negotiate what you're willing to do sexually before you and your partner get too turned on.
- Birth control pills, cervical caps, implants, and diaphragms may prevent pregnancy, but they cannot guard against HIV or other diseases.
- Regardless of how you or your partner acquired the virus (through unsafe sex, contaminated drug injection equipment, transfusion, etc.), you can still transmit or acquire it sexually now.
- Remember, "it's not who you are, but what you do" that transmits this virus. Reducing your number of partners may put you in contact with fewer people who may have HIV or another sexually transmitted disease, but making all of your behaviors safer is the best way to avoid reinfection or infecting someone else.

The best way to avoid transmission of HIV is to avoid activities that include penetration. If you decide to have intercourse, using a latex condom with a water-based lubricant is the best way you can protect yourself and your partner from HIV and other diseases. Your local Red Cross office, public health department, or AIDS service organization can give you literature and instruction about condoms and their use. Many public health clinics provide condoms free of charge.

There are also prelubricated "female" condoms, designed to be inserted into the vagina instead of over a man's penis. Many people also use this condom rectally, although its safety during anal sex has not been determined. The female condom resembles a combination condom/diaphragm, composed of a thin polyurethane sheath with a flexible ring at each end. Couples taking part in trials of these products liked them as well as or better than traditional male condoms.

Female condoms are widely available in drug stores and many public health clinics. If you have Public Aid, you can get a prescription for free female condoms to redeem at your local pharmacy.

Some people's partners refuse to use condoms or follow other safer sex practices. They may protest the loss of sensation or the birth control aspects, deny their risk in transmitting or acquiring the virus—or simply not care about your or their own safety. If this is true in your case, and you don't feel you can safely negotiate some compromise (such as abstinence, intercourse alternatives, or at least using spermicide alone), seek help outside the relationship. Find a supportive friend, social worker, or counselor who can help you explore your options or provide a space for you to think on your own. AIDS service organizations and battered women's shelters are often good places to start.

Because HIV is a sexually transmitted disease, knowing you're HIV-positive will almost certainly color your feelings about sex. If you've never been comfortable with your sexuality, or had feelings of guilt or inadequacy, your diagnosis will tend to magnify those negative emotions. Even if you've always been very confident and open sexually, you may still have some unexpected reactions. Intimacy becomes a very complicated issue with both new and established partners. You may feel less desirable or lovable. You might be tempted to withdraw from others completely—or have the opposite reaction, using indiscriminate sex as an "escape."

The main thing to remember is, your reactions are normal and permissible. You're coping with a significant loss in the only way you know how. It's perfectly okay to feel angry or sad or confused at first. Your sexuality is a big part of your identity as a human being. With HIV in the picture, you'll have to rethink that identity a bit, maybe come to grips with a new one—and that's not an easy process.

There are several things you can do to begin to deal with sexual confusion and change. If you're married or involved in a relationship, your spouse or partner may want to do them with you.

I came out in 1982; I finally started living as a gay person. In 1986, I tested positive. One of my first reactions was, wait a minute—this isn't fair! These other people have been running around screwing everything in sight for twenty years, and they're still healthy—and I finally get to the party and all the beer is gone, and all I get to do is clean up the place!

CHARLIE

The problem with screwing someone else when you have this virus is, you're packing a loaded gun in your pants. And all that lies between you and killing another person—the safety on the gun—is a little piece of rubber. The problem is, knowing all that while you're having sex can take a lot of the fun out of it. Knowing that if you actually have any care or love for this other person, the risk is pretty great—it's a scary thought. My sex drive isn't a bit diminished, but I've lost my desire to have sex for that reason.

ADAM

> We can rewrite the history of this epidemic in our community, one man and one woman at a time. We are infected one at a time; we can break this silence one at a time. Tell someone you care about that you love them, then get them to talk explicitly and openly about sex. Our sharing can launch an epidemic of HIV prevention that no CDC campaign could ever touch.
>
> STEVE WAKEFIELD
> FORMER EXECUTIVE DIRECTOR,
> TEST POSITIVE AWARE NETWORK

> I had a friend who slept with this girl, or he wanted to. I got mad at him. I said, "I'm your friend, and I'm living proof that anybody can get this disease! Can't you think before you act? Do you even love her? You don't even know each other that well. It's not my decision, but I'm telling you as a friend, be careful. You guys have a big talk before you do this. You know how to use a condom, don't you?" When he said, "Yeah, yeah," I told him, "Don't say yeah, yeah. You better use one!"
>
> GINA (AGE 16)

1) *Acknowledge and deal with the loss you're feeling.* Talking to a therapist or going to a support group may help. You can also check out couple's groups, where sex is always a big topic. Explore your changing feelings about your body and sexuality, both alone and with your partner.

2) *Establish your own "bottom line" with regard to safer sex.* Decide with your partner what you are and aren't willing to do, and how much risk you're willing to accept. It may take a lot of work, a lot of exploration with your partner to get beyond the "all or nothing" mindset. Many couples think, "If we've done it without a condom for this long and one of us is still negative, a few more times probably won't matter." But it takes only one unprotected encounter to transmit HIV. While the ultimate goal can be consistent protection for you and your partner, recognize that the journey there may take a while.

3) *Begin to explore new ways to express your sexuality.* Previously, you may have equated penetration with sex—considering all activities leading up to intercourse as secondary to the "main event." But human beings are capable of a huge range of sexual enjoyment and communication. The safer sex "do not" list is much shorter than the "do" list of fun, exciting, and low risk activities. You can have a lot of fun experimenting with a wealth of things you may not have considered before.

In your sexual explorations, don't neglect your need for love and affection. Without communication and emotional sharing, the mechanics of sex can become just that—mechanical.

4) *Find new ways to communicate.* Talking with a partner about sex can be extremely difficult. However, it's essential if you're to arrive at mutually comfortable decisions about risk and new ways of pleasuring. Shelly Ebbert, Administrator of the Grundy County Health Department (Illinois), offers some advice on how to begin:

When you're dealing with such an intimate subject, you want to take the time to do it right. Talking in a neutral place helps. Having this discussion in bed is probably not a good idea.

Feeling safe in your environment, feeling private and protected, is important. You have to make sure you won't be interrupted. If you have children, you may want to take them to a relative's for a while. You'll have some privacy and won't need to worry about who is listening.

It may be helpful to get a book with pictures. That way, you can begin to develop a common vocabulary. Ask your partner: "What do you call this? Is it okay if I touch you there? Do you want me to touch you there?" You have to come to a common language, and one that's explicit enough so there's no misunderstanding. Phrases like "down there" or "between your legs" aren't enough.

Finally, a sense of humor is extremely important to any discussions about sex—acknowledging how weird this is to talk about. Because it's hard to look your lover in the face and say, "I'm infected," or "I can't have sex with you anymore the way we used to." It's hard to put that much of yourself on the line.

5) *Don't shut yourself off from sexual feelings.* You may decide, in the face of HIV, to abstain from sex altogether, temporarily or permanently. Despite the messages society sends us, many people are quite comfortable without sexual relationships. However, it's important to approach celibacy as a choice, not an escape or form of self-punishment. If you have been very sexual in the past and a sense of fear or shame because of your HIV is what is driving your decision now, celibacy may not be a good option for you. Studies have shown that people who try to change their sexuality because of shame are very likely to fail, and when they do they're less likely than others to practice safer sex. If you're considering celibacy as an option, talk it through with someone you trust who knows you well and can help you be certain it's the right decision for you.

When our outreach workers talk to younger gay men in the bars, some of the men say they don't need condoms because they aren't going to date anyone over 30. The perception is that if they just partner with someone their same age, they are safe—"Only older gay men have AIDS." But according to the hard core CDC numbers, 40% of all gay men in this country between the ages of 19 and 39 will become HIV-positive by the time they're 40 years old. So you still have a good chance, based on current statistics, of becoming infected. Putting arbitrary age limits on who you'll sleep with is no substitute for latex condoms.

DEBORAH STEINKOPF
Executive Director, BEHIV—
Better Existence with HIV

People wonder, "Can I have sex now? Is safe sex really safe? Can I infect people—am I dangerous?" It suddenly becomes a very death-loaded thing. You've hooked up the concept of death with sex—two powerful, major life issues. People become very scared, which is understandable. The thing to do is be as safe as possible. You may be feeling the very thing that should be life-affirming and joyful and interchanging love has now become a means of death for you. But it's the <u>virus</u> that causes the disease, not sex. Sex is just a mode of transmission. Sex does not equal death.

"GARY"

Safer Sex Resources

Many local health departments and HIV care clinics offer free prevention counseling to people with HIV and their partners. Local community organizations may offer safer sex information, group education, counseling, and peer support to keep practicing safer sex. The Illinois AIDS Hotline is a good place to start looking for resources.

Illinois AIDS Hotline
800-243-2437–Hotline staffed 8 a.m.-11 p.m., 7 days/week
800-782-0423–Hearing-impaired TTY/TDD
• Confidential safer sex information and referrals to programs near you. English/Spanish.

American Red Cross/ Mid-America Chapter
43 East Ohio Street
Chicago, IL 60611
312-440-2000
312-440-5216—FAX
• Educational services and programs, brochures, and community presentations. HIV/AIDS instructor training for language-specific and culturally sensitive presentations. English, Spanish, American Sign Language. Serves Cook and surrounding Illinois counties; call for referrals to other Illinois chapters.

CDC National AIDS Clearinghouse
800-458-5231—English/Spanish
800-243-7012—Hearing-impaired TTY/TDD
9 a.m.-7 p.m. Mon-Fri (Eastern time)
• Free safer sex brochures in English and Spanish.

Chicago Women's AIDS Project
5249 North Kenmore Avenue
Chicago, IL 60640
773-271-2242
773-271-2618—FAX
• Group STD/HIV prevention programs and counseling for women. Free.

Coalition for Positive Sexuality
PO Box 191
Chicago, IL 60613
773-604-1654
• Distributes "Just Say Yes" safer sex pamphlet for adolescents. English/Spanish.

Condomania, Mail Order Division
7306 Melrose Avenue
Los Angeles, CA 90046
800-9CONDOM (926-0636)
213-934-9784—FAX
http://www.condomania.com
• Mail order latex and polyurethane condoms, lubricants, and other safer sex supplies, including hard-to-find items.

ETR Associates
PO Box 1830
Santa Cruz, CA 95061
800-321-4407
• Safer sex brochures for people living with HIV, gay men, women, injection drug users, and partners. English/Spanish.

Gay Men's Health Crisis
129 West 20th Street
New York, NY 10011
212-337-1950
212-337-1975—FAX
• Safer sex materials and videos for gay men. English/Spanish.

Planned Parenthood, Chicago Area
14 East Jackson Boulevard, 10th Floor
Chicago, IL 60604
312-427-2276
312-427-2275—Hotline
312-427-0802—FAX
• Provides HIV/STD risk reduction education and counseling, family planning, gynecological services, and HIV counseling and testing for women and male partners of clients. Seven locations throughout the Chicago area. Spanish-speaking staff at some locations. Public Aid accepted.

Reimer Foundation
3023 North Clark Street, Suite 1000
Chicago, IL 60657
773-935-SAFE (935-7233)
773-281-4844—FAX
• Safer sex literature in English and Spanish specifically for men who have sex with men. Organizes distribution of condoms. Free.

Stop AIDS
909 West Belmont Avenue
Chicago, IL 60657
773-871-3300
773-871-2528—FAX
• Prevention education, outreach, safer sex discussions, workshops, and testing buddy program. Prevention programs for substance users and persons in recovery. Lesbian and bisexual women's programs. English/ Spanish (Mexican, Puerto Rican). "Stop AIDS" is a program of the Howard Brown Health Center. Free.

Stop AIDS–African-American Program
1718 East 75th Street
Chicago, IL 60649
773-752-7867
773-752-9695—FAX
• HIV counseling and testing, education and outreach to the African-American community. Safer sex discussions, workshops, and testing buddy program. Free.

Stop AIDS—Latino/a Program
1352 North Western Avenue
Chicago, IL 60622
773-235-2586
773-235-2662—FAX
• Offers HIV/AIDS education and outreach to the Latino community. Safer sex discussions and workshops. English/Spanish (Mexican, Puerto Rican). Free.

Books and Publications

The Good Vibrations Guide to Sex
Winks, Cathy and Anne Semans
Cleis Press, 1995
Mail order: Cleis Press, 412-937-1555
• Explicit resource with basic information and ideas for safer sexual relationships. Covers a wide range of topics in a positive way. Includes a good list of other safer sex books and resources.

The New Joy of Gay Sex
Silverstein, Charles, and Felice Picano
HarperCollins, 1992
Mail order: HarperCollins, 800-331-3761
• Explicit manual for gay men covers many safer sex and sexuality topics in an encyclopedia format.

The Lesbian Sex Book
Caster, Wendy
Alyson Publications, 1993
Mail order: Alyson Publications, 800-253-3605
• Clear and explicit safer sex resource, covering many lesbian sexuality topics in encyclopedia format.

The Complete Guide to Safe Sex
Book (1992) and Video (1988)
Mail order: Institute for the Advanced Study of Human Sexuality, 415-928-1133

Making It: A Woman's Guide to Sex in the Age of AIDS
Patton, C. and J. Kelly
Ithaca, NY: Firebrand Books, 1987
• Available in English and Spanish.

Safe Encounters: How Women Can Say Yes to Pleasure and No to Unsafe Sex
Whipple, Beverly and Gina Ogden
New York: McGraw-Hill, 1989

Safer Sexy: The Guide to Gay Sex Safely
Tatchell, Peter
London: Freedom Editions, 1994
Mail order: The Sexuality Library, 800-289-8423, or e-mail: goodvibe@well.com
Internet catalog: http://www.goodvibes.com

Videos

"The Gay Man's Guide to Safe Sex," and "Getting It Right: A Young Gay Man's Guide to Safe Sex"
Terrence Higgins Trust
Mail order: Focus International, 800-843-0305
e-mail: Sex_Help@focusint.com
Internet catalog: http://www.hip.com/focus
• Explicit British safer sex videos.

Using a Computer and Modem

Safer Sex Page
http://www.cmpharm.ucsf.edu~troyer/safesex.html
• Offers brochures, articles, and video and audio clips on safer sex. Information is geared to the needs of adults, teens, parents, and other groups. Maintained by an individual, this site also provides links to other sexuality-related sites on the Internet.

Gay Men's Health Crisis (GMHC) on the Web
http://www.gmhc.org/
• A good source of information on safer sex, living with AIDS or HIV, and more. Links to other sites.

My gynecologist called me at home and told me everything was all right with the pregnancy, so far, so good, but that one test came back problematic. I knew which one it was. It was pretty devastating. I mouthed "HIV" to my husband. He thought he gave it to me, but it turns out he's not positive.

I don't believe in abortion. I thought of it only because my physician told me to terminate the pregnancy—over the phone! He told me I should terminate the pregnancy because I would "succumb quicker"—those were his words. He said my T-cell count would drop by 20%. He failed to tell me that all women's counts do that during pregnancy, and then they come back up. I learned the real story at WITS.

My own personal advice is, never abort if you're HIV-positive and pregnant if you feel you could take care of the child. In my case I am so happy I didn't abort! It gives you a reason for living, a new lease on life. It's a joy.

EVIE

HIV in Newborns and Children

In almost all cases, a baby born to a woman who is HIV-positive will test positive for HIV antibodies at birth. However, the standard antibody test used for determining the presence of HIV in adults is meaningless in babies. Infants don't have a complete immune system, and while theirs is developing, nature lends them Mom's antibodies. Standard tests can't tell us whether the HIV antibodies present in an infant's blood were produced by mother or baby. Therefore, an antibody test cannot be used to determine the presence of HIV in babies until at least 15–18 months of age. By then, all the antibodies being produced are the infant's alone.

A laboratory test called Polymerase Chain Reaction (PCR) can be used much earlier than the antibody test to get a reading on an infant's HIV status. Ask your doctor or pediatrician about it. A culture is another way to test for the virus early on.

As time goes on, the mother's antibodies gradually disintegrate while the baby's immune system develops independently. If at 18 months of age a baby still has significant HIV antibodies in its blood, doctors can be fairly certain the baby has been infected by the virus. If the blood sample is free of HIV antibodies, they can safely assume the baby is not infected.

This process of a noninfected infant changing from HIV-positive to HIV-negative status is called "seroconversion." Researchers now believe that without intervention, about 3 out of 4 babies born to HIV-positive mothers will seroconvert to negative, turning out to be uninfected by the virus. There seems to be a higher rate of perinatal (birth-related) transmission of HIV in women who become infected during pregnancy, those whose viral load is high, and those whose disease is more advanced at the time they give birth. Researchers are studying what other factors may increase or decrease the chance that an HIV-positive woman will pass on HIV to her newborn.

Without intervention, at least 1 out of 4 infants will pick up their mother's infection, either in the womb, during childbirth, or through breast feeding. However, if a pregnant woman is taking AZT orally during the second and third trimesters of pregnancy, and intravenously while giving birth, and her newborn receives the drug for the first six weeks of life, the risk of the child being infected is reduced from 1 in 4 to 1 in 12. Ask your obstetrician about this and any other experimental studies underway that might be options. You can also contact:

CDC National AIDS Clearinghouse
800-458-5231—English/Spanish
800-243-7012—Hearing-impaired TTY/TDD
9 a.m.-7 p.m. Mon-Fri (Eastern time).
• Request the brochure, "Pregnancy and HIV: Is AZT the Right Choice for You and Your Baby?" Available in English, Spanish, and Haitian Creole.

There are clinical signs a doctor can observe in an infant which occur more commonly (though not exclusively) in HIV-infected children. These include:

- swollen glands or enlarged organs
- failure to thrive (difficulty gaining weight)
- frequent infections
- severe or chronic diarrhea
- thrush (a fungus) in the mouth or diaper area
- certain types of pneumonia
- neurological problems or slow development of motor skills (or loss of developmental milestones).

Along with a doctor's observation of symptoms, laboratory testing may be used to confirm a diagnosis of HIV or AIDS in an infant. A low T cell count, low platelet count, or anemia are some of the markers that are monitored.

Any one of these symptoms or markers by itself does not necessarily signal HIV infection. However, several of them occurring in extreme, chronic, or unexplainable form are often a reliable sign that the baby is HIV-infected or has AIDS (especially when the mother is known to be infected).

About 20% of HIV-infected infants don't live beyond the first four years of life. Life expectancy for those who make it that far looks a lot like that of adults, when aggressive measures are taken to prevent and treat infections. Many children born infected with HIV live until the age of nine or ten, and some are now teenagers.

Common childhood illnesses such as chicken pox or measles can be deadly for children with an immune system weakened by HIV. It's important to avoid these illnesses, and to receive notification when a child may have come in contact with infectious diseases in a child care or school setting, so that appropriate preventive medications can be prescribed. Since you can't always know what health conditions might be a problem for your child, be sure you feel comfortable enough with your health care provider to call with questions or concerns that may seem minor.

Immunizations should be administered to children with HIV as with all children. However, in immune-compromised children it is recommended to use vaccines with "killed" instead of live virus samples. An exception is the mumps/measles/rubella (MMR) immunization—a live virus vaccine that can be given to HIV-infected infants.

The majority of children with HIV face special neurological problems such as learning disabilities, speech disorders, developmental delays or loss of developmental milestones, and more. An HIV-infected child should be monitored by a trained specialist. Early interventions, including developmental, therapeutic, medical, and educational services, can make a marked difference in the child's functioning.

There are likely services near you that can provide early developmental intervention. Work with your child's health care provider, school district, case manager, or a social service agency to obtain interventions in a convenient setting.

Video

"Caring for Infants and Toddlers with HIV Infection" and "Caring for School Aged Children with HIV Infection"
Mail order: Child Welfare League of America, 800-407-6273
• Compassionate videos address rewards and fears of caring for children with HIV. Highlights many issues of daily living, medical care, day care and school.

(Note: For additional information and assistance, see the resource listings for women, children, teens, and caregivers in Part 1 of this book.)

Having Children

Women of childbearing age are the fastest-growing group of people with AIDS. Many of these women will have to decide whether having a baby is an option they want to pursue given their HIV status (or that of their partner).

Pregnancy is extremely stressful to any woman's immune system. Almost all women experience a significant, although temporary, drop in their T cells during pregnancy. If your T cells are already well below normal due to HIV infection, the further drop you undergo could make you vulnerable to life-threatening illness during or after pregnancy.

Maybe, like many other women, you learned you were HIV-positive when you found out you were pregnant. For some, this means learning that the man in their life or a child is also infected. You may be thinking you have to make an impossible decision, right when everything seems to be up in the air. If you've discovered in this way that you're HIV-positive, try not to make any quick decisions. You need to be as calm as possible before deciding about anything, and taking care of yourself is the first step.

The risks involved for both mother and baby must be weighed very carefully against the rewards of becoming a parent. Many women choose to terminate a pregnancy if they are HIV-infected. If you are deciding whether to continue or begin a pregnancy, you'll need to talk at length with your doctor about the clinical facts for you and your baby. Get a second or third opinion if you wish.

You'll have to ask yourself some difficult questions, too. Are you willing to go through the uncertainty about the infant's HIV status? Are you prepared to get the medical care you and your baby will need during pregnancy and afterward, and to deal with any addiction you may have? How well will you cope if the child turns out to be infected? Are you willing to gamble that you won't become ill yourself during pregnancy or after giving birth? How will your decision impact you and your family?

I found out I was HIV-positive when I found out I was pregnant. I was, like, 21 weeks along and on drugs. At the time, it didn't shock me—I thought, I don't really want to live anyway. I'm not having a good life. I thought about terminating the pregnancy, but at that point every dime went to drugs.

I went to an AIDS clinic. They told me there was a 15–25% chance my baby would have it. I figured when he was born they'd take him away, throw me in prison. But they gave me a chance.

I don't regret having Phillip. I stay clean because of him. He's my high—the best thing that ever happened to me.

The real shock came when we found out Phillip was infected, because he's so healthy. I try not to dwell on it, but sometimes bad thoughts come. I think way ahead, instead of one day at a time. Like, what happens if he goes to school and other kids are mean to him? He'll never be able to get married. When I get way ahead of myself like that, I get depressed and crazy. I have to be careful, because that would be a good excuse to go and get blasted.

CHRISTINE

Obviously, there is no one answer for all HIV-positive women who find themselves pregnant or wanting to be pregnant. *This decision is yours alone, and you must trust yourself to do what is best for you.* Take some time, and talk it over with someone you trust. Talk to as many people as you need to, to get all the information and emotional support you can to feel certain about your decision.

If you are not HIV-infected yourself but the man you are with is, you'll have additional things to think about. By trying to conceive with an HIV-positive man, you place yourself at serious risk of infection. At present, there are no natural or artificial procedures that make it safe for you to conceive. Researchers have experimented with a procedure known as "sperm washing," whereby efforts were made to remove the virus from the man's semen before artificially inseminating the woman. So far, this procedure hasn't worked—and at least one of the women in the study became HIV-infected as a result.

Artificial insemination from an uninfected male is one option. But keep in mind that a man's negative antibody test does not prove he hasn't become infected since the test was taken. Similarly, he could have become infected shortly *before* taking the test, but was not yet showing antibodies at the time blood was drawn. Only repeated HIV tests taken over a period of six to twelve months, while no risk behavior is taking place, can assure the potential sperm donor is uninfected.

As an alternative to bearing children yourself, you can also consider adoption. However, if you or your spouse reveal your positive HIV status, your application may be denied.

If you're determined to try and conceive a child despite your own or your partner's HIV infection, it's best to talk to a counselor before attempting to conceive. Try to understand why this is so important to you, and why you're willing to undertake such serious risks. While it's your right to become pregnant and have a baby by any means you choose, this is not a decision to be made lightly or impulsively. You may also want additional information about HIV-positive children. Contact one of the organizations listed in Part I of this book, under the sections "Resources for Women" and "Resources for Children."

If you've always counted on having kids, finding out you won't can be a tremendous blow. If you decide that having children is not an option, you may also find counseling to be of value.

If you do decide to become pregnant, or if you're pregnant now, one of the questions you'll want to ask yourself is whether to have a C-section. Whether there is any advantage to children born to HIV-positive women who choose a cesarean section over vaginal delivery is one of the hottest issues in OB/GYN care today. Proponents of C-sections over vaginal births say that the reduced amount of blood to which the newborn is exposed may cut back the risk of transmission from mother to baby.

Probably the greatest single loss I had right when I found out I was positive and for about a year afterward was the fact that I'd never be able to have children of my own, from me. I don't think about it as often now, because I've pretty much resigned myself to the facts.

ADAM

I have three children from two other women. My wife doesn't have any kids. So that comes up—how much she'd like to have a child with me, so in the event that I die, she'd have our child. We haven't really done too much with that, in terms of finding out how or if that's possible. Maybe I'm selfish, because I have kids already; but my thought was not to do anything to put her or a baby at risk. Even if it's 50/50, to me, that's too much. A lot of us with AIDS are always looking out to protect other people, rather than ourselves.

GEORGE

After being told at age nineteen that I had tested positive for HIV, and then told to keep silent, I was further told that there would be certain things I couldn't do anymore, including having children. But a week after my diagnosis I found out that I was already pregnant.

Against everyone's advice, I decided to go through with the pregnancy because I very much wanted to experience the miracle of giving birth. I took it as a sign that things were not always as they appeared. I had faith. By choosing to go through with the pregnancy, I was choosing life. I put the fate of my unborn child in God's hands.

SHARI

My personal feeling is, it's a woman's right to become pregnant. Professionally, however, I feel she has to get all the information she possibly can and weigh all the pros and cons. It's important to make an <u>informed</u> decision, not a blind or half-baked one.

DR. HARVEY WOLF
CLINICAL HEALTH PSYCHOLOGIST

To date, there is no strong indication that this is true, and surgical C-sections are more stressful to the mother than vaginal births. What may be advisable in vaginal deliveries is the use of an antiseptic douche during the birth process to reduce the amount of maternal secretions to which the infant is exposed. Talk with your health care provider to get more details about the issues involved in choosing the birth procedure.

(For additional information and assistance, see the resource listings for women and children in Part 1 of this book.)

Alcohol and Other Drug Use

Now that your immune system is under attack, it's a good idea to look at all the substances you're putting into your body—food, drink, chemicals, drugs and medications—and determine whether you want to keep putting them into your body. Tobacco, alcohol, caffeine, and other drugs can further damage or destabilize an already-weakened immune system. If you've made a commitment to practice safer sex, drugs and alcohol can interfere with that commitment.

Certain people and publications will suggest that the only course to take is to quit using mood-altering substances immediately and forever. You will hear that HIV-positive people should "rid their body of all toxins" or "avoid drugs and alcohol." The arguments often take on moral overtones.

Complete and instant sobriety may sound like a noble goal, but none of us is perfect and change is never easy. Trying to go "cold turkey" on everything all at once is a good way to set yourself up for failure. Instead, do the best you can each day, and recognize that recovery is not a magical event, but a lifelong process involving a lot of struggle and hard work.

Some of the literature takes a very hard-nosed approach, suggesting that any use is abuse and calls for treatment. However, the distinction between "use" and "abuse" can be made only by you, the individual. One way to make that distinction is to sit down and ask yourself a few basic questions: What is my relationship to the substance I am using? Is my use of this substance causing problems for me or others close to me? Is it affecting me physically, mentally, emotionally, or spiritually in ways I don't like? Is it detracting from my ability to function or get along with others? Do I feel as though I'm losing my sense of values or identity?

You can also pose these questions about yourself to an addictions counselor or another trusted person in your life and ask for that person's honest impressions. Listen without challenging, and accept this feedback as a starting point in your self-evaluation.

Be aware that denial is a key factor in alcohol and drug addiction. If you find yourself vigorously denying you have a problem, despite much evidence to the contrary, take that into account as you proceed.

If through this process you decide you do have a substance abuse problem and would like to make a change, you have several options. You can get individual counseling, join a support group or 12-step program, or enter a program at a specialized addiction treatment facility on an inpatient or outpatient basis. Ask your doctor or a local AIDS service organization for referrals.

The support group option is relatively inexpensive, readily available, and offers scheduled sessions that shouldn't disrupt your life too much. 12-step groups are always free to participants (though a small voluntary donation may be requested). Meetings may be organized to address a single issue (such as narcotics use) or multiple issues (such as HIV and drug/alcohol use). Meetings are held at a variety of day and evening times.

Access to formalized addiction treatment at a medical facility may depend on your ability to pay. If you are working, your employee assistance program and/or health insurance may provide for treatment. If you don't have insurance or other financial resources to cover it, your choices will be more limited. You may have to wait a long time to enter the program of your choice. In addition, checking into an addiction treatment facility can be difficult to manage with a family and/or job commitments. However, you may decide the potential benefits of such a program outweigh the expense and inconvenience.

If you have to wait for admission to an appropriate treatment facility and are nervous about the wait, talk to the admissions counselor about what steps you can take in the meantime. The counselor may suggest participating in a day program, attending 12-step meetings in your area, or speaking daily with a therapist to help you stick with your decision.

Sometimes, people who are already working a program of recovery will discover they're HIV infected—and wonder, "What's the use? Why should I bother to continue the struggle?"

Although everyone needs to find their own answer to that question, many point to their philosophy in recovery of living "one day at a time." They truly want what their recovery gives them *today*, finding that life is best lived and cherished in the present moment. A life potentially shortened by HIV has that many fewer days in which to experience all that recovery has to offer. To the extent that recovery is bringing something positive to your life, the biggest argument for continuing is HIV.

The bottom line is, don't give up on something you feel is working for you. If that "something" is recovery, fine. If it is continuing to use a particular substance that isn't causing you or anyone else in your life problems, that's your choice, too. Whichever path you take, remember that you're a unique and valuable person with the right to choose how you will live your life.

I think in terms of not much longer than today. Tomorrow, maybe next week. My plans don't go out that far. That's part of the 12-step program I do, live for today. When I look real far into the future it gets me scared. For one thing, I might not be here. It just really brings the focus off what I should be looking at—which is in the moment. Looking ahead or backward is always looking away from what's going on. You learn that in a 12-step program, in my case Narcotics Anonymous, and it's really true.

If I look into the future and say to myself, "I can never, ever get high again"—it's all over. I fail before I even start. That's where "one day at a time" comes in. It works; I think that's why I'm still here today.

GEORGE

One safety note: if you *are* planning to use injection drugs, you can protect yourself and others from HIV and other blood-borne diseases by following these guidelines:

- Always use sterile drug injection equipment.
- If you have to share, clean the syringe and needle by doing the following as soon as possible before and after use: flush with water, then fill with bleach straight from the bottle, shake or tap to the count of sixty. Repeat this procedure three times, then flush again with water.
- Discard used needles/syringes safely. Some cities have needle-exchange programs, where you confidentially receive an unused needle when you turn in used ones.

Syringe Exchange Programs

Many communities now have syringe exchange and other harm reduction programs for injection drug users. Call the Illinois or CDC National AIDS Hotline for confidential referrals to local programs.

CDC National AIDS Hotline

800-342-2437—English
800-344-7432—Spanish
800-243-7889—Hearing-impaired TTY/TDD
• 24-hour toll-free hotlines providing confidential information, referrals, and educational materials to all.

Illinois AIDS Hotline

800-243-2437—Hotline staffed 8 a.m.-11 p.m., 7 days/week
800-782-0423—Hearing-impaired TTY/TDD
• Referrals to HIV and general health and social services throughout Illinois. Up-to-date information on HIV transmission, HIV counseling and testing sites. Offers information, risk and harm reduction, and support resources. English/Spanish.

The Illinois programs listed below offer free needle and syringe exchange, sterile injection supplies, condoms, and other risk reduction materials. These agencies provide information about safer injecting, health education, and referrals to a wide range of services.

Chicago Recovery Alliance

PO Box 368069
Chicago, IL 60636
773-471-0999
773-471-1240—FAX
• Also provides HIV prevention information, literature, condoms, detox, and referrals for treatment of chemical dependency or HIV. Many sites throughout Chicago and suburban Cook County. Call for locations and times. English/Spanish.

When my dad died, I smoked four packs a day. Generally when I'm stressed, I smoke a lot more. Since HIV and AIDS, it's a very stressful situation, I just smoke more—what can I say? I smoke a lot, and that's it. Without a doubt, giving it up would be even <u>more</u> stressful.

You'll read a lot of conflicting stuff. For instance, I've read everything in the world from smoking pot is good for you, to smoking pot reduces your T cells. You have to make those decisions yourself. The doctor can recommend and say all sorts of things, but you have to decide if you're going to do them.

ADAM

When I found out about my HIV, I really didn't deal with it. It was like, "Yeah, okay, what's next? Why does everything gotta happen to <u>me</u>?" I finally developed some self-esteem around the table, in recovery. I have a lot of people who are real close to me now.

A lot of good things have happened to me since I've been in recovery. That's not just me—that's my higher power. I take it one day at a time with HIV, just like in my recovery.

KAREN

Chicago Health Outreach
1015 West Lawrence
Chicago, IL 60640
773-275-2060
773-275-3689—FAX
• Various sites in Chicago; call for locations and times. English/Spanish.

Harm Reduction Outreach
623 7th Street
Rockford, IL 61104
815-961-1269
• Six sites in Rockford; call for locations and times.

Be aware that if you are using nonprescribed illegal drugs for medicinal purposes (such as smoking marijuana to ease pain or stimulate appetite), you are breaking the law. Although there have been cases where the courts have allowed such usage to be a defense to possession charges, and some police may look the other way, there is no legal requirement for them to do so. Keep this risk in mind when deciding whether to use illegal substances. For more information, contact:

National Organization for the Reform of Marijuana Laws
1001 Connecticut Avenue NW, Suite 1010-C
Washington, DC 20036
202-483-5500
202-483-0057—FAX
http://www.natlnorml.org/

> I found out I should have done this and that with the bleach and the needles after it was already too late and I had AIDS. Even if I <u>had</u> known to do it, I don't know that I would have. At different times when I was using, I'd be so into the feeling of getting high or needing a fix, I wouldn't care where the needles came from. If I was in a room with a couple of other fellows, as it got passed around, I would just use it. Of course, I knew not to share needles twenty years ago because you can get other things blood-to-blood. I caught hepatitis and syphilis sharing needles. Today, knowing what I know—I believe I'd think twice.
>
> GEORGE

After one of my fairly serious suicide attempts, I was sort of lying there and somebody asked me if this was really how I wanted to be remembered. I kind of went back and thought about all of the things I'd been told throughout the years that I was never going to do: "You're never going to get a good job, because you don't go to school." "You're not a good parent, not a good wife." All of that stuff about me being sort of a derelict…a "less-than-the-rest-of-society" kind of person.

I finally reached a point that I knew in recovery I had some sense of dignity and some sense of…that somehow, I fit in somewhere. Not that I fit in all the time—I still don't. I don't deal with the AIDS factor very well; I try to avoid it at all costs sometimes. But the longer that I try to deal with recovery and have that self-respect and dignity, the easier it is to see why I need to take care of myself and be involved with people.

I think that learning to live with AIDS is a lot like going through the recovery process. It's identifying and accepting and asking for help, and then accepting the help. I feel if I didn't work on my recovery, then I certainly wouldn't be working on wanting to live or feel better.

Compared to a year ago, there have been so many more high points and senses of connection and purpose in my life. There are struggles, but I've never been totally able to just say—forget it. And that is what has been different: that internal survival skill is so much bigger than it used to be.

SANDI

There are some things we know, medically. We know that alcohol, heroin, cocaine, and other drugs do have negative effects on the immune system. This is one of the things that is black and white. Alcohol, heroin, cocaine, and marijuana kill off T cells, and cocaine helps the virus to proceed at a faster rate. How does a person use a line of cocaine and not cause harm to their health? They don't.

THOMAS
DUNNING, CADC
ALCOHOL AND DRUG HIV
PREVENTION SPECIALIST,
STOP AIDS

Finding Chemical Dependency Treatment and Support

National Drug and Alcohol Treatment Referral Routing Service
U.S. Department of Health and Human Services
800-662-HELP (662-4357)—24-hour Hotline
• Confidential referrals to local substance abuse treatment and recovery programs anywhere in the U.S. Free.

Illinois Referrals

Illinois Alcoholism & Drug Dependence Association
937 South Second Street
Springfield, IL 62704
800-252-6301—8 a.m.-5 p.m. Mon-Fri
• Confidential referrals to substance abuse treatment and recovery programs, including 12-step programs, in Illinois. Free.

Interventions Central Intake
140 North Ashland Avenue, First Floor
Chicago, IL 60607
312-850-9411
• Information and referrals for substance abuse and treatment programs. Physical exams assess overall health plus drug screening, urine tests, and detox evaluations. No eligibility requirements. Free. English/Spanish.

Illinois Treatment and Recovery Programs

Listed below is a sampling of chemical dependency treatment and recovery programs located in Illinois. Many HIV service agencies have support groups and other services for substance users and people in recovery. Check the listings under "Support Groups and Mental Health Services" (located above), and "Local Hospitals and HIV Clinics" (in Part 3 of this book).

Alcoholism and Drug Dependence Program (ADD)
Lutheran Social Services—Central Intake
4840 West Byron
Chicago, IL 60641
773-282-7693
773-282-3916—FAX
• Eight sites in the Chicago metro area and one in McHenry County. Refers to ADD substance abuse treatment programs, including inpatient, outpatient, halfway house/residential aftercare, detox facility, and counseling services. For those with alcohol or other drug abuse/dependency problems, and their families. Men's and women's residential services. Sliding scale fees. Public Aid accepted. English/Spanish.

Alcoholics Anonymous AIDS Awareness of New Town Alano Club
4407 North Clark Street
Chicago, IL 60613
773-271-6822
• AA and other 12-step meetings specific to gay and lesbian recovering alcoholics and addicts. Several AIDS-related groups for recovering people.

Association House of Chicago
2150 West North Avenue
Chicago, IL 60647
773-276-0084
773-276-7395—FAX
• Residential and addiction recovery programs for the economically, mentally, and/or physically disabled. English/Spanish.

Branden House
800 Bramble
Manteno, IL 60950
800-244-0996
815-468-6558—FAX
• Inpatient treatment for chemical dependency. Sliding scale fees.

Brass Foundation
8000 South Racine
Chicago, IL 60620
773-994-2708
773-994-6024—FAX
• Substance abuse treatment and rehabilitative services for adolescents and adults. Methadone maintenance. HIV counseling and testing. Public Aid accepted. Sliding scale fees.

Bridge House
3016 Grand Avenue
Waukegan, IL 60085
847-662-4124
847-662-4227—FAX
• Halfway house for chemically dependent adults. Sliding scale fees. English/Spanish.

Center for Addictive Problems
609 North Wells
Chicago, IL 60610
312-266-0404
312-266-8169—FAX
• Individual and group counseling. Methadone maintenance, on-site 12-step meeting. Physician on site daily. HIV support and referral for clinic members. Set fee includes all services. English/ Spanish.

Clean Start—Illinois Masonic Center for Addiction Medicine
919 West Wellington Avenue
Chicago, IL 60657
773-477-2000
773-477-2002—FAX
• Multilevel chemical dependency treatment center sensitive to gay/lesbian issues. Detox and outpatient intensive programs. Private insurance and Medicare Accepted. English/Spanish.

Cook County HIV Primary Care Center
1835 West Harrison Street
CCSN 1268
Chicago, IL 60612
312-633-3005
312-633-3002—FAX
• Provides medical care and substance abuse treatment. Support groups for HIV-positive people in recovery. Free. English/Spanish.

Cook County Hospital Women and Children's HIV Program
1835 West Harrison Street
CCSN 1200
Chicago, IL 60612
312-633-5080
312-633-4902—FAX
• Provides inpatient and outpatient care for HIV-positive adults and children, including chemical dependency counseling. On-site child care available. English/Spanish.

Duane Dean Recovery Project
700 East Court Street
Kankakee, IL 60901
815-939-0125
815-939-1249—FAX
• Outpatient substance abuse treatment services and recovery support.

El Rincon Community Clinic
1874 North Milwaukee Avenue
Chicago, IL 60647
773-276-0200
773-276-4226—FAX
• Methadone treatment for heroin addiction. Public Aid accepted. English/Spanish.

Family Guidance Center
737 North LaSalle, Suite 300
Chicago, IL 60610
312-943-6545
312-943-9431—FAX
• Outpatient methadone treatment for men and women age 23 and older. Methadone and drug-free programs for pregnant women. Special programs for pregnant and breast-feeding women. HIV counseling and testing. Sliding scale fees. Public Aid accepted. English/Spanish.

Garfield Counseling Center
4132 West Madison
Chicago, IL 60624
773-533-0433
773-533-6288—FAX
• Residential treatment and rehabilitation for chemically dependent injection drug users. HIV case management, counseling and testing. English/Spanish.

Gateway Foundation—Northwest
2855 North Sheffield Avenue
Chicago, IL 60657
773-862-2279
773-929-5780—FAX
• Individual counseling and intensive 10-week program for those with HIV/AIDS who have a history of substance abuse. Public Aid accepted. English/Spanish.

Gateway Foundation—South
2615 West 63rd Street
Chicago, IL 60629
773-476-0622
773-476-0859—FAX
• Women's group, outpatient substance abuse treatment, and basic aftercare. Accepts pregnant women. Public Aid accepted.

Harbor Light Alcoholism and Drug Dependence Service
1515 West Monroe Street
Chicago, IL 60607
312-733-0500
312-421-6930—FAX
• Psychiatric outpatient treatment center for drug and alcohol abusers. Medical clinic includes an intensive rehabilitation unit offering 30-day treatment for male alcoholics, as well as legal, dental, and information referral services. Halfway house and adult residential services available. Sliding scale fees. English/Spanish.

Haymarket House
108-120 North Sangamon
Chicago, IL 60607
312-226-7984
312-226-0638—FAX
• Provides substance abuse detox, case management, residential and outpatient services for men and

women, prenatal/postnatal counseling, education, and HIV test counseling. English/Spanish.

Healthcare Alternative Systems—North
2755 West Armitage Avenue
Chicago, IL 60647
773-252-3100
773-252-8945—FAX
• Intensive outpatient chemical dependency treatment and aftercare services. HIV/AIDS case management in English or Spanish, and HIV counseling and testing for chemical dependency clients. Chemical dependency support groups. Sliding scale fees. Public Aid accepted.

Healthcare Alternative Systems—Residential Programs
Offices at:
1949 North Humboldt
Chicago, IL 60647
773-252-2666

4534 South Western Avenue
Chicago, IL 60609
773-254-5141
773-254-5753—FAX
• Residential chemical dependency treatment programs for Spanish-speaking men. HIV counseling and testing. Sliding scale fees. Public Aid accepted. English/Spanish.

Howard Brown Health Center
945 West George Street
Chicago, IL 60657
773-871-5777
773-871-5843—FAX
• Alcohol/drug abuse counseling and support for current users and people in recovery. "AIM Project" offers group programs for gay and bisexual men about substance use and safer sex. English/Spanish.

Illinois Department of Alcoholism and Substance Abuse (DASA)
100 West Randolph Street, Suite 5-600
Chicago, IL 60601
312-814-3840
312-814-2419—FAX
312-419-8432—Hearing-impaired TDD/TTY
• Coordination of alcohol and other drug treatment services. Offers grants to community-based and statewide service agencies in the areas of treatment, prevention, and HIV/AIDS in women. Sliding scale fees. Public Aid accepted.

Interventions
140 North Ashland Avenue
Chicago, IL 60607
312-633-4990
312-663-9059—FAX
• Substance abuse assessment and treatment, outpatient and residential detox, HIV counseling and testing, and case management. Free.

Interventions
26991 Anderson Road
Wauconda, IL 60084
847-526-0404
847-526-0472—FAX
• Residential rehabilitation for adolescent females.

Interventions Crossroads
3401 West 111th Street
Chicago, IL 60655
773-239-1400
773-239-8131—FAX
• Outpatient substance abuse treatment services for adolescents and adults. Sliding scale fees. Public Aid accepted.

Lake County Alcoholism Treatment Center
2400 Belvidere Road
Waukegan, IL 60085
847-360-6540
847-360-3696—FAX
• Outpatient detox and short-term rehabilitation services for the chemically dependent. Transportation and child care for those in outpatient women specific programs.

Lutheran General Hospital Addiction Treatment Program
1700 Luther Lane
Park Ridge, IL 60068
847-696-6050
847-698-4068—FAX
• Offers a full range of addiction treatment, including detox, partial hospital, day and night intensive outpatient, and continuing care.

Near North Health Service Corporation
1276 North Clybourn
Chicago, IL 60610
312-337-1073
312-337-7616—FAX
• Outpatient substance abuse treatment services, primary care, and HIV counseling and testing. Programs for African-Americans, Latinos/as, gays and lesbians, and injection drug users. English/Spanish.

Northern Illinois Council on Alcohol and Substance Abuse (NICASA)—Women and Children's Center
2031 Dugdale
North Chicago, IL 60064
847-785-8660
847-785-8665—FAX
• Intensive outpatient substance abuse treatment services for children and women age 18 years

and older. Day care, transportation, residential halfway house. Four sites. Sliding scale fees. Public Aid accepted. English/Spanish.

Omni, Incorporated Initiative
4004 West Division
Chicago, IL 60651
773-278-6106
773-486-7773—FAX
• Substance abuse and housing programs for persons with HIV/AIDS. Referrals to other services.

Peer Services, Inc.
906 Davis Street
Evanston, IL 60201
847-492-1778
847-492-0320—FAX
• Outpatient counseling for substance abuse, including methadone when indicated. HIV education, outreach, and support groups available. Sliding scale fees for substance abuse treatment, no charge for HIV services. English/Spanish.

Renz Addiction Center
76 Fountain Square Plaza
Elgin, IL 60120
847-742-3545
847-742-3559—FAX
• Drug and alcohol abuse treatment and prevention programs. English/Spanish.

St. Catherine's of Genoa Catholic Worker
842 East 65th Street
Chicago, IL 60637
773-288-3688
• Transitional residence for homeless HIV-positive men and women. All residents are required to have a case manager and/or be in a substance abuse program. Length of stay is assessed monthly. Also provides hospice housing. Free.

Serenity House
891 South Route 53
Addison, IL 60101
630-620-6616
630-620-7924—FAX
• Men's and women's halfway house offering intensive outpatient care and family and parenting counseling. HIV counseling and testing. Sliding scale fees.

Share Program
1776 Moon Lake Boulevard
Hoffman Estates, IL 60194
847-882-4181
847-882-4299—FAX
• Outpatient and inpatient treatment for alcohol and chemical abuse, detox, and rehabilitation. HIV counseling and testing with DuPage County Health Department. Sliding scale fees. English/Spanish.

South Suburban Council on Alcoholism and Substance Abuse
1909 Cheker Square
East Hazel Crest, IL 60429
708-957-2854
708-957-2895—FAX
708-957-3106—Hearing-impaired TTY/TDD
• Inpatient detox programs for men and women. Residential rehabilitation, youth and adult outpatient services, anonymous and confidential HIV counseling and testing, and case management. Sliding scale fees.

Travelers & Immigrants Aid—Rafael Center
4750 North Sheridan Road, Suite 200
Chicago, IL 60640
773-989-0049
773-989-1935—FAX
• Substance abuse programs, including residential recovery house and support groups for current substance users and recovering persons. Comprehensive HIV/AIDS services including case management, mental health, support groups, and residential housing for people with HIV/AIDS. Free. English/Spanish.

The Way Back Inn
104 Oak Street
Maywood, IL 60153
708-345-8422
708-345-6978—FAX
• Transitional living facility for adult males recovering from alcohol and substance abuse, and for those diagnosed with mental illness and substance abuse. Sliding scale fees.

UIC Community Outreach Intervention Project
Offices at:
4650 South Martin Luther King Drive
Chicago, IL 60653
773-536-4509
773-536-2306—FAX

4407 North Broadway Avenue
Chicago, IL 60640
773-561-3177
773-561-8813—FAX

5218 West Division Street
Chicago, IL 60651
773-379-1137
773-379-1424—FAX

1612 North Kedzie Avenue
Chicago, IL 60647
773-252-4422
773-252-1153—FAX
• The UIC Community Outreach Intervention Project offers HIV/AIDS and substance abuse referrals, HIV prevention and education, HIV counseling

and testing for substance users and their partners, case management, and peer support. Call for services at each site. English/Spanish.

**Veterans Administration Medical Center—
North Chicago**
3001 Green Bay Road
North Chicago, IL 60064
847-688-1900
847-578-3863—FAX
• Range of services for eligible veterans including substance abuse treatment.

**Veterans Affairs Department—
Edward Hines V.A. Hospital**
5th Avenue at Roosevelt Road
Hines, IL 60141
708-343-7200
708-216-2410—FAX
• Range of services for eligible veterans including substance abuse treatment.

**Western Clinical
Health Services**
326 North Michigan Avenue
Chicago, IL 60601
312-251-5020
312-251-0628—FAX
• Outpatient methadone treatment and case management.

**Woodlawn Organization
Substance Abuse Services**
1447 East 65th Street
Chicago, IL 60637
773-493-6116
773-288-5871—FAX
• Inpatient substance abuse treatment for adult, African-American males who are HIV-positive or at high risk. Length of stay is 30 days. Case management, AA/NA meetings, non-medical detox for adults (5-day stay). Intensive outpatient services available. Free.

Video

"AIDS and Addiction"
Mail order: Newist,
800-633-7445
• This 3-part video chronicles the difficult decisions faced by HIV-positive people who reached out for recovery from addiction.

HIV and Homelessness

If you're on the street or staying in a shelter or warming center, you are probably under a lot of stress. You may be focused on your daily survival, have trouble eating well or taking care of yourself. You may find yourself among other people who are also run down and in poor health. You may be using illegal drugs or selling your body to get by. These factors can put you at risk for developing full-blown AIDS earlier than you might otherwise.

If you are HIV-positive, no matter what else is going on in your life, do yourself a favor by making your health a top priority. With good care you can feel a lot better, and be better equipped to control the damage HIV does to your body.

To start with, try to have tuberculosis (TB) and other health screenings on a regular basis. Work with your doctor to control any problems. If you're given medication for TB or some other condition, take it exactly as your doctor prescribes, even when you feel better. If you don't finish all your medicine, the disease may quiet down for a while only to come back again, resistant to treatment.

If you shoot IV drugs, use only clean needles, and consider seeking treatment to help you stop using. Practice safer sex, and contact a social service organization about obtaining regular meals, vitamin supplements, and emotional support.

For many people, learning they're HIV-positive enables them to make changes they've long wanted to make. For some, this could mean finding a permanent place to live. If this is true in your case, remember that other people have gone through what you are going through. Your life is not over; don't give up! You deserve to have a safe place to call home, and there are people and agencies who can help you find it.

If you don't have a working relationship with a case manager or social worker, now's a good time to develop one. Some agencies that provide HIV case management have special programs to assist homeless people and families. Call one of the agencies listed under "Housing Assistance" or "Case Management and Related HIV/AIDS Services," both located in Part 5 of this book. Or contact:

Department of Health and Human Services
800-654-8595
312-744-5000
312-744-3996—Hearing-impaired TTY/TDD
• 24-hour emergency service refers to city-sponsored homeless shelters, domestic violence shelters, and other emergency services in Chicago. Assists with transportation to shelters, if needed. Intake and referrals during normal business hours at local community service offices. Call for locations. Free. English/Spanish.

In any community, you can always go to the local police department or hospital emergency room. They will let you stay inside while they help you locate emergency shelters.

HIV in Prison

Being incarcerated means you've forfeited certain freedoms, but it does not mean you've lost your basic human rights. You have a right to educate yourself about HIV and other health concerns, and to receive appropriate medical care. You have a right to fair and humane treatment by employees of the correctional facility. You have the right to receive protection from abuse by your fellow inmates. You have a right to keep your health information private. HIV is not spread through casual contact; therefore, as long as you don't present a health risk to others (by having an active case of TB, for example), you should have equal access to institutional programs, job training opportunities, the library, visiting room, and recreation facilities.

Although authorities don't like to admit it, there is sexual activity and drug use in jails and prisons. This can put non-infected inmates at risk for contracting HIV. In Illinois alone, more than 100 incarcerated individuals become HIV-positive each year. This life-threatening problem is being addressed by prison advocacy groups. No matter what crime a person has committed, no one deserves to become HIV-infected. If you are HIV-positive when you enter prison, be aware that unsafe behavior on your part can expose others to HIV. It also can expose you to new strains of the virus that can make your own illness worse.

You can help protect yourself and others by abstaining from sex and needle sharing, or by practicing safer sex and refusing to share drug paraphernalia unless it's been disinfected. (See the earlier section on "Alcohol and Other Drug Use" for details.) You may be able to get condoms through the clinic at your facility or from HIV prevention groups that visit or mail packages. Many prisons have formal policies banning sexual or drug-related activity, but will allow condoms, dental dams, or bleach kits to be passively distributed at neutral sites within prison walls.

If condoms aren't available or if you're tempted to have sex without them, keep in mind that you're jeopardizing your own health by doing so. Potential partners who claim to be HIV-negative could be lying, in denial, or unaware of their own infection. Repeated re-infections of HIV and other sexually transmitted diseases can lead to rapid progression of your disease.

If you feel that rape is a real possibility, ask to be placed in protective custody until the threat is diminished. Contact your attorney, the ACLU, or other prison advocacy groups if you're abused, discriminated against, or mistreated. If you've been assaulted, speak immediately (within a few hours) with your doctor about medications that may reduce the risk of HIV transmission.

You can help prevent the spread of HIV in prison and create a better environment for those who are already HIV-positive by encouraging people to become educated about the disease. Campaign to have speakers, training sessions, literature, and prevention materials brought to your facility. Encourage the prison librarian to carry relevant books and to schedule discussions on HIV, chemical dependency, sexuality, and health. (Note: Many of the HIV treatment newsletters listed in this book will be mailed free to incarcerated persons.) Speak with the clinic supervisor about how prevention activities can be increased, and write to HIV advocacy organizations for more ideas. Encourage strong treatment programs at your facility, and support those inmates who make use of them.

No matter how you feel right now or how anyone else would like you to feel, remember: you are not alone! You're a valuable human being who deserves care and good health. Even if you've done things that you regret, you can make a new start. Reach out to a counselor or HIV specialist for help and support. Try to view your diagnosis as a wake-up call—a reminder that each and every day of your life is precious.

(Note: If you haven't yet read Part 2 of this book, you might want to turn to the essay, "Positively Positive." In it, author Edward Rothas talks of his experiences living with HIV in prison.)

Prisoner Resources

Following is a list of resources that inmates can use to empower themselves in the area of HIV/AIDS. (Please be aware that the agencies and organizations listed do not accept collect calls unless otherwise noted.)

All Care, Inc.
961 Clark Street, Suite 304
Denver, CO 80218
• A national organization that provides educational materials and information for prisoners and correctional facility staff. Write for free resources directory.

American Civil Liberties Union (ACLU)—National Prison Project (NPP)
1875 Connecticut Avenue NW, Suite 410
Washington, DC 20009
202-234-4830
e-mail: infoaclu@aclu.org
Web site: http://www.aclu.org/index.html
• The ACLU's National Prison Project is dedicated to the preservation of the civil liberties guaranteed citizens by the Constitution. Within NPP, the "AIDS in Prison Project" serves as a resource center for educational and advocacy assistance surrounding HIV/AIDS in correctional facilities. The project maintains a collection of articles, including studies done on inmates with HIV/AIDS, statistics, problems within correctional facilities, and policies. The project assists HIV/AIDS correctional support groups and peer education programs, and maintains a list of referrals for inmates, their families and friends, and HIV/AIDS service organizations.

National Women's Law Center
11 DuPont Circle NW
Washington, DC 20036
202-588-5180
Web site: http://essential.org/afi/nwlc.html
• Provides a networking point for women and attorneys to work on legal matters concerning women, such as spousal abuse, obstetrical rights, discrimination, child abuse, and the rights of incarcerated women, including AIDS-related issues.

Osborne Association—AIDS in Prison Project
135 East 15th Street
New York, NY 10003
212-673-6633
• Information for prisoner activists and others on how to start an HIV support group in prison, how to obtain adequate medical treatment for detainees held in a county jail, and how to serve HIV-positive prisoners in community-based organizations. Conducts research and recommends policy regarding HIV-positive inmates and persons on parole. The project has established an AIDS/HIV clearinghouse and a bilingual hotline for inmates and former inmates. Staff and peer counselors provide inmates and former inmates, their advocates, family members, and friends with information on HIV prevention and treatment, TB prevention and treatment, discharge planning, inmate support groups, and medical parole.

Osborne Association—AIDS in Prison Project Internet Resource
http://www.aidsnyc.org/aip/links.html
• Lists Internet resources and national organizations that provide information, advocacy, and support for and about prisoners with HIV. Links to other sites.

Prison Activist Resource Center (PARC)
PO Box 3201
Berkeley, CA 94703
510-845-8813
e-mail: PARCER@igc.org
• PARC is a volunteer-run project that serves as an information clearinghouse on such areas as control units, women in correctional facilities, and activist and legal work publications in the United States and Canada, statistics, correctional facilities conditions, and AIDS. The project uses publishing and communications resources to sustain existing activist projects and get new ones off the ground. Demonstrations, action alerts, educational presentations, campaigns, and statistical research are among the resources used. News and information on crime and correctional facilities is available through Peace Net's Prison Issues Desk; queries can be made to the desk via e-mail. PARC provides Internet newsgroups and a listserv for the discussion of correctional issues. Electronic delivery of documents can be requested.

Prisoners with AIDS Rights Advocacy Group
PO Box 2161
Jonesboro, GA 30227
770-946-9346
• Provides advocacy and legal referrals for all 50 states, Canada, and Puerto Rico. Publishes quarterly newsletter, "PWA Rag."

Books and Publications

"Alive and Kicking!"
425 South Broad Street
Philadelphia, PA 19147
215-546-2120
• This newsletter details current news about the AIDS pandemic, often approaching issues from an advocate's point of view. Regular features include memorials, personal stories by PWAs, columns relating to incarcerated persons' and women's issues, letters to the editor, news briefs, and a calendar of events.

Be Good to Yourself: A Resource Guide for Inmates Living with HIV
Published by AIDS Project Los Angeles
1313 North Vine Street
Los Angeles, CA 90028
213-993-1600
• Manual providing self-help guidelines for incarcerated persons who are HIV-positive. Focuses on techniques they can use in everyday situations to maintain their health, despite having little control over their own care and mental, physical, and emotional well-being. (Note: A photocopy of this material is available from the CDC National AIDS Clearinghouse Document Delivery Service. Write PO Box 6003, Rockville, MD 20849, or call toll-free, 800-458-5231. Price: $7.15.)

"CorrectCare"
2105 North Southport, Suite 200
Chicago, IL 60614
312-528-0818
• Newspaper discussing issues related to health care delivery in correctional facilities. Also covers news of the publishing organization, including guidelines and position statements. Provides a conference calendar and list of job opportunities.

"The Keepers' Voice"
1333 South Wabash
PO Box 53
Chicago, IL 60605
312-996-5401
• Journal focusing on health issues and education/prevention programs within correctional facilities, both national and international.

"The Kite"
1525 Santa Barbara Street
Santa Barbara, CA 93101
805-899-3820
http://www.silcom.com/~chc
• Covers topics pertinent to the rights of incarcerated persons with HIV/AIDS and their families.

"The National Prison Project Journal"
1875 Connecticut Avenue NW, Suite 410
Washington, DC 20009
(202) 234-4830
• Features articles on the rights of incarcerated persons in correctional facilities. Health issues, legislation affecting incarcerated persons, and legal briefs of important cases are discussed extensively.

"Progress Notes"
1525 Santa Barbara Street
Santa Barbara, CA 93101
805-899-3820
http://www.silcom.com/~chc
• Contains information pertaining to the education and medical treatment of incarcerated persons.

"PWA Newsline"
50 West 17th Street, Suite 316
New York, NY 10011
212-647-1415
• This magazine looks at a variety of issues affecting PWAs. It studies advances in treatment as well as holistic therapies and touches on advocacy for minorities, inmates, and gays and lesbians, including safer sex. Also includes letters to the editor, memorials, and a directory of services.

Resource listings adapted with permission from the March/April, 1997 issue of "Positively Aware," the newsletter of Test Positive Aware Network. For more information, call 773-404-8726.)

Hygiene

The rules of good hygiene apply equally to people living with or without the virus. Remember that HIV and AIDS are not spread through casual contact. There are no reported cases of the virus or disease being transmitted via touching, hugging, shaking hands, or kissing; sharing clothing, dishes, silverware, or living quarters; on surfaces at home, work, or elsewhere; or through the air, food, or an insect bite.

There are two key reasons for you to be concerned about cleanliness (besides aesthetics). The first is to avoid contact with bacteria or other organisms that can cause you to become ill. The second is to avoid transmitting the virus to others.

To avoid being infected by disease-causing organisms:
- follow safer sex and drug injection guidelines (see the "Sex" and "Alcohol and Other Drug Use" sections earlier in Part 4).
- watch what you eat (see "Food Safety").
- wash your hands before eating or smoking.
- wash your hands after using the toilet, touching your own or others' blood or body fluids, changing diapers, or handling raw food.
- wear gloves when gardening indoors or out or cleaning up after people or pets.
- don't walk outdoors barefoot.
- throw away old, stale food and disinfect the inside of your refrigerator regularly to control mold.
- stay away from people with measles, shingles, or TB. However, there's very little risk of getting sick by going out in public or being in a crowd.
- be very cautious when traveling, especially to underdeveloped countries, wilderness areas, campsites, or caves. Drink only bottled water and be careful of what you eat. Consult your doctor before committing to travel in countries where vaccinations are required.

To avoid transmitting HIV to others:
- follow safer sex and drug injection guidelines.
- do not donate blood, plasma, sperm, tissue, or organs.
- don't share any sharp implements such as razors, tweezers, tattooing or ear piercing equipment, or needles that could come into contact with blood or other body fluids. The National Hemophilia Foundation also suggests avoiding needle stick injuries by never recapping, bending, or breaking needles after use. Dispose of them by putting them into puncture-proof containers (hard plastic or metal), especially if children are around.
- don't share toothbrushes, toothpicks, water picks, or dental floss.
- clean up any spills of your own or other people's blood, vomit, urine, feces, or other body fluids with antibacterial soap and water. Then disinfect with a weak bleach/water solution. Use one cup of bleach to nine cups of water; mix fresh before using and throw away at the end of the day.

- add a cup of bleach to the wash water when laundering clothes or linens soiled with blood, semen, or other body fluids. (It is not necessary to use bleach in all of your laundry.)
- Many health care professionals feel that no special care need be taken in diapering HIV-infected infants where no blood is present. In day-care settings, or where blood or a rash are present or there is some other reason for concern, use the same universal precautions recommended for anyone handling body fluids: keep a barrier such as a glove or cloth between yourself and body fluids, and wash your hands after contact.

At home, I wouldn't want the kids to use each other's toothbrushes because your gums could be sensitive and there could be some bleeding, and we have kids in the family who are not infected. I never worry about them doing things together, though, or using the same utensils. We do the laundry the same for everybody.

I have all these boxes of gloves and I use them mostly for cleaning up after the dogs. I've only needed to use gloves around the kids maybe three or four times in the past seven years. There was only one incident that was a bloody accident. I would use the gloves for doing my daughter's central line care, because that was a sterile procedure. But for anything else, not really.

TERRY RUCKER
Foster Parent

Pets

Who will stick with you through your hardest days, help you fight both stress and discrimination, keep you alert and connected with the world, refuse to let you lose your sense of humor, and help you out of even the darkest of moods? Pets animate your home like friendly spirits, giving unconditional support and love.

Studies of ill pet owners have shown that spending time with animals can bring measurable health benefits and positively affect survival. For people with AIDS who sometimes find themselves fighting social isolation as well as physical illness, the affection of a pet can be especially meaningful.

Yet many people with HIV have been counseled to give up their pets because animals can carry disease-causing organisms that are dangerous to those with a weakened immune system. You don't have to give up your pet, but you do have to be more careful around animals now. (For the record, you cannot give HIV to your pets.)

The following advice from the organization Pets Are Wonderful Support (PAWS) will help you care for and enjoy your animal companions in the safest possible manner.

About Cats

1) *Toxoplasmosis.* Cats can carry toxoplasmosis and transmit it to people through their feces. Many people are infected with this organism and never know it, because a healthy immune system renders it harmless. Most HIV patients who develop toxoplasmosis are actually experiencing a "reactivation" of something they already had, but which didn't make them sick until their immune system deteriorated. Thus, removing cats from "at risk" households will have little effect on the number of new cases seen with HIV disease.

It's still important to prevent the cat from becoming infected by following safe pet guidelines. Cats can be screened for toxoplasmosis by a veterinarian.

2) *Feline Leukemia Virus (FeLV) and Feline Immunodeficiency Virus (FIV).* Both these viruses are contagious among cats, but neither has been shown to infect humans. However, these diseases suppress the cat's immune system, making it more susceptible to other conditions that it could pass on to you.

3) *Cat Scratch Disease.* This disease has been reported in people with AIDS. It appears to be most commonly acquired from kittens; thus, declawing an older cat will be unlikely to lower the risk. Still very uncommon in people with AIDS, cat scratch disease is treatable. Keep your cat's nails trimmed, monthly. If you get scratched, clean the wound with a tamed iodine solution such as Betadine™, and call your physician for further advice. Do not let your cat lick any wounds you may have.

About Fish

Be cautious around aquarium water to avoid acquiring unusual infections. Be especially careful if you have cuts or sores on your hands.

About Dogs

Dogs carry some diseases that could be spread to you. The risk is probably greater if they drink out of the toilet.

About Birds

Birds carry some diseases that can be transmitted to people, but they're considered safe pets, especially if you are careful. All new birds should be checked by an avian veterinarian. Mycobacterium Avian Complex (MAC) is a disease seen in people with AIDS, but is not typically transmitted to people directly from a bird. The infection is found everywhere in the environment, and as the immune system deteriorates, one becomes prone to this infection.

For crying out loud, people, do not all of a sudden abandon your cherished, loved pets! I've heard, "Oh my God, I've got to get rid of my cat/dog/bird!" That's hogwash, and if you're a pet person, the thought can be very traumatic. Just be careful, that's all. My three cats have been a wonderful source of comfort and support. It would take a hell of a lot to make me give them up.

JIM

I feel sorry for all the people, who early on in the days of AIDS, were scared into getting rid of their pets. Pets are very, very important. Animals can be your best friends, especially for kids who find it difficult to express themselves sometimes. I would never take a pet away from anybody. The rule in our house is, nobody touches the litter but me.

TERRY RUCKER
FOSTER PARENT

Safe Pet Guidelines

1) *Hygiene.* Wash your hands, especially before eating or smoking. Keep your pet and its living area clean. Groom your pet and trim its claws monthly. Eradicate fleas and cockroaches. Avoid contact with your pet's vomit, feces, urine, blood, or saliva. Wear gloves and clean up messes with a disinfectant. Better yet, have someone not at risk clean it up.

   Keep the litter box away from the kitchen and eating areas. Change the litter daily, using a new disposable plastic liner each day. (It takes the toxoplasmosis parasite at least 24 hours to become infectious.) If possible, have someone who's not at risk change the litter. Don't dump the litter! The resulting dust could possibly infect you. Twist-tie the liner closed and place it in the garbage. Disinfect the litter box at least once a month by filling it with boiling water and letting it stand for five minutes. Always wash your hands after cleaning the litter box.

2) *Preventive Veterinary Medicine.* Keep all pet vaccinations current. At least once a year, take your pet in for a checkup. Contact your veterinarian at the first sign of possible illness in your pet, such as persistent coughing, sneezing, losing weight, or persistent diarrhea.

3) *Animal Bites.* Tend to any animal bite right away. Rinse the wound with cold running water. Disinfect with a "tamed iodine" such as Betadine™ solution (not Betadine™ soap), readily available at drugstores. Contact your physician to get further advice.

4) *Your Pet's Diet.* Feed your pet commercial pet foods only, never raw meat or unpasteurized milk. Don't let your pet eat its own or other animals' feces, and keep them from drinking from the toilet bowl or rooting through the garbage. Keep your dog on a leash for walks to help control scavenging. Don't allow your animals to hunt. Cats can catch toxoplasmosis from eating birds and rodents. If your cat must go outdoors, place a double bell on its collar to help scare off potential prey.

5) *Adopting New Pets.* New pets present more of a risk because their health history is often sketchy at best. All new pets should be examined by your veterinarian, who may want to run tests to screen for diseases and parasites. Puppies and kittens are more likely to be infected with diseases, especially if they have diarrhea or are strays. Be cautious with them.

6) *Pets to Avoid.* Some animals have been found to be more likely to carry diseases that could spread to humans. These include strays, sick, wild, or exotic animals, animals with diarrhea, and monkeys.

Adapted from "Safe Pet Guidelines," by Pets Are Wonderful Support (PAWS). For more details, contact:

Pets Are Wonderful Support (PAWS)
539 Castro Street
San Francisco, CA 94114
415-241-1460
415-252-9471—FAX
9 a.m.-5 p.m., Mon-Fri (Pacific time)
• Request the brochures "Safe Pet Guidelines" and "Questions You May Have about Toxoplasmosis and Your Cat." Referrals to PAWS chapters throughout the U.S.

NAPWA Fax
National Association of People with AIDS
202-789-2222—FAX
• Offers the fax publication, "Toxoplasmosis and Your Cat." Request the "Living with HIV" fax catalog of fax documents in English. A Spanish catalog is also available. You must be at a fax machine to use the NAPWA Fax service.

PART 5

Getting through the Runaround

1. Insurance
    - Health Insurance
    - Disability Insurance
    - Life Insurance
    - Insurance and Benefits Information

2. Government Assistance Programs
    - Case Management
      Finding a Case Manager
    - Going It Alone: A Few Pointers for Navigating the System
    - Lessons from the Front Lines
    - Social Security Administration Programs
    - Illinois Department of Public Aid Programs
    - Housing and Rental Assistance
    - Housing, Food, Transportation, and Other Resources

3. Financial Planning

4. Your Legal Rights
    - Finding and Working with an Attorney
    - Legal Assistance

The financial and legal aspects of living with HIV can be overwhelming. Even the most educated among us may feel intimidated by complicated insurance forms, public assistance applications, and legal documents—not to mention the agencies and people who generate them.

Still, to live successfully with HIV, you will need to overcome your fear of these matters. It's vitally important for you to learn about your insurance options, and the benefits and protections to which you're legally entitled. Whether you "dive in" and do your own research or find a case manager to guide you through these murky waters, it'll help to have an overview of the basics. We've outlined some of the key things you'll need to know about insurance, government assistance programs, financial planning, and legal issues so you'll have a base from which to start.

It was not by whim that we entitled this section, "Getting through the Runaround." There often is a maddening amount of red tape involved in dealing with bureaucracies. As you begin making calls and visits to get information or apply for benefits, you may find yourself being put on hold, shuttled from department to department, or given conflicting answers. One of Murphy's Laws seems to be that whatever time you present yourself, the *only* person who can handle your question will be either out to lunch, on vacation, or "away from her desk" for an unknown time.

To get what you're after, you'll have to be persistent. You may need to call several different places or work your way through multiple layers of people to get accurate information. If you reach someone who doesn't know the answer to your question (or doesn't seem to know what they're talking about), don't hesitate to ask politely to speak with a supervisor. (Hostility will get you nowhere, but sometimes the best strategy is to *start* at the top.)

Realizing all this going in—and doing your best to maintain a sense of humor about it—can help make the process a little less infuriating. You'll find that most insurance and benefits workers really do want to help you get what you're entitled to. Remember that the person on the other end of the line is a human being just trying to do his or her job.

When you talk to Social Security or Public Aid personnel, don't be afraid to be open and honest about your situation. You needn't worry that they will notify the government or your employer that you have AIDS, or that you are planning to go on disability and leave your job. If nothing else, they simply don't have time for that sort of thing—not to mention that it would be illegal.

Above all, don't let the system get to you too much. Unlikely as it may seem at times, it's there to serve you—not defeat you. Don't forget that you have a right to contest decisions that don't go in your favor. Ask for written information on how to file an appeal.

1. INSURANCE

Insurance is a critical resource for people living with HIV. However, getting and keeping affordable coverage can be a difficult proposition. Finding the best protection for the lowest price will take some homework on your part.

The following pages address some of the most commonly asked questions on health, life, and disability insurance.

Health Insurance

At what point should I start looking into my insurance options?

Immediately. Don't wait until you're sick to find out what coverage you have or don't have.

If you don't have health insurance now, you'll want to figure out how you can get it. If you do have coverage, it's crucial for you to keep it as long as possible. In the May, 1991 issue of "Positively Aware," insurance industry expert Franklin Thomas asserted that "HIV-infected people almost have to live their lives according to the requirements of remaining insured." Brent Nance, a Los Angeles-based private insurance consultant, added in the same issue:

> *Insurance considerations are extremely serious, and deserve a thorough, detailed investigation and analysis. People have to get aggressive, read their existing policies if they have them, and ask questions when they don't understand. They have to understand the options available to them, and plan in advance how to obtain and maintain quality health insurance.*

Why should I go through all this bother to try and get insurance? Won't Medicaid and other public assistance programs take care of me if I'm sick?

Not necessarily. Depending on your circumstances, you may find yourself in the frustrating position of being "not disabled enough" or "too wealthy" to qualify for government benefits. You also may be unwilling or legally unable to dispose of your assets in order to become eligible. Although it's a hassle, finding some way to obtain new insurance or extend existing coverage can be far safer and less devastating to you, financially, in the long run. As a further protection, you may want to start putting some money away in an interest-bearing account to cover unforeseen future expenses.

What types of health insurance are available?

Generally speaking, there are individual policies and group plans. Individual policies are purchased directly from insurance companies by self-employed or non-employed people, those who work part-time or at small firms that don't offer health benefits, or those wanting to improve upon inadequate group coverage.

Group plans are commonly offered by employers as part of their standard employee benefits package. The employer may contribute all or part of the monthly premiums (money paid to the insurance company in exchange for coverage). Group plan premiums typically are much lower than individual policy premiums since the risk is spread among many people. Group health insurance also can be obtained through many unions and trade associations.

Some companies offer a choice among several different types of group plans. "Health maintenance organizations" (HMOs) or "preferred provider organizations" (PPOs) usually do not have a "pre-existing conditions" clause, which means your HIV-related claims are payable from the *first* day of coverage. Other "standard" plans may require you to wait 6 to 12 months before they will cover such expenses. During that waiting period, you would be insured only for accidents or "new" illnesses not related to your pre-existing conditions. After that period is up, you'll receive full coverage for *all* medical treatment the plan allows. In short, *pre-existing conditions clauses in your insurance plan don't mean you'll never be insured for your HIV disease—only that you'll have to wait a while for coverage.*

If you've been on your employer's group health plan for a long time, you probably will have no trouble filing claims or receiving benefits. However, if you've just taken a new job or if your employer has recently changed insurance carriers, your coverage may be limited for a time. Talk with the people in charge of benefits at your job, or to the insurance company directly, if you aren't sure what you're covered for. (You may want to check with your insurance company anonymously, and be very cautious about revealing your HIV status to benefits advisors on the job.)

Can the insurance company force me to be tested for HIV?

Not if you're already a member of an established group. If your employer were to change insurance carriers, the new company could require *everyone* in the "new group" to undergo medical screening for one or more conditions, including HIV. However, that carrier could not refuse coverage to selected individuals based on the results. *Nor can a carrier ever legally reveal medical information or test findings on individual workers to their employer.* An insurance carrier can choose not to continue covering any group when it's time to renew the policy, or charge higher rates for a group with an HIV-positive member. Any risk classification is lawful if it is based upon actuarial data.

What if I switch jobs or join a new group plan?

The insurance company still cannot require you as an individual to submit to an HIV test as a condition for joining the group. However, it can require you to provide a medical history. This may involve answering questions on an application or giving the carrier access to your medical records. Insurance companies do this to uncover disabilities or pre-existing conditions that may affect the start date of coverage for these conditions. But keep in mind:

- smaller group plans (fewer than 10 persons covered) usually require the most thorough investigation of group members. The plans of larger organizations may do only a cursory screening or none at all. When changing jobs, "bigger tends to be better."
- the application form may ask whether you have ever been diagnosed with ARC (AIDS-Related Complex) or AIDS. If you are only HIV-positive and have never been "officially" diagnosed with ARC or AIDS by a doctor, you can truthfully (and legally) answer no. However, you may be asked if you've ever been diagnosed with a blood disorder, sexually transmitted disease, or some symptom of HIV disease you may have had. In those cases, you'll have to answer yes. If the application then asks for further explanation, answer as truthfully as you can (or seek legal advice before turning in the application).
- in order to protect yourself in the future, it's recommended that you *always* tell the truth on any application for insurance. If the carrier finds out later that you lied, it can cancel your policy and take legal action against you.
- regardless of what the insurer uncovers about your health, it cannot lawfully refuse to insure you as a new member of the group.

Then you're telling me I *can* switch jobs?

Certainly—if you're *very* careful not to jeopardize your health coverage during the transition.

If you have a choice in the matter, your best option is to try for a transfer within the same company. That way, your coverage will remain intact. If you dislike your job but a transfer isn't possible, and you decide the company's benefits are simply too good to give up, consider counseling to find ways to cope better with your present position.

If you do decide to seek employment elsewhere, you'll want to be strategic in selecting the company to which you move. The reality is, your ultimate choice of employer may come down to a decision between benefits packages, rather than corporate cultures or advancement opportunities.

Whatever you do, don't drop your insurance! If you lose that, you are in big trouble with this disease.

"SAM"

There are so many people who are not getting the medical care they should because they're afraid to file a claim, and that's <u>wrong</u>.

CHARLIE

Don't let your insurance company get away with anything! Remember, they're making money from you. A lot of people are intimidated by their insurance company, which the insurance companies love. You have to make demands if you expect to get any service.

JOE

I've talked to people in support groups who finally decided they were tired of hiding this from their insurance company, and just one day said, "I'm going to submit this claim and I don't give a damn what happens after that." But I'm not at that point yet.

"RALPH"

In moving to a new job, you'll want to consider:

- the size of the firm. Besides offering less intrusive medical screening in their group plans, only companies with 20 or more employees can provide an extension of your benefits through COBRA should you leave. (More on COBRA later.)
- whether the firm offers an HMO or PPO plan—and if not, the length of the pre-existing conditions clause in its standard health plan. Larger companies' plans tend to have shorter waiting periods.
- your present state of health. If you've been tested for HIV anonymously and there is no evidence of your condition in your medical records, you'll be better off in the event the new group plan insurer wants to examine them. Also, if your T cells are high and you've never been ill or on HIV medication, you may feel better about gambling with coverage waiting periods.

Will I risk my group coverage if I make an HIV-related claim?

The answer to that is a qualified "probably not." Some people are afraid that if they submit a claim for an HIV-related drug or a T cell test, that will "tip off" the insurance company (and possibly their employer) about their positive HIV status. They worry that by running up too many "telltale" bills, their insurer may drop them or their employer may fire them.

Most of the time, these fears are unfounded. If you're already enrolled in your employer's group plan, didn't lie on your application, have paid in your required share of the premiums, and have met the plan's requirements for pre-existing conditions, your insurer cannot legally:

- deny you benefits or drop you for submitting a claim.
- raise your individual premiums relative to those of the group (though they may try to raise the group premium rates at some point in the future).
- reveal any details to your employer about you, your illness, or the exact nature of your claims.

Nor can your employer fire you or make you opt out of the company's benefit plan just because you're HIV-positive or submitting sizable claims. In most cases, there's no sense paying for tests or treatment out-of-pocket when your insurance will cover them without penalty to you or your job.

There *are* precautions you can take to make sure you're fully protected. When you submit your first HIV-related claim under the plan, enclose a note to the insurance company stating that your claim, treatment, and medical condition are confidential information, not to be disclosed to anyone outside that company or to your employer. Keep a copy of this note with your insurance records. This will give you some legal backup in case your condition is ever disclosed against your wishes.

Insurance companies' vision of the person with AIDS is not that of a human being. Their vision is dollar signs, as in, "This person is a guaranteed future claim. This is a person who's maybe going to have three hospitalizations, huge bills—and we know that, that's a fact." And it may not be a "fact," you may never have any of those things happen to you. But to them, any person with AIDS is a person who is not cost-effective. No matter how much they talk about, "We are a humanitarian insurance company," they're always aware of the dollar signs. They're out to make dollars and to spend as few dollars as possible. So if you come in and they can figure out how to get rid of you because you have an AIDS diagnosis, they're going to try to do it.

The problem is, people don't realize insurance companies can't just get rid of anyone they want to. And that's what those companies are counting on, that you won't know your rights or act upon them.

MICHELLE MASCARO
POLICY ASSOCIATE,
AIDS FOUNDATION OF CHICAGO

It was very helpful to me to talk to the AIDS Legal Council of Chicago to find out what my options were, in terms of going and staying underground for my care. Insurance is very unstable these days; there's a lot of discrimination around HIV and a lot of rigmarole around pre-existing conditions and things of that nature. It just seemed advisable, as long as I don't require a lot of intensive treatment, to keep this out of my medical records as long as possible. I think it's better to keep my options open.

I realize this may change at some point. I may have to come out from underground. But as long as I can stay there and am comfortable doing so, I'm going to do it. It's important to think out in advance what is morally and ethically right. I had some struggles with that; but a doctor put it to me: "Is it more important to you to preserve yourself, or preserve the system?" Looking at it that way helped a lot. To me, if you need to screw the system, then screw the system. 'Cause it's gonna screw you.

"RALPH"

Is there any benefit to keeping my HIV status out of my medical or insurance records?

There is if you're anticipating changing jobs in the near future, or if you want to continue working in an HIV-sensitive field like teaching or health care. Once the details of your condition "get into the computer," there's no getting them out.

However, there may come a time when you can no longer absorb your medical expenses yourself, become noticeably ill, or simply grow tired of the cloak-and-dagger routine. Then, you may find it useful to talk with a lawyer or private insurance consultant to see what the ramifications would be for revealing your condition.

What else do I need to know about filing claims?*

It's important to keep good records—documents, claims, and all communications with your employer, insurance company, hospital, and doctors. You may want to set up a special file which will allow easy access to bills, letters—anything and everything pertaining to your insurance. A diary or log can help you keep track of phone calls. [See the Appendix of this book for a Contact Form to copy and use in documenting such calls.] Should a question arise regarding your insurance, you'll need as much information and documentation as possible.

What do I do if my insurance company refuses to pay my claim based on pre-existing conditions?*

The burden of proof for pre-existing conditions is with the insurance company. If the situation cannot be resolved between you, your doctor, and your insurance carrier, seek advice from your lawyer or the advocacy program of your local AIDS service organization.

*Sections adapted with permission from Living with AIDS: A Guide to Resources in New York City, published by Gay Men's Health Crisis. For information, call 212-807-6655.

I'm covered under an employee benefit plan rather than a group insurance plan. Are there any differences I should know about?

Very possibly. Employer-funded plans are not required to play by the same set of state rules that insurance companies are. For instance, where an insurance carrier cannot arbitrarily set lower lifetime benefit caps for people with HIV, an employer-funded plan *may* be able to discriminate in this fashion. However, employers are still not legally permitted to fire or penalize workers under these plans simply because they submit an HIV-related claim. When in doubt, get competent legal advice.

If I leave my job and don't transfer right away to another one, what happens to my insurance?

If your company employs 20 or more workers, you probably will be eligible for coverage under COBRA (the federal Consolidated Omnibus Budget Reconciliation Act of 1986). COBRA allows you to continue your same group health benefits for up to 18 months, with the possibility of an 11-month extension if you are disabled. You also have the option to continue benefits for your insured dependents. However, you will be responsible for signing up for the program and paying the premiums yourself—up to a maximum of 102% of the cost.

Your employer is obligated to inform you of your COBRA continuation rights within 14 days after you leave your job. You'll have 45-60 days after that notification to opt for COBRA coverage. Premiums will be due retroactively to the last date you were covered by your employer.

To what kinds of coverage does COBRA apply?*

COBRA covers standard and HMO medical, dental, prescription drug, and vision benefits to the extent that they exist in your present group plan. Life and disability insurance are not included.

Are all group plans covered by COBRA?*

No. Your employer must have 20 or more employees. Or, if you are working for a company under a union-negotiated contract signed prior to July 1, 1986 then you are not covered by COBRA until your contract is renegotiated. COBRA coverage also does not apply to not-for-profit religious organizations or agencies of the federal government.

* From <u>Living with AIDS</u>, Gay Men's Health Crisis.

I work for a company with fewer than 20 employees. Is COBRA the only continuation plan available?

Not necessarily. Some small group health insurance plans offer a similar continuation option. Check with your employer to see if that option exists in your case. Many smaller firms have set up COBRA-like programs.

What if my group plan isn't eligible for COBRA or a COBRA-like extension?

You have the option of converting your group plan to an individual plan with your former company's insurance carrier. However, you must act within 30 days of leaving your job or you will lose your rights to make the change.

While your individual conversion coverage probably won't be as good as your group coverage, and will undoubtedly have higher premiums, it may be the best you can do at this time. Find out from your former employer what steps you need to take to convert your plan. Be sure to get the names and addresses of all the insurers who need to be notified of your intention to convert (in some plans, there are more than one).

Most group insurance contracts also have an "extension of benefits" provision. If you are disabled at the time you leave your job, you will continue to receive benefits for the period of time outlined in your insurance policy. At the end of that period, you will have to convert to an individual plan and begin paying premiums if you want continued coverage. If you can't afford them and are eligible for Medicaid, that program may pay your premiums if you apply in advance.

Suppose I can't afford the premiums to keep my COBRA or other group insurance coverage. What then?

As an Illinois resident, you may be eligible for assistance from the state. The Continuation of Health Insurance Coverage (CHIC) program helps pay health insurance premiums for people who had to leave their employment, but will continue to receive health benefits through the COBRA plan. Applicants must currently be covered by a group plan that covers prescription drugs and must meet income eligibility levels. For information, contact:

Illinois Department of Public Health
Continuation of Health Insurance Coverage (CHIC) Program
HIV/AIDS Section, First Floor
525 West Jefferson
Springfield, IL 62761
800-825-3518
217-785-8013—FAX
800-547-0466—Hearing-impaired TTY/TDD (non-hotline)
8:30 a.m.-5 p.m. Mon-Fri

Let's say I can get a COBRA extension. What should I do when it expires?

Before your COBRA period ends, make arrangements to convert to individual coverage as described above. If you let your COBRA-extended insurance run out before acting, you will be denied the privilege of converting—or may only be able to do so by answering health questions that can cause you to be turned down for coverage.

What if I go back to work for a different company during the COBRA extension period. Will I be picked up by a new group plan?*

As long as your new company includes at least 10 employees on its group plan, you probably will be able to enroll in the new plan without answering too many medical questions. Although you may be subject to a pre-existing condition waiting period, you will once again be covered. You may retain your COBRA policy to cover you through the new plan's waiting period, but you'll have to continue paying your COBRA premiums and report your dual coverage to the new insurer. You should also be prepared to handle a gap in coverage should your COBRA extension expire before the end of the new plan's waiting period.

What if I go back to work after the COBRA period has ended. Will I be insured?*

As described previously, you will be entitled to enroll in your new group plan. If you have converted your extended group plan to an individual plan, consult with an insurance specialist to help decide whether or not to give up your individual policy at this time. If you can afford to keep up the premiums, your combined coverage under the two plans may be better than your coverage under the new group plan alone (especially if there is a waiting period for benefits).

What happens if the company I worked for ceases to exist? Will my COBRA extension continue?*

Unfortunately, no. If a company closes, the insurance plan ends, and therefore, COBRA extension ends. However, if the company changes plans, you go to the new plan.

* From <u>Living with AIDS</u>, Gay Men's Health Crisis.

What other coverage options are available to me?

That will depend largely on your employer. Many people who've decided to leave their jobs due to AIDS-related illness have persuaded their employers to extend life and health coverage voluntarily. This not only reduces the individual's premium expenses, but buys them additional time later under COBRA. Some employees also have negotiated "creative" ways to leave the firm gradually—perhaps by taking an extended medical leave of absence—before terminating officially or retiring. In some cases, this allowed them to keep full or partial benefits coverage as a continuing employee while absent from work.

You should be aware that the federal Family and Medical Leave Act (FMLA), which applies to companies that have more than 50 employees, may entitle you to up to 12 weeks of unpaid leave for medical reasons. The FMLA generally applies after a worker has been on the job for one year.

What are my chances for getting an individual health policy on my own, as opposed to through a conversion?

Virtually nonexistent. These days, most companies screen individual applicants very carefully. If you apply for a policy, you may be asked to take a blood test and/or submit an exhaustive medical history. It's a "catch-22"—if you refuse to comply, your application will be denied. If you reveal you are HIV-positive, your application also will be denied.

In the latter case, it is also likely that the insurance company will notify the Medical Information Bureau (the insurance industry's central data bank) of its findings and decision to turn you down. Although the Bureau cannot legally reveal the reason you were turned down, other insurers you apply to can find out you've been rejected. On that basis alone, they also may decline to insure you.

I already have an individual health policy. Is there any way my insurance company could drop me or refuse to honor my claims?*

Possibly—if your insurer claims "material misrepresentation." This means that, by examining your medical records, your insurer has discovered a fact about which you either failed to inform them or answered incorrectly on your application for insurance. They may claim that they would never have issued your policy (or issued it at that premium level) had they known about the "misrepresented" fact. Policies with higher benefit ceilings, lower deductibles, and shorter waiting periods for pre-existing conditions are the most likely to be investigated.

A common example of material misrepresentation is failure to report that you saw a particular physician for a particular ailment, such as a sexually transmitted disease. But an insurer may cling to any omission of fact as material misrepresentation in an effort to reject your claim and cancel your policy. That's why it's important that you be honest on all applications for insurance.

When material misrepresentation is claimed, your insurance company will return your policy along with a check for the amount you have paid in premiums. *Before cashing the check*, seek legal counsel to determine if you have grounds for contesting your insurer's actions. By cashing the check, you accept their claim and will have no further recourse.

Should I continue to pay insurance premiums even if it appears that my insurance company is going to deny coverage?*

Yes. In order to maintain your policy, it is imperative that you pay the premiums within the time frame specified on your bill. Your insurance company is not required to tell you that your policy has lapsed for nonpayment, and can drop you for being "delinquent."

* From <u>Living with AIDS</u>, Gay Men's Health Crisis.

Is there a limitation on how long a carrier is allowed to claim material misrepresentation?

The standard "contestability clause" in most individual policies is two years. After that time, the carrier cannot deny claims or cancel your policy for application "irregularities" they failed to uncover. Check your own policy for its time limit in this regard. Be aware that the law permits insurers to drop policyholders at *any* time if they are found to have obtained coverage fraudulently (by lying).

What should I do if I can't get group or individual health coverage through any means?

You still may be able to obtain coverage through the Illinois Comprehensive Health Insurance Plan (CHIP) program for "uninsurable" state residents. If you've been denied insurance within the last nine months because of your HIV/AIDS condition, or can provide adequate proof of that condition, CHIP probably will admit you to the program. (CHIP is also available to Illinois residents who've been denied insurance for medical reasons other than HIV.)

There are two separate CHIP plans, available to Medicaid-eligible and non-eligible persons and their families. Be aware that CHIP premiums and out-of-pocket co-payments can be hefty, depending on the plan and deductible level you choose. Due to high demand, the wait to get into the program may be up to eight months. If you apply today, you may not start receiving benefits for a year or more.

To get an application for CHIP coverage, contact any agent licensed to sell insurance in Illinois. Or contact:

Illinois Department of Public Aid
Illinois Comprehensive Health Insurance Plan (CHIP)
400 West Monroe Street, Suite 202
Springfield, IL 62704
800-367-6410
8 a.m.-5 p.m. Mon-Fri

Also call this number to ask any question about the CHIP program before signing on, and to inquire about any aspect of your policy, claims, or coverage after signing on.

You'll be required to submit your application with documentation about your health status and first premium payment enclosed. The program will notify you of your acceptance or denial within 45 days of the date they receive your completed application. If you're accepted, your "place in line" to begin receiving CHIP benefits will be calculated from the date you *applied*, not the date you were accepted. To find out after acceptance when you can expect to begin receiving benefits, call:

CHIP Board of Directors
800-962-8384

In the unlikely event you are denied coverage under CHIP, the program is required to explain the reason in writing. You will then have the opportunity to protest the decision.

Disability Insurance

What is private disability insurance?

These group or individual plans pay cash benefits to policyholders who become disabled through illness or injury and are unable to work. They provide only a portion of your former income, but that can help pay some of the bills if you have no money coming in. Policies vary widely on their definition of "disability" and on how quickly they begin to pay benefits after a claim. Some plans provide benefits for a few weeks, others for a lifetime. Consult your own plan to see what applies in your case.

How does group disability insurance work?*

Group policies may offer either short- or long-term benefits, or both. These group plans usually integrate with public plans (such as State Disability, Worker's Compensation, or Social Security). When you file a claim for disability benefits with your group plan, you'll want to simultaneously file for Social Security Disability Insurance, or SSDI. (You can find more details on SSDI in the section on Government Assistance Programs.)

Am I allowed to convert my group disability to an individual plan if I become unemployed?*

No. If, however, you are disabled at the time your employment ends, you will not be denied benefits. Generally, this applies even if you have not met the full waiting period specified in your plan. Review your plan, especially the sections concerning termination and end of coverage.

Bear in mind that filing for disability may affect your group health and life insurance benefits. Review your plans carefully and consult with your personnel department or insurance carrier before filing, if you have any questions.

* From Living with AIDS, Gay Men's Health Crisis.

What are the odds of my obtaining a private individual disability policy?

Frankly, your chances of success are very small. Almost any company you approach about obtaining a policy will require you to take a blood test for HIV—and will turn you down if you refuse or test positive. Your best bet is to try and get coverage on a group plan, either through work or a trade union or association. Unfortunately, not all employers offer disability as part of their benefits package.

I thought I'd be doing all sorts of charity work, but I'm "employed" full-time fighting AIDS and trying to be well. I'm busy with an art project, doing calls and paperwork to keep my benefits, meeting with my attorney, keeping appointments with doctors and HIV service agencies, et cetera. You really do have to redesign yourself. I never would have believed I'd be living like this at age forty! You have to grapple with the whole structure of things.

Disability is like retirement, only without the benefits. I've had to ask myself, "What is it that I truly value?" For me, it's family, and trying to keep my relationships intact. I want to be healthy and last a long time.

"SPARKY"

Life Insurance

I currently don't have any life insurance. Can I get coverage?*

If you are HIV-positive or have been diagnosed with AIDS, it's unlikely that you will be able to obtain an individual life insurance policy. [Note: As this book goes to press, there is at least one company test-marketing an individual term life product to HIV-positive people. Proposed premiums are high, and coverage is limited. Depending on the outcome of this company's "experiment," other insurance providers may eventually jump on the bandwagon. Ask your case manager or an AIDS organization in your area if there are any life insurance companies currently offering policies to people with AIDS.]

If you go to work for an employer that provides group life insurance coverage, read carefully the section of your benefits booklet which describes the plan's exclusions, limitations, and pre-existing conditions. Also be cautious of insurance offers that do not require you to answer health questions; some are of questionable value.

I have life insurance coverage under my group plan at work. Is there any way I might lose my coverage as long as I'm employed by the company?*

No. As long as you are enrolled in the group plan, your coverage cannot be terminated for any reason, including changes in your health status.

What if I become disabled and leave my job?*

In most cases, you probably will be eligible for a group life conversion policy or a no-cost group life extension. In the case of a conversion, you can apply for any policy as long as the amount of coverage is not greater than the amount of coverage you had under the group policy. You have 30 days from the date of your employment termination to convert your policy, and you will be responsible for paying the premiums yourself.

However, some plans do not have these provisions and will cancel life insurance when an employee goes on disability. Check your policy to see which scenario applies to you.

I'm leaving my job, but am not disabled. What happens to my group life policy?*

You are entitled to convert it to an individual policy. Notify your insurance company in writing of your intent to convert. You will then be responsible for paying the premiums yourself.

> *I think what is happening, because of the new treatments, is that the kinds of resources that were not made available to people with AIDS are becoming available. Life insurance is one. There may be some changes in health insurance availability, too. There is certainly a growing perception that people with HIV are going to be around a lot longer than they have been in the past. The door is opening up for them to help with long-term planning for their loved ones.*
>
> DEBORAH STEINKOPF
> EXECUTIVE DIRECTOR, BEHIV—
> BETTER EXISTENCE WITH HIV

What if I have an individual life insurance policy and become disabled. How will this affect my insurance?*

If your policy includes a disability premium waiver, your insurer will waive (stop) premiums for as long as you meet their definition of disability. You will remain covered under the policy but will not have to pay the premiums as long as you are disabled.

If no such waiver is included in your policy and you are unable to pay the premiums yourself, an alternative may be to borrow against the policy's cash value or dividends. Or, ask a family member or friend to pay your premiums.

* From Living with AIDS, Gay Men's Health Crisis.

I accidentally let my individual life insurance coverage lapse. Is there any way I can retrieve it?

That depends on your policy. Some plans have generous "grace periods" or "reinstatement rules" that allow delinquent policyholders to pay up the premiums and have full coverage restored without medical screening. Review your policy carefully or contact your insurer to find out whether this applies in your case.

Are there companies that buy life insurance policies for cash?

The technical term for such transactions is "viatical settlement." There are at least 50 viatical companies in the United States that will buy out life insurance policies for 55-80% of the death benefit. By making such a company your sole beneficiary, you can receive an immediate cash payout to help cover your expenses. You will need to provide medical records, life insurance policy and other information to the viatical company or to a company that acts as a seller's representative or broker. Under federal legislation passed in 1996, income from viatical settlements is not subject to income tax.

Before you contact a viatical company or broker, first contact your current insurance carrier to see if your policy can be used as collateral for a loan, or if they offer "living" or "accelerated" benefits. While loan advances are not taxable, you will have interest payments to make. Some insurance companies require that you cancel all policies that you hold with them, including health, before your policy can be viaticated. Have a tax consultant review your situation and make a recommendation.

If your insurance carrier doesn't offer these choices, you'll have to contact a viatical company or broker. Be careful. For the most part, these companies are new and not yet regulated. Only a handful of states regulate such investments, and they do so very loosely. Make sure that any company you contact is financially sound. You can contact your state insurance commissioner to see if any complaints have been filed against the company in question. In Illinois, call:

Illinois Department of Insurance
320 West Washington Street, 4th Floor
Springfield, IL 62767
217-782-4515
217-782-5020—FAX
217-524-4872—Hearing-impaired TTY/TDD
• Accepts complaints about insurance companies doing business in Illinois. Also offers insurance information and referrals.

Be aware that the sale of your policy could disqualify you from receiving public assistance. If the assistance program imposes a cap on your income or other resources, its benefits may be reduced or terminated for a period of time. Check with the program in question or your case manager.

At present, there are no rules for minimum settlements and companies differ. It pays to shop around. Get bids from at least three companies, or contact a seller's broker who will try to maximize your payout. These brokers, acting as middlemen, usually charge fees. Ask them to disclose the cost to you upfront. If they resist doing so, find another broker who is more straightforward. Remember, you are not obligated to accept any offer at any time.

Are there additional life insurance options for veterans?

Yes. Active-duty service personnel have 120 days after discharge (or up to a year if they're totally disabled) to convert their group life policy to a non-renewable 5-year term policy. At the end of that term, they have the option to convert to an individual plan. No medical exam is required in either case. Veterans who were disabled while in the service also may be eligible for low-cost or free term life policies with face values of up to $10,000. Veterans can purchase these any time after discharge, regardless of their health. For details, contact:

Department of Veterans Affairs—Veterans Service Division
800-827-1000
8 a.m.-4:00 p.m., Mon-Fri
(except federal holidays).

How can I get more information?

To get answers to your personal insurance-related questions, we recommend contacting/consulting:

- your personnel department or benefits advisor at work;
- your insurance agent or carrier directly; and/or
- your local AIDS service organization. AIDS organizations can provide you with up-to-date reference materials, and often sponsor workshops and seminars on insurance-related matters.

Insurance and Benefits Information

Illinois Department of Public Aid
Illinois Comprehensive Health Insurance Plan (CHIP)
400 West Monroe Street, Suite 202
Springfield, IL 62704
800-367-6410
8 a.m.-5 p.m. Mon-Fri
• Insurance plan for eligible HIV-positive Illinois residents who have been denied health insurance and who are not eligible for other coverage. Call for application and information about wait lists and premiums.

Illinois Department of Public Health—HIV/AIDS Section
AIDS Drug Assistance Program
525 West Jefferson, First Floor
Springfield, IL 62761
800-825-3518
217-785-8013—FAX
800-547-0466—Hearing-impaired TTY/TDD (non-hotline)
8:30 a.m.-5 p.m. Mon-Fri
• AIDS Drug Assistance Program provides certain AIDS-related drugs to eligible Illinois residents. Call for eligibility requirements and drugs currently available through the program. Referrals to HIV/AIDS-related services in Illinois. English/Spanish.

Illinois Department of Public Health—HIV/AIDS Section
Continuation of Health Insurance Coverage
(CHIC) Program
525 West Jefferson, First Floor
Springfield, IL 62761
800-825-3518
217-785-8013—FAX
800-547-0466—Hearing-impaired TTY/TDD (non-hotline)
8:30 a.m.-5 p.m. Mon-Fri
• CHIC Program pays COBRA premiums for eligible persons who leave employment and will continue to receive health insurance through the COBRA plan. Call for income and other eligibility requirements. Referrals to HIV/AIDS-related services in Illinois. English/Spanish.

Illinois Director of Insurance
320 West Washington Street, 4th Floor
Springfield, IL 62767
217-782-4515
217-782-5020—FAX
217-524-4872—Hearing-impaired TTY/TDD
• Accepts complaints about insurance companies doing business in Illinois. Also offers insurance information and referrals.

Illinois Insurance Information Service
800-444-3338
9 a.m.-4 p.m. Mon-Fri
• Consumer information hotline answers questions about all types of insurance and offers help to those having trouble with an insurance company. Provides free educational literature and factual information about companies. Funded by the Illinois insurance industry.

"The COBRA Continuation Options: Questions and Answers."
"Clearinghouse Review,"
April, 1988
• Available in any good law library.

The AIDS Benefits Handbook
McCormack, Thomas P.
New Haven:
Yale University Press, 1990.
Mail order: Lambda Rising Books, 800-621-6969
• Includes a brief but helpful section on health and life insurance, in addition to in-depth information and advice on obtaining all manner of public benefits.

"Taking Charge: The HIV Planning Guide"
Mail order: Impact AIDS, 505-995-0722
• Booklet provides an overview of insurance coverage, public entitlement programs, and legal resources.

Using a Computer and Modem

Marty Howard's HIV/AIDS HomePage
http://www.smartlink.net/~martinjh/
• Compiled by an individual, this is an exhaustive list of HIV/AIDS-related links. Includes Social Security information.

Viatical Settlements

NAPWA Fax
National Association of People with AIDS
202-789-2222—FAX
• Several viatical settlement publications available by fax, including frequently updated lists of viatical settlement companies. Request the "Living with HIV" fax catalog of fax documents in English. A Spanish catalog is also available. You must be at a fax machine to use the NAPWA Fax service.

2. GOVERNMENT ASSISTANCE PROGRAMS

If you are diagnosed with AIDS, the government considers you to be "medically disabled." Disabled persons automatically qualify for benefits under one or more government assistance programs. This is true whether or not they have actually been sick or unable to work. However, if you haven't been "officially" diagnosed with AIDS, but can get your doctor to document the fact that your HIV-related ailments seriously impair your ability to function or earn a living, you may still be able to get some disability benefits.

Government assistance programs are a valuable resource for people disabled by HIV disease—especially those with limited financial resources. Entitlement programs can provide income, medical coverage, and help with the basic necessities of life.

In seeking and applying for assistance, you may choose to work with a personal case manager, or "go it alone" through the system.

Case Management

In case management, HIV-infected persons and their families link up with a social worker who is a professional "problem solver" in the HIV service area. Your assigned case manager will do an intake interview with you to determine what your needs are. You will then work together on an ongoing basis to get whatever medical, legal, emotional, and/or financial assistance you require throughout your illness.

Your case manager can tell you about new or unfamiliar programs, introduce you to agencies where you're not known, help you apply for and get the benefits you're entitled to, and intervene on your behalf in the event of problems. Instead of making many phone calls trying to get a question answered or mix-up straightened out, you simply call your case manager and she or he does the rest.

You will not be a passive participant in this process, however. The idea is not just to sit back and let someone else make the decisions or do all the work for you. You can only assure yourself of effective care by working with your case manager on a regular, ongoing basis, by being very honest and clear about your needs, and by conscientiously working on the plans you and your caseworker have set.

At times, your case manager might confront you on certain things—so your relationship won't always be completely harmonious. There's a theory that if a social worker has only clients who love him or her, that person is probably not the best social worker. There is some challenge involved. But you should, in general, have a sense that this person has your well-being in mind, and that they are respectful and accepting of you—which doesn't necessarily mean they're accepting of all your choices or opinions.

Every case manager has a different philosophy. There are some guiding ethical principles they go by—that social work should be client-led and beneficial to the client. But for the most part, people

---

One of the biggest questions you have when you are first diagnosed is, "How am I going to pay for this disease? How can I afford to have this—and are they going to let me die because I don't have any money?"

"MARIE"

You find out more from people who are in the HIV community. For instance, I found out that with Public Aid, if you file an appeal within 10 days, they can't cut you off until a decision is made. They'll tell you the deadline is sixty days, but after the first ten days they can cut you off while making the decision. Little stuff like that, you learn from talking to people.

CHRISTINE

are going to make judgment calls. If they feel like you're using them or working against them in some way, it's not going to be a very productive relationship.

Case management quality can vary widely. Some case managers are more effective and easier to work with than others. If you don't feel comfortable with the first person you're assigned to, request a switch. Remember, *you are the client*. Case managers and the agencies they contact are in place to provide service to *you*. If you have problems with your case manager or other HIV services that you can't resolve, you may want to contact your Regional HIV/AIDS Care Consortia Coordinator (the numbers are listed in Part 1). In Chicago, there is a consumer line to help resolve complaints about HIV services:

HIV Services Consumer Access Line
312-747-9650—English/Spanish
8:30 a.m.-4:30 p.m. Mon-Fri

Case managers can help you access:
- Illinois Department of Public Aid or Social Security Administration programs;
- support groups for PWAs, family, friends, and caregivers;
- special grants, rent subsidies, and financial assistance for outstanding bills;
- in-home services for disabled individuals such as meal preparation, laundry, shopping, and bathing;
- medical and home health services;
- food and nutrition programs;
- legal services such as powers of attorney, property wills, and living wills;
- housing alternatives;
- child care and respite services;
- resources for complementary therapies; and/or
- substance-abuse treatment programs.

> *It's important that people don't look at their case manager as someone who's going to manage their life. The case manager is a person who <u>assists you</u> in managing your life with HIV.*
>
> *What's good about case management is that it provides a centralized way for you to organize yourself and get information. The case manager works with you if you go to the hospital, and throughout the course of whatever's going on with you.*
>
> *There are two basic "stages" of case management. The first stage is right after clients test HIV-positive. They want to know what resources are out there. They need to get themselves together in some kind of structured way. At that point, those people generally have a job and are still healthy.*

Look for service providers who treat you with respect and especially who respect the choices you make in your life. Look for people who are willing to go with you as peers on a journey, rather than as guides.

Each person's way of dealing with HIV is unique. For some people a certain amount of information will be comforting. For others, the same information will be anxiety-provoking. That's why it's so important to work with someone who will take the time to get to know you and your ways of responding.

HIV hits at the heart of what life is all about. It's a fertile field for getting at our existential issues: death, guilt, isolation, responsibility, the meaning of life. When a person confronts HIV, it pushes you up against those issues, and so it offers you a way to really grow and change, if you want to use it that way. The way you deal with practical issues is intimately intertwined with the whole way you deal with life.

JOAN PALMER
FORMER COORDINATOR OF
SOCIAL WORK, WITS,
UNIVERSITY OF ILLINOIS
AT CHICAGO

They don't need to worry about applying for Social Security or anything like that yet. They might want to use a case manager to help them assess their overall picture, and to get things in place in the event that some day, they want to get into the social services system.

The case manager also helps in this early stage with things like setting up durable powers of attorney for health care and living wills, and also getting clients any kind of help they need in the community, whether it's hooking them up with a physician or a support group or what have you.

The second stage of case management tends to occur when people get really sick and can no longer work. They have to start looking at how they can get on disability, which is something the case manager is well equipped to help with. Sometimes people drop into case management for the first time at this stage because up until now, they've been handling things by themselves pretty well. However, navigating the social service programs can often go a lot more smoothly when you're working with someone who knows all the ins and outs.

MICHELLE MASCARO
Policy Associate,
AIDS Foundation of Chicago

Anything a client tells a case manager is kept strictly confidential. That's <u>any</u> case manager. There are all sorts of forms we give our clients explaining the nature of confidentiality, which they have to sign off on. However, it's a two-way street—our clients have to sign a confidentiality pledge, too. That means if they come here for a support group, they promise they aren't going to talk about who came to that group when they go out with friends the following night.

We also get a release of information form signed any time our case managers need to work with outside agencies on a client's behalf. We don't do <u>anything</u> without the client's permission or approval. It's by definition a "safe interaction." Anything you tell a case manager is protected information—just like in a doctor/patient or lawyer/patient relationship. Only in cases where there's a suspicion of child abuse or neglect is a social worker mandated by law to report it. Drug use, most illegal activity, sexuality issues…a client can disclose any of these to a case manager without fear of repercussions.

DEBORAH STEINKOPF
Executive Director, BEHIV—
Better Existence with HIV

If you have a choice, pick your case manager in the same way you would go about picking a doctor. This handy person, if motivated and not burned out yet, can help guide you through almost any minefield.

Remember, though, case managers are not a breed of super people. Some know more than others. In fact, some of them are downright useless. It's like picking a bad doctor—some of 'em walk in, write a prescription, then walk out again without even looking at you. But with the caseworkers who <u>are</u> good, you feel like you're on a game show, and you've just won a brand new car, a new Amana refrigerator, and a year's supply of AZT. They can pretty much find anything. They're like the Shell Answer Man of AIDS—the good ones have all the answers to all your questions.

ADAM

I had been working on the HIV Planning Council, and I knew the definition of a case manager, I knew we were funding them; but I really didn't <u>know</u>, from a personal standpoint, that it's absolutely impossible to get through the morass of bureaucracies and agencies and forms without a case manager. I needed one to deal with all of Michael's stuff. I don't know how people make it without someone. It gets pretty desperate.

JOE

Finding a Case Manager

For referrals to case management programs throughout Illinois, contact your region's HIV/AIDS Care Consortia Coordinator (listed in Part 1 of this book). Or call:

Illinois AIDS Hotline
800-243-2437—Hotline staffed 8 a.m.-11 p.m., 7 days/week
800-782-0423—Hearing-impaired TTY/TDD
• Referrals to HIV case management, and health services and general social services throughout Illinois. English/Spanish.

Referrals in Cook County

AIDS Foundation of Chicago
411 South Wells, Suite 300
Chicago, IL 60607
312-922-2322
312-922-2916—FAX
312-922-2917—Hearing-impaired TTY/TDD
• Provides referrals to Chicago-area case management agencies. English/Spanish.

Outside Illinois

CDC National AIDS Hotline
800-342-2437—English
800-344-7432—Spanish
800-243-7889—Hearing-impaired TTY/TDD
• 24-hour toll-free service with a database of more than 19,000 organizations can help people in any U.S. state or territory identify state and local resources.

Using a Computer and Modem

Test Positive Aware Network
http://www.tpan.com
• Site includes full listings from the "Chicago Area HIV/AIDS Service Directory," including case management agencies. National resources and state hotlines for persons outside of Illinois.

You may also directly call one of the case management agencies listed below. If you prefer to have a case manager where you receive HIV primary care or substance abuse treatment services, check the listings under "Local Hospitals and HIV Clinics" (located in Part 3 of this book) and "Finding Chemical Dependency Treatment and Support" (in Part 4) to see which offer case management.

Case Management and Related HIV/AIDS Services

AIDS Care Network
221 North Longwood, Suite 105
Rockford, IL 61107
815-968-5181
815-968-3315—FAX
• Case management, financial assistance, volunteer services, buddy program, and referrals. Support groups, including substance abuse/HIV group.

AIDS Ministry of Illinois
68 North Chicago Street, Suite 240
Joliet, IL 60432-4380
815-723-1548
815-740-5910—FAX
• Provides case management, DORS, referrals, advocacy, education, housing assistance, support groups.

Ascension Respite Care Center
1133 North LaSalle Street
Chicago, IL 60610
312-751-8887
312-751-3904—FAX
• Serves families of HIV-affected individuals. Offers case management, individual counseling for family members, mother's support groups, and food pantry.

Better Existence with HIV (BEHIV)
PO Box 5171
Evanston, IL 60204
847-475-2115
847-475-2820—FAX
• Case management, including DORS; domestic assistance; financial assistance for rent and utilities; food pantry. "Safe Start" program assists homeless persons with an AIDS diagnosis who have a mental illness and/or use substances. "Safe Start" program assists homeless persons with an AIDS diagnosis who have a mental illness and/or use substances. Serves northern Chicago and north/northwest suburbs. Free. English/Spanish.

Catholic Charities
126 North Desplaines Street
Chicago, IL 60661
312-655-7715
312-263-4290—FAX

Catholic Charities—Southwest Suburban
10661 South Roberts Road
Palos Hills, IL 60465
708-430-0428
708-430-0502—FAX

**Catholic Charities—
West Suburban**
1400 South Austin Boulevard
Cicero, IL 60804
708-209-1110
708-209-1124—FAX
• Case management, counseling, and emergency assistance with basic needs, including rent, food, clothing, and shelter. Information and referrals. English/Spanish.

**Catholic Charities—
Lake County**
671 South Lewis Avenue
Waukegan, IL 60085
847-249-3500
847-623-6750—FAX
• Comprehensive case management for those with HIV/AIDS and their families. Emergency financial assistance for housing, food, and transportation, DORS in-home services, professional and volunteer support. Free. English/Spanish.

**Chicago House and
Social Service Agency**
PO Box 14728
Chicago, IL 60614
773-248-5200
773-248-5019—FAX
• Provides case management to clients in their residences and to the community. Sliding scale fees. English/Spanish.

Chicago Women's AIDS Project
5249 North Kenmore Avenue
Chicago, IL 60640
773-271-2242
773-271-2618—FAX
• Counseling, case management, financial assistance referrals, support groups for women, and individual counseling for children and teens of parents living with HIV/AIDS. Also offers child care, second-hand clothing, buddies, social events, massage therapy, speakers bureau, peer advocacy, and STD/HIV prevention programs. Free.

Circle Family Care
4909 West Division Street,
3rd Floor
Chicago, IL 60651
773-921-8100
773-921-4428—FAX
• Provides case management and other HIV services from a Christian perspective.

**Community Counseling
Centers of Chicago**
4740 North Clark Street
Chicago, IL 60640
773-769-0205
773-769-0344—FAX
• Case management and counseling. Also offers transportation, referrals to low-cost housing, home-delivered meals, substance abuse treatment, support groups, nursing home or hospice care, and home health care. English/Spanish.

Community Response
225 Harrison Street
Oak Park, IL 60304
708-386-3383
708-386-3551—FAX
• Comprehensive support services for people with HIV/AIDS and their loved ones. Provides case management, food, long- and short-term housing assistance, referrals to mental health counseling, health and nutrition teaching, peer-led support groups, volunteer services and companions. Free. English/Spanish.

**Comprension y Apoyo a
Latinos en Oposicion al
Retrovirus (CALOR)**
2015 West Division Street
Chicago, IL 60622
773-235-3161
773-772-0484—FAX
• Case management and support groups for Spanish-speaking persons with HIV. Information on HIV-related issues, alternative therapies, and benefits. Free. English/Spanish.

**Cook County Department
of Public Health**
1010 Lake Street, Suite 300
Oak Park, IL 60301
708-445-2530
708-445-2130—FAX
708-445-2406—Hearing-impaired TTY/TDD
• Case management for northwest, west, south, and southwest suburban Cook County. Also provides dental services, anonymous and confidential HIV counseling and testing, health education, and referrals to physicians and other services in suburban Cook County. Free. English/Spanish.

**Cook County HIV
Primary Care Center**
1835 West Harrison Street
CCSN 1268
Chicago, IL 60612
312-633-3005
312-633-3002—FAX
• Case management, substance abuse and mental health treatment, housing referrals, financial assistance, food and transportation assistance. Other services available through the Cook County Hospital Women and Children's HIV Program. Free. English/Spanish.

Crusader Clinic
120 Tay Street
Rockford, IL 61102
815-968-0286
815-968-3881—FAX
• HIV/AIDS program provides case management, nutritional assessment, HIV primary care clinic, dental care, HIV counseling and testing, assistance with medications, financial assistance, substance abuse counseling, legal assistance, and DORS. Sliding scale fees. Public Aid accepted. English/Spanish.

DuPage County Health Department AIDS Program
111 North County Farm Road
Wheaton, IL 60187
630-682-7979, ext. 7310
630-462-9439—FAX
• HIV case management for residents of DuPage County, referrals to physicians, housing, and other services in DuPage County. Also provides free anonymous and confidential HIV counseling and testing, support groups, TB testing, health education, and transportation to appointments for those with HIV. English/Spanish.

Erie Family Health Center
1701 West Superior Street
Chicago, IL 60622
312-666-3488
312-666-5867—FAX
• HIV case management, primary care, and referrals. Confidential HIV counseling and testing. Public Aid accepted. English/Spanish.

Fox River Valley Center for Independent Living
730 West Chicago Street
Elgin, IL 60123
847-695-5818
847-695-5892—FAX
847-695-5818—Hearing-impaired TTY/TDD
• Case management, information and referrals, deaf services, housing referrals, independent living skills counseling, peer counseling and support, personal care assistant training, transportation, DORS, and training on using public transportation. Free. English/Spanish.

Garfield Counseling Center
4132 West Madison
Chicago, IL 60624
773-533-0433
773-533-6288—FAX
• HIV case management, HIV counseling and testing. Residential treatment and rehabilitation for chemically dependent injection drug users. English/Spanish.

Haymarket House
108-120 North Sangamon
Chicago, IL 60607
312-226-7984
312-226-0638—FAX
• Provides substance abuse detox, case management, residential and outpatient services for men and women, perinatal counseling, education, and HIV test counseling. Public Aid Accepted. English/Spanish.

Hemophilia Foundation of Illinois
332 South Michigan Avenue, Suite 1720
Chicago, IL 60604
312-427-1495
312-427-1602—FAX
• HIV case management, education and counseling for those with hemophilia. Financial counseling and DORS. English/Spanish.

Howard Area Community Center
7648 North Paulina Street
Chicago, IL 60626
773-262-6622
773-262-6645—FAX
• HIV case management, DORS, and other assistance services for low-income Rogers Park residents. Free. English/Spanish.

Howard Brown Health Center
945 West George Street
Chicago, IL 60657
773-871-5777
773-871-5843—FAX
• HIV case management, primary care, STD and HIV testing and counseling, support groups, substance abuse counseling, and referrals for legal and other assistance. English/Spanish.

Interventions
140 North Ashland Avenue
Chicago, IL 60607
312-633-4990
312-663-9059—FAX
• Case management, substance abuse assessment and treatment, detox, HIV counseling and testing. Free.

Lawndale Christian Health Center
3860 West Ogden Avenue
Chicago, IL 60632
773-521-5006
773-521-2742—FAX
• Case management, pastoral care, primary outpatient care,

transportation, support and referrals. Sliding scale fees. English/Spanish.

Love & Action Midwest
107 South Hi Lusi
Mount Prospect, IL 60056
847-392-3123
• Interdenominational Christian ministry provides spiritual, emotional, and physical support for HIV-impacted persons. Professional and volunteer services, home visits, support groups, volunteer training. Free.

Lutheran Social Services of Illinois
1144 West Lake Street
Oak Park, IL 60301
708-445-8341
708-445-8351—FAX
• "Second Family" program assists HIV-positive parents in making long-term plans for their children. Prospective adoptive "second families" trained and licensed. Support group for Gay/Lesbian parents affected by HIV, and case management for parents. "Positive Care" program places state wards with HIV/AIDS, and works with families in reuniting children with their parents. The program also offers medical care, parenting classes, and support groups. English/Spanish. Free.

Madison County AIDS Program (MADCAP)
2016 Madison Avenue
Granite City, IL 62040
618-877-5110
618-876-4952—FAX
• HIV case management, DORS, advocacy, information and referrals to local physicians and other services, financial assistance, home services, meals on wheels, anonymous HIV counseling and testing, lending library of HIV-related books and materials. Support groups for women, heterosexuals, and gay men. English/Spanish.

Minority Outreach Intervention Project (MOIP)
1579 North Milwaukee Avenue, Suite 314
Chicago, IL 60622
773-276-5990
773-276-3002–FAX
• Case management services to African-American and Latino gay and bisexual men who are HIV-positive or at risk. Peer support groups and prevention education for HIV-positive African-American men. Free. English/Spanish.

Open Door Clinic
164 Division Street, Suite 607
Elgin, IL 60120
847-695-1093
847-695-0501—FAX
847-695-8893—Hearing-impaired TTY/TDD
• Case management and information on support groups. Also offers anonymous and confidential HIV counseling and testing, STD testing/treatment, nutritionists, HIV primary care in Aurora and Elgin. Free. English/Spanish.

Pilsen Little Village Community Mental Health Center
2007 South Blue Island Avenue
Chicago, IL 60608
312-226-5864
312-226-7367—FAX
• HIV case management, health education, and a drop-in center for persons with HIV and their families. English/Spanish.

Southern Illinois University School of Medicine Clinics
751 North Rutledge
Springfield, IL 62702
217-782-0181
217-782-5504—FAX
• Comprehensive HIV services including case management, social services, primary care, dental care, and nutritional assessments.

Travelers & Immigrants Aid—Rafael Center
4750 North Sheridan Road, Suite 200
Chicago, IL 60640
773-989-0049
773-989-1935—FAX
• Comprehensive HIV/AIDS services including case management, mental health, HIV support groups, residential housing for people with HIV/AIDS. Substance abuse programs, including residential recovery house and groups for current substance users and recovering persons. Free. English/Spanish.

Treatment Alternatives for Safer Communities (TASC)
1500 North Halsted Street
Chicago, IL 60622
312-787-0208
312-738-8933—Health Services Manager
312-738-9260—FAX
• Provides HIV case management, individual counseling and education for men and women detained at Cook County Jail and youth at Cook County Juvenile Temporary Detention Center. Free. English/Spanish.

UIC Community Outreach Intervention Project
4407 North Broadway
Chicago, IL 60640
773-561-3177
773-561-8813—FAX
• Case management and primary care clinic for people with HIV. HIV/AIDS and substance abuse referrals, prevention education, HIV counseling and testing, peer support. Free. English/Spanish.

University of Illinois at Chicago
Community Health Project
4650 South Martin Luther King Drive
Chicago, IL 60653
773-536-4509
773-536-2306—FAX
• Case management, referrals, comprehensive HIV primary care, dental services, clinical trials, HIV counseling and testing, and prevention education. English/Spanish.

West Towns Visiting Nursing Service
6438 West 34th Street
Berwyn, IL 60402
708-749-7171
708-749-7185—FAX
• Case management, homebound mental health care, home-based hospice, bereavement, and spiritual support. Public Aid accepted. English/Spanish.

Westside Association for Community Action (WACA)
3600 West Ogden Avenue
Chicago, IL 60623
773-277-4400
773-277-0270—FAX
• Case management, substance abuse programs, and prevention education.

Will County Health Department
501 Ella Avenue
Joliet, IL 60433
815-727-8670
815-727-8852—FAX
815-727-8690—Hearing-impaired TTY/TDD
• Case management and referrals. Also provides anonymous and confidential HIV counseling and testing and primary care. English/Spanish.

Going It Alone: A Few Pointers for Navigating the System

If you decide to apply for public benefits yourself, you probably will find that a strategic, organized approach will help cut down on the runaround. When dealing with the various entitlement agencies:

1) *Don't wait to apply for programs you're eligible for.* The longer you put off applying, the longer you'll have to wait for benefits. Some programs have delays ranging from a few weeks to many months after you're accepted.

2) *Apply in person if at all possible.* Although it can be a hassle, it really does speed up the process significantly. If you're unable to visit the office in person, ask if you can apply by mail or phone.

3) *Always call ahead to see if you need to make an appointment.* If you just walk in, you may not get to apply for assistance that day—and you'll have wasted valuable time and transportation resources in the process.

If the office only takes applicants on a first come/first served basis, the least hectic times to go in are usually mid-week and mid-month. Try to get there right when they open to get a low number. Otherwise, you may find yourself waiting for several hours. If you can't get in first thing in the morning, be prepared to have your visit take the better part of the day. Arrange child care, wear comfortable clothing, and bring snacks and something to read or work on while you wait.

The public aid application process can be a very stressful experience. The trick is to be prepared for that stress, and plan to take care of yourself physically and mentally as you go through the system.

One hint: if you're comfortable telling the receptionist when you sign in that you're applying for benefits because you have AIDS, you may get seen earlier and be on your way sooner than if you offered no explanation.

4) *Make sure you have all the required documents with you before you make the visit.* It's no fun waiting in line for several hours only to find out you need one more form of I.D. or a different kind of income statement. Remember, you can never have too much documentation. At the very least, you'll want to gather your birth certificate, passport, or baptismal certificate; Social Security card; recent lease and rent receipts (or cancelled checks for those expenses); W-2 or income tax return for the previous year; and your three most recent bank statements. However, the exact list of documents needed will vary from program to program. Call to check out exactly what is required before you go.

Also, *never mail or give an original of a personal document to anyone.* If they lose it, you may not be able to replace it or be left with no

---

For anyone who's just starting to enter the realm of public assistance programs, I tell them, "You really need to focus on your situation and not listen to other people's horror stories. We don't know what the other person's situation was. We don't know if they provided accurate information. We don't know if what they're saying is a distortion of what actually took place." So take the information you hear at a meeting or at a support group, but always filter it through with "What is my situation?" Don't automatically anticipate the worst.

MICHELLE MASCARO
POLICY ASSOCIATE,
AIDS FOUNDATION OF CHICAGO

extra copy. Make copies and take them with you or ask the caseworker to make photocopies of everything while you wait.

5) *Be prepared to back up income and expense claims with written proof.** For instance, if you share an apartment, you must be able to show that you and your roommate(s) share all costs (rent, utilities) equally and that you purchase and prepare food separately. If you're no longer working, you must show some means of current support. This may be in the form of savings or loans from family or friends. You will be asked to provide letters from those who are loaning you money stating the amounts of the loans and that they expect to be repaid when your benefits are in place (regardless of whether this is actually the case).

* From <u>Living with AIDS</u>, Gay Men's Health Crisis.

6) *Keep records of your encounters with entitlement agencies.* Whenever you call or visit an agency to apply for benefits, or follow up or ask for information, it's a good idea to keep a log. (See Appendix D for a sample form to use.) Record what was discussed, what you learned, and what "next steps" there are, if any. Write down the name and title of everyone you talk to in case you have to get in touch with them again. Then store that notebook along with any and all benefits-related receipts, paperwork, or correspondence in a large, expandable file folder or shoe box. That way, you'll have everything you need in one place.

Lessons from the Front Lines
Contributed by Adam

I've been slipping and sliding around the AIDS world of red tape for quite awhile now. Being an impatient person by nature, and cheap by necessity, I have had to figure out the quickest and least expensive ways to get what I need for my health care and livelihood.

When Northwestern Memorial Hospital in Chicago decided to relieve me of getting my AZT for free, at a time when I had no money, no insurance, or any other financial means, I had to scramble. Instead of just giving up and doing without my medication, I started making calls. At that time, my only chance to get free drugs and doctor care was at Cook County Hospital. I spent a lot of time on the phone to that place.

Calling a major public hospital and reaching the right person or department is like calling the Pentagon in Washington, DC. It's tough to get anything accomplished. Still, I was fast running out of my AZT and had no choice. Through sheer persistence and force of will, I got myself an audience with one of the founding physicians of the already-overcrowded AIDS clinic and persuaded him to take me on as a patient. *Lesson #1: It's your life on the line. Don't give up.*

This was many years ago, and things have changed, so I can't pick on CCH as much as I used to. Probably the worst thing about it now is the waiting. I won't even talk about the hospital; staying overnight is like a scene from your worst nightmare. On the other hand, if you go to the AIDS clinic there, you will get good help from medical professionals for all areas of your body. Best of all, with only a little hassle, you can get your life-saving drugs for free (depending on your income). So you have to wait five hours to get your medications—that's the breaks. The way the system is set up, your time is their "money." *Lesson #2: Learn to deal with it. Cultivate ways to amuse yourself to make the waiting more tolerable.*

Insurance makes life much easier, but it costs so damn much money. Therefore at times, it's better to just learn to skirt the system. For instance, most people don't think you can pick your own doctor, especially at a "free clinic." You can. Check them out, find out who the nurses and clerks like the most, then give that doctor a try. If it doesn't work out, try again. Be honest with the person you settle on, that's how you'll get the best help.

Clinical trials are another way to get free health care and medications. Some studies pay for all of your blood work, doctor care, and drugs. I've even heard of some studies you stay with from cradle to grave; even if you're no longer taking the study drugs, they keep paying 100% for your care and medications. This is one hell of a deal, but do check the fine print before getting involved in any study. You can find out from your doctor if you qualify for one of these programs.

I think of this book you're reading as a manual for AIDS survival, but there are many more out there you'll want to look at. At my last visit to a major bookstore, I counted about 35 books on AIDS. Although most of them were about getting through this disease in the emotional sense, there were still plenty available on how to "work" the financial aspect. The key thing is, try not to become overwhelmed by all the information out there. Go after one thing that you need, see it through, then move on to the next thing to help you survive. It can be inebriating to try to read too many books or apply to too many AIDS programs. I have found myself at times with so much good information, in such large quantities, that I end up using none of it. *Lesson #3: Learn to be focused and only work on one need at a time.*

Incidentally, I'm not suggesting you actually go out and buy any of those books. Your local library can get almost any book published, including out-of-print ones, through interlibrary loan. It may take a few weeks to track down a particular book, but then you can read it for free and photocopy any pages containing information you want to keep. Same thing with newsletters and magazines. Why pay for a subscription when many will send out their publication free to people with HIV? AIDS service organizations also subscribe to one or more newsletters, and have current and back issues sitting around for you to read/copy. If you want to get your hands on a technical or medical journal that won't give out any freebies, ask your doctor if s/he subscribes, or ask the library of a nearby dental or medical school if they subscribe. Most public and many private schools will let you look at their collections on the premises at no charge. *Lesson #4, and this is a biggie: Never crack open your wallet unless you believe you've exhausted every other angle.*

What else is out there? Study the resources in this book and you can probably find anything you need. Throughout this country, there are federal, state, county, township, and community-based programs with money that need you so they have a reason to exist. There are also the much-harder-to-find private and business providers of help (like the big drug companies). Don't be shy when writing or calling any of the sources that you find. Don't be rude when they are, however. Remember, *you* are the expert in many cases, not them. That bugs the hell out of them, so try to be patient.

You can get information and services from so many sources, even though much of the hype does not apply to you. If you are a straight male who got the virus through sex, there is no reason on earth that you can't call up the National Hemophilia Foundation or the Gay and Lesbian Task Force. By the same token, don't think you won't be welcome at a place like Catholic Charities if you're not Catholic. You can be a Muslim fundamentalist or practice Wicca, and they will still help. Organizations like these can give you information and advice on how to get insurance, free food, legal advice, applications for drug trials, emergency housing, emergency money, and so on. If they can't help you directly, they'll know someone who can.

If you're not working, you should apply for SSDI or SSI. If you're eligible for SSDI it pays more, and after a year they give you a Medicare card. If they turn you down on your first or second try, keep going at it. Remember that Social Security must pay you all the way back to your *first* application. Some people end up with very large, one-time back payments. If you've worked in your life, these moneys are owed to you. *Lesson #5: Apply early, apply often.*

It has always been my position that I am deathly ill and have no money or resources. I make this known to hospitals and clinics so I can see a doctor before the next century, and so when the hospital social worker (finance department) comes for money, I can tell them it's time to get creative concerning my visit. If federal money was used in the building of the hospital, by law they must accommodate you. They won't like it, and they may say I don't know of what I speak. But if you tell them you can't sell your car for medical reasons and you must pay your rent and utilities, and still have enough left over to buy a few morsels of food, they will go into the dusty old rule books and then miraculously come back to you and say there is a way.

This happens most of the time, if not all of the time; so if you know what hospital you'll be using in an emergency, check up on its policies. Also, if you are hospitalized due to AIDS, ask your doctor to give you some extra medication to take home so you'll save money on buying prescriptions. *Lesson #6: As in business, ask for the moon and the stars, or just a great deal more than you need, and you will probably get what you can live with.*

I can tell you from my own experience, it's possible to have AIDS and not spend every cent you have. Think of it as US vs. THEM. It may sound a little paranoid, but you must take care of your health first and foremost. If you find a new, handy money-and-time-saving scam, share it with as many people as you can. By "scam," I don't mean anything illegal (necessarily)—just a way to slip around a stupid obstacle or series of obstacles. Over time, work up your attack plan for all these things. Remember that in most cases, the person who cares and worries about your health and welfare the most is not a doctor, case manager, bureaucrat, or even a relative. It's *you*.

True fact: finding your way through the maze can be entertaining if you sell yourself on the right way to do it. It's good for your health to have something to do, and taking care of yourself is a very important thing to do. Once you've come out of the maze and know some of the so-called "secrets," you will attain the status of guru, and people will come to seek out your wisdom. This is a wonderful thing. It feels great to truly help another person with AIDS, and meanwhile those T cells keep rising.

Good luck, and remember patience…that's the most important lesson of all.

Social Security Administration Programs

1) *Social Security Disability Insurance (SSDI)*. If you've had a paying job or been self-employed, you've probably been contributing to the Social Security system in the form of federal FICA or self-employment taxes. If you have to leave your job or occupation due to disability, you automatically qualify for income through SSDI (provided you paid in enough taxes to accrue benefits). This income is not "charity" or a handout, but money you paid in over time that will be paid back to you now that you're disabled.

   SSDI is the highest paying benefit program that exists. The amount of money you receive each month is calculated based on your lifetime average earnings under Social Security before you became disabled. Still, the SSDI income you'll receive will be only a small portion of what you made at your job. (That's one reason why many people with AIDS who can continue to work still do so.)

   SSDI is not a need-based program. You aren't limited in terms of the amount of assets or property you may own or income you may draw from private (non-wage earning) sources. The only qualification is that you worked long enough and recently enough under

Social Security to be insured. The people at the Social Security office can tell you whether you qualify, and how much you can expect to receive each month you're "on disability."

SSDI benefits are paid for as long as you're disabled. The program is not considered a permanent form of disability coverage. You may decide you're able to go back to work at some point, or find some way to change or adjust your work habits such that you'll no longer need benefits. However, if you remain disabled for the rest of your life, you'll continue to receive SSDI income.

There are also allowances under SSDI for "trial work situations," during which you can draw some benefits while you attempt to make the transition back into productive employment. This is a very complicated process, however. If you go this route, you will probably want to seek the advice of an experienced case manager.

The biggest downside to SSDI is the long waiting period involved—five months from the date you become disabled or the last day you worked until you become eligible, then another full month before you receive your first check. If your savings and other assets are limited, you may qualify for other assistance while you're waiting for SSDI to kick in. Your case manager can help you plan for gaps in financial and insurance coverage.

Apply for SSDI at your local Social Security office. Before starting the process, call Social Security or ask your case manager to find out what documents you need to prove how much and how long you paid into the system. You'll also need proof of your AIDS diagnosis or HIV-related disability (probably in the form of a letter from your doctor).

Even if you're not sure whether you actually want to go on disability soon, it's recommended that you apply for SSDI. You can always withdraw your application if you decide you're well enough to keep working.

For more information on SSDI, or the location of the Social Security office nearest you, call:

Social Security Administration (Illinois)
800-772-1213 (English/Spanish)
7 a.m.-7 p.m., Mon-Fri

If you live outside Illinois, check the government listings in your phone book, under "Social Security Administration."

Be sure to have your Social Security number near the phone. The people who answer can respond to questions, send application materials, and make appointments for you at your local Social Security office.

Books and Publications

NAPWA Fax
National Association of People with AIDS
202-789-2222—FAX
• Dozens of insurance and benefits publications available by fax, including guides to SSI, disability, and Medicaid benefits. Request the "Living with HIV" fax catalog of fax documents in English. A Spanish catalog is also available. You must be at a fax machine to use the NAPWA Fax service.

"A Guide to Social Security and SSI Disability Benefits for People with HIV Infection"
Mail order: CDC National AIDS Clearinghouse
800-458-5231—English/Spanish
800-243-7012—Hearing-impaired TTY/TDD
• Available in English and Spanish. Free.

2) *Supplemental Security Income (SSI)*. SSI is a federal income program for needy disabled people, regardless of whether they've ever been employed. SSI cash payments are substantially lower than SSDI payments. The amount of assets and property you can own and still qualify for SSI is strictly limited. In addition, you must be a U.S. citizen or legal alien to qualify.

Children may qualify for SSI if they are "on the record" of a person receiving disability or retirement benefits from Social Security, and are eligible for benefits through age 18 if a parent has died. Applications for children must include a birth certificate, social security number, and income of the parent or guardian. Children are also eligible for disability benefits if they meet certain criteria or if they have an impairment that reduces their ability to do things that children of a similar age normally do. Children with AIDS are "presumed eligible" until their application has been considered, and they can receive benefits faster than if they went through the normal eligibility review.

If you qualify for SSI, you automatically qualify for basic health care coverage under Medicaid. (For a description of this program, see the section on "Illinois Department of Public Aid Programs.")

If you have low or no income and few assets and are applying for SSDI, SSI can provide some money to tide you over through the five-month SSDI waiting period. Or, if you've been on General Assistance through the state of Illinois, when you become disabled, you'll switch over to SSI.

Once you're accepted, SSI benefits don't take nearly as long to get as SSDI benefits. However, it may still take several weeks before your first check arrives. When you apply for SSI, ask about other short-term assistance programs to help fill in the gaps. In Illinois, these programs may include:

- Presumptive Supplemental Security Income. Presumes the applicant will qualify for SSDI. Takes 4-6 weeks for persons with a confirmed AIDS diagnosis.
- Interim General Assistance. Small cash loans that you will have to repay. Loaned amounts will be deducted from your first SSI check.
- State Supplemental Payments. Small additional monthly cash grants for special expenses. Availability to qualified SSDI and SSI recipients determined on a case-by-case basis.

The latter two programs are administered through the Illinois Department of Public Aid. The intake worker at the Social Security office will give you a letter of introduction to take to the Public Aid office. This letter will verify that you have applied for SSI.

For more information, contact the Social Security Administration or:

Illinois Department of Public Aid
624 South Michigan Avenue
Chicago, IL 60605
800-252-8635
8:30 a.m.-4:45 p.m. Mon-Fri
- Information and eligibility requirements for Interim General Assistance and State Supplemental Payments. English/Spanish.

3) *Medicare.* Medicare is a federally-sponsored medical insurance program for people 65 or older and for people who have been getting Social Security disability benefits for two years. Eligible applicants automatically receive hospitalization, hospice, home health care, and skilled nursing facility coverage under Medicare "Part A." They may also elect to pay a small additional monthly premium for Medicare "Part B," which covers basic medical and some in-home health care. (For disabled persons who request "Part B," the premium is deducted from their SSDI checks.)

Special programs are in place to help low-income people participate in Medicare. The Illinois Department of Public Aid can provide assistance in paying for premiums (for both Parts A and B), deductible expenses, and co-insurance charges.

Medicare does not pay for drugs and medications. These may be covered under private insurance plans, Medicaid, or through the Federal AIDS Drug Assistance Program.

On the plus side, Medicare is a good health care plan. On the minus side, it takes a long time to kick in—*thirty-one months* from the time you become disabled and apply for SSDI:

- 5-month-plus-1 waiting period for SSDI to begin, plus—
- 24 months (2 years) of SSDI payments required, plus—
- 1 additional month after receiving the 24th SSDI check before Medicare coverage begins.

The best thing to do is to apply for Medicare at the same time you apply for SSDI—and then forget about it while you maintain other forms of health coverage. Again, your case manager can help you plan ahead and sort through your insurance options.

For more information about Medicare, call:

Medicare Hotline
800-638-6833
8 a.m.-8 p.m. (Eastern Time), Mon-Fri

Social Security Administration (Illinois)
800-772-1213 (English/Spanish)
7 a.m.-7 p.m., Mon-Fri

Illinois Department of Public Aid (IDPA) Programs

IDPA programs provide cash payments, food stamps, and help with medical bills for qualifying individuals. Some of the key Illinois programs include:

- Aid to Families with Dependent Children (AFDC)
- Aid to the Aged, Blind, or Disabled (AABD)
- Refugee and Repatriate Assistance (RPA)
- General Assistance (GA)
- Medicaid (MediPlan)
- Medical Assistance No Grant (MANG)
- Special Pregnant Women and Children Programs (AFDC)
- Food Stamps (FS)
- Women, Infant, and Children Supplemental Food Program (WIC)
- Illinois Department of Rehabilitation Services (DORS)

Cash Programs

Cash programs are meant to help people meet basic needs. These programs help clients pay for food, shelter, utilities, and other non-medical expenses. People who qualify for cash also get medical coverage.

The four cash programs are:

1) *Aid to Families with Dependent Children (AFDC)*. The AFDC cash program provides money to qualifying families with dependent children, and to some pregnant women. These families receive a Medicaid (MediPlan) card for help with their medical needs.

2) *Aid to the Aged, Blind, or Disabled (AABD)*. AABD is a cash program for qualifying individuals. AABD recipients also receive a MediPlan card. There are several sub-programs within AABD.

For instance, AABD(A) helps people who are at least age 65; AABD(B) helps those who are blind as defined by the Social Security Administration (SSA); AABD(D) helps individuals who have been found by SSA to be disabled.

A person who is financially eligible can receive AABD when they are denied SSI because of income and are at least 65 years of age, or have been found to be blind or disabled by IDPA.

3) *Refugee and Repatriate Assistance (RPA)*. The Refugee Resettlement Program (RRP) provides assistance to the following individuals:

- those admitted to the U.S. as a "refugee," "asylee," or "conditional entrant";
- resident noncitizens who were formerly refugees;
- Amerasian immigrants and close family members from Vietnam admitted through the Orderly Departure Program; and/or
- Cubans or Haitians granted parole or issued a valid form I-94 on or after April 21, 1980.

The Repatriate Program provides assistance for up to 90 days to U.S. citizens who moved to another country and were then sent back to the U.S. for various reasons. Only those referred by the Department of Health and Human Services can receive help from this program.

4) *General Assistance (GA)*. Individuals who do not qualify for AFDC, AABD, or RRA may receive cash and limited medical benefits through the state's General Assistance (GA) program. In Chicago, this program is run by IDPA. Outside the city, townships that receive state funds run the program based on IDPA policy.

There are two types of General Assistance. Family and Children Assistance (GA-FCA) serves eligible families that do not qualify for AFDC or RPA, except in cases where the family was refused help through these programs because they failed to cooperate, or because they received a lump sum payment. Transitional Assistance serves eligible individuals who do not qualify for AABD or RPA and do not receive SSI, except for the same exclusions listed for GA-FCA (above).

Other Illinois Programs

1) *Medicaid (MediPlan)*. Medicaid provides assistance for people who need help paying their medical bills. The program is sponsored jointly by the federal government and individual states. Thus, benefit levels and eligibility requirements vary from state to state. If you were turned down for Medicaid in another state, apply again in Illinois (or any other state you might move to). There's nothing to lose by applying, and you just might qualify.

If you already receive money through another Public Aid program, you are eligible for Medicaid (otherwise known as MediPlan). If you do not already receive money from Public Aid, but need help paying your medical bills, you still may be eligible for Medicaid. If you are pregnant, you may be eligible for immediate coverage under Medicaid before you apply for assistance at your Public Aid office.

Soon after you qualify, you will receive a MediPlan card (also known as a Medicaid "green card"). You can present this card to hospitals, doctors, dentists, optometrists, clinics, and pharmacies that accept Medicaid reimbursement for their services. Medicaid patients must go to a medical provider who is approved to participate in the program, and who has agreed to accept IDPA payment.

For more information on Medicaid (MediPlan) benefits and/or eligibility requirements, call:

Illinois Department of Public Aid
800-252-8635 (English/Spanish)
8:30 a.m.-4:45 p.m. Mon-Fri

2) *Medical Assistance No Grant (MANG)*. MANG programs serve individuals who qualify for medical assistance but have enough income and assets to meet basic needs. Certain participants are also eligible for a monthly MediPlan Card. Depending on the individual's assets and income, a "spend-down" may apply. IDPA does not pay medical expenses used to meet spend-down. (Contact your case manager or IDPA for details on what spend-down currently entails.)

Noncitizens with an emergency medical need may qualify for the MANG program. They do not have to be in this country lawfully, nor do they need a Social Security number. However, they must meet all income, asset, and other rules of the AABD or AFDC program.

Special AABD MANG programs are also in place to help disabled adult children, qualified severely impaired individuals, and others who receive Social Security Disabled Widow/Widowers' benefits and meet eligibility criteria.

3) *Special Pregnant Women and Children Programs (AFDC)*. IDPA has special medical programs for eligible pregnant women and their children. These programs have higher income standard than the regular AFDC program. They are for pregnant women who are not eligible for AFDC or MANG, but do qualify for the "Healthy Start" program.

4) *Food Stamps.* The Food Stamp program is a federal nutrition program run by IDPA according to U.S.D.A. eligibility guidelines. If you are on SSI, GA, or AFDC, or if you are on SSDI and are sufficiently needy, you may automatically qualify for Food Stamps. *Ask for Food Stamps when you apply for any assistance program.* You can also apply for Food Stamps at any Public Aid office if you're not on one of these programs but still have low or no income.

   Food Stamps cover only food, and may not be used for tobacco, alcohol, paper or cleaning products, pet food, and some ready-to-eat foods.

5) *Women, Infant, and Children Supplemental Food Program (WIC).* WIC is a program of the Illinois Department of Public Health. It assists low-income pregnant and nursing women, high-risk infants, and children considered to be at risk with food coupons and nutritional education and guidance. You need not reveal your HIV status to receive assistance. Call your local health department for a referral.

6) *Illinois Department of Rehabilitation Services (DORS).* The DORS Home Services Program offers in-home health care, respite care, meals, medical equipment, and living assistance aimed at keeping the sick or disabled HIV-positive person out of the hospital or long-term care facility. To apply for DORS, you must first apply for Medicaid. Even if you don't qualify financially for Medicaid (or if you have other insurance resources), you may still qualify for the DORS portion of Medicaid. Contact:

   Illinois Department of Rehabilitation Services (DORS)
   6200 North Hiawatha Street, Suite 300
   Chicago, IL 60646
   773-794-4800
   or:
   Illinois Department of Rehabilitation Services (DORS)
   623 East Adams, PO Box 19429
   Springfield, IL 62794
   217-782-2093

Housing and Rental Assistance

Many people living with AIDS find it hard to pay for adequate housing. Prolonged illness inevitably means health care and living expenses will be higher while income will often be lower, due to disability. The National Commission on AIDS has reported that up to one-half of PWAs are either homeless or in imminent danger of becoming so.

Eventually, you may find that your needs include rental assistance, housing support services, or even intermediate care or hospice facilities. Federal funds have been appropriated through the Housing Opportunities for People With AIDS (HOPWA) program to provide rent subsidies, advocacy, support services, and representation in housing-related legal cases. The grants are not a permanent solution, but they can get you through some tough times. Compensation can range from one month's rent or security deposit to 3- to 6-month subsidies.

To apply, you'll need to provide proof of your HIV-positive status or AIDS diagnosis, monthly rent expenses, income, and living-arrangement information (i.e., if a partner, spouse, or roommate is helping share expenses).

Most communities have programs that provide shelter, food, meal delivery, transportation, clothing, case management, counseling, emergency financial assistance, homebound services, or other forms of assistance to eligible residents, including persons with HIV.

Here are some other easy ways to find the services you need:

- Call the human services division of your local township, county, or village. Ask about available services and eligibility requirements.
- Talk to an HIV case manager at any AIDS service organization. Most will be glad to provide you with referrals, even if you're not their client.
- Check the agencies listed under "Case Management and Related HIV/AIDS Services" (earlier in this section), "Local Hospitals and HIV Clinics" (located in Part 3), or resources for specific clients (such as women, children, or people of color—see the listings in Part 1). Many AIDS service organizations provide comprehensive assistance with food, shelter and other basic needs.
- Look in the yellow pages under "Social Service Organizations," or call your local United Way office.

Housing, Food, Transportation, and Other Resources

Housing Assistance

Access Living
310 South Peoria Street,
Suite 201
Chicago, IL 60607
312-226-5900
312-226-2030—FAX
312-226-8976—Hearing-impaired TTY/TDD
• A center for independent living, serving people with disabilities. Peer counseling, "Transition to Independence" program, education, advocacy, domestic violence program, personal assistant training, and referrals. English, Spanish, American Sign Language.

AIDS Care
315 West Barry
Chicago, IL 60657
773-935-4663
773-935-4662—FAX
• Long-term housing for people with advanced HIV disease. Continuum of care through personal physicians and outside agencies. Residents are provided with case management, food, and basic necessities, as well as pastoral care and counseling. Public Aid accepted.

AIDS Legal Council of Chicago
220 South State Street,
Suite 1330
Chicago, IL 60604
312-427-8990
312-427-8419—FAX

Outreach program office at:
Cook County Hospital
1900 West Polk Street,
Room 634-635
Chicago IL 60612
312-733-8026
312-633-8651—FAX
• Legal advice and service in housing and landlord/tenant law, among other areas.

AIDS Ministry of Illinois
68 North Chicago Street,
Suite 240
Joliet, IL 60432-4380
815-723-1548
815-740-5910—FAX
• Provides transitional housing to promote independent living. Long-term rent subsidies for those with mental illness and AIDS.

Asian American AIDS Foundation
4750 North Sheridan Road,
Suite 429
Chicago, IL 60640
773-989-7220
773-989-7769—FAX
• Housing through Asian House. Free. Multilingual (Asian languages).

Association for Individual Development
765 Orchard Avenue
Aurora, IL 60506
630-859-1291
630-859-2994—FAX
• Serves HIV-positive individuals who are homeless and/or substance users. Also serves persons who are developmentally and/or physically disabled or mentally ill. Case management, prevention services, and education. English/Spanish.

Association House of Chicago
2150 West North Avenue
Chicago, IL 60647
773-276-0084
773-276-7395—FAX
• Residential programs for the economically, mentally, and/or physically disabled. Shelter for women. Emergency shelter. Legal services. English/Spanish.

Austin People's Action Center
5931 West Corcoran Place
Chicago, IL 60644
773-921-2121
773-626-4911—FAX
• Housing assistance with sliding scale fees.

Better Existence with HIV (BEHIV)
PO Box 5171
Evanston, IL 60204
847-475-2115
847-475-2820—FAX
• Financial assistance for rent and utilities. "Safe Start" program assists homeless persons with an AIDS diagnosis who have a mental illness and/or use substances. Serves northern Chicago and north/northwest suburbs. Free. English/Spanish.

Bonaventure House
PO Box 148187
Chicago, IL 60614
773-327-9921
773-327-9113—FAX
• Residential service for PWAs offering case management, assistance with residential health care and hospice services, support groups, pastoral care, and transportation to doctor appointments. Sliding scale fees.

Casa Central
1401 North California
Chicago, IL 60622
773-276-1902
773-276-0465—FAX
• Transitional housing for families, adult day care, foster care, day care, domestic violence programs, and assistance with necessities for families. Sliding scale fees. English/Spanish.

Catholic Charities
126 North Desplaines Street
Chicago, IL 60661
312-655-7715
312-263-4290—FAX

**Catholic Charities—
Southwest Suburban**
10661 South Roberts Road
Palos Hills, IL 60465
708-430-0428
708-430-0502—FAX

**Catholic Charities—
West Suburban**
1400 South Austin Boulevard
Cicero, IL 60804
708-209-1110
708-209-1124—FAX
• Emergency assistance with basic needs, including rent and shelter. Information and referrals. English/Spanish.

**Catholic Charities—
Lake County**
671 South Lewis Avenue
Waukegan, IL 60085
847-249-3500
847-623-6750—FAX
• Emergency financial assistance for housing, food, and transportation. Free. English/Spanish.

**Chicago House and
Social Service Agency**
PO Box 14728
Chicago, IL 60614
773-248-5200
773-248-5019—FAX
• Three long-term housing facilities and scattered site apartments, each geared toward a different stage of HIV disease. Eligibility based on diagnosis, need, ability to live in a group setting, and willingness to abide by rules banning drug/alcohol use. Provides case management to clients in residence as well as the community. Sliding scale fees. English/Spanish.

The Children's Place
3059 West Augusta Boulevard
Chicago, IL 60622
773-826-1230
773-826-0705—FAX
• Temporary residential home for children from birth-5 years. Services available to natural or foster parents and siblings. Free. English/Spanish.

**Community and Economic
Development Association of
Cook County (CEDA)**
224 North Desplaines Street
Chicago, IL 60601
312-207-5444
312-207-6943—FAX
• Emergency housing, food, weatherization, and utility payments for HIV-positive residents of suburban Cook County. Free. English/Spanish.

Community Response
225 Harrison Street
Oak Park, IL 60304
708-386-3383
708-386-3551—FAX
• Long- and short-term housing assistance. "Shelter Plus Care" program pays most rent and utilities, plus intensive case management for eligible homeless persons. Free. English/Spanish.

**Community Supportive
Living Systems, Inc.**
10837 South Western Avenue,
Suite 2
Chicago, IL 60643
773-239-0501
773-239-9309—FAX
• Provides transitional, second stage, and permanent housing for low-income males age 18 years and over with HIV/AIDS. Independent and assisted residential housing, scattered site apartments. Case management, social services. Sliding scale fees. Public Aid accepted.

Cornerstone Services, Inc.
800 Black Road
Joilet, IL 60435
815-774-3660
815-727-6661—FAX
• Residential, vocational, group and individual counseling and financial assistance to persons with HIV/AIDS. Free.

**Department of Health
and Human Services**
800-654-8595
312-744-5000
312-744-3996—Hearing-
impaired TTY/TDD
• 24-hour emergency service refers to city-sponsored homeless shelters, domestic violence shelters, and other emergency services in

Chicago. Assists with transportation to shelters, if needed. Intake and referrals during normal business hours at local community service offices. Call for locations. Free. English/Spanish.

DuPage County Health Department AIDS Program
111 North County Farm Road
Wheaton, IL 60187
630-682-7979, ext. 7310
630-462-9439—FAX
• Help in accessing housing and utility assistance.

Fox River Valley Center for Independent Living
730 West Chicago Street
Elgin, IL 60123
847-695-5818
847-695-5892—FAX
847-695-5818—Hearing-impaired TTY/TDD
• Housing referrals and independent living skills counseling. Free. English/Spanish.

Genesis House
911 West Addison Street
Chicago, IL 60613
773-281-3917
773-281-0961—FAX
• Shelter and housing referrals for women who have been or are involved in prostitution. On-site residence program for women who have gone through a detox program and are in recovery. Free.

Genesis House— West Side Satellite
743 South Sacramento
Chicago, IL 60612
773-533-8701
773-533-8705—FAX
• Referrals to shelters for women who have been or are involved in prostitution.

Greater Community AIDS Project
PO Box 713
Champaign, IL 61824
217-351-2437
• Transitional housing and support services for those with HIV/AIDS and their loved ones.

Kelzer Care Center
5129 South Throop Street
Chicago, IL 60609
773-268-8438—Voice/FAX
• Transitional housing for males for up to one year. Case management and nutritional service.

Legal Assistance Foundation of Chicago
343 South Dearborn Street, Suite 700
Chicago, IL 60604
312-341-1070
312-347-8311—HIV Housing Law Project
312-341-1041—FAX
312-431-1206—Hearing-impaired TTY/TDD
• Legal counseling and advocacy for low-income persons with HIV/AIDS in all housing-related matters. Legal services in civil law matters to Chicago residents unable to afford legal counsel. Free. English/Spanish.

Omni, Incorporated Initiative
4004 West Division
Chicago, IL 60651
773-278-6106
773-486-7773—FAX
• Substance abuse and housing programs for persons with HIV/AIDS. Case management. Referrals to other services.

New Phoenix Assistance Center
7624 South Phillips, #1A
Chicago, IL 60649
773-978-6322
773-978-6056—FAX
• Scattered site housing available for females j233 with HIV/AIDS over age 21. Call for eligibility screening. Sliding scale fees.

Northern Illinois AIDS Resource Center
4505 North Main Street
Rockford, IL 61103
815-633-1660
815-633-1790—FAX
• Staffed residential housing program with access to support services, including AA/NA meetings, home delivered meals, legal services, mental health counseling, and home health services.

Public Action to Deliver Shelter (PADS)
773-737-7070—Southwest Chicago PADS
708-681-5517—Tri-Village PADS (Maywood)
708-754-4357—South Suburban PADS (Cook County)
630-682-3846—DuPage PADS
630-897-2165—Hesed House (Aurora)
847-622-5476—Northwest Suburban PADS (Cook County)
847-249-0737—PADS Place (Lake County)
• Shelter, transitional housing, and resources for homeless persons. Sites in many communities throughout the Chicago metropolitan area. Call for locations and availability of participating shelters. Free.

St. Catherine's of Genoa Catholic Worker
842 East 65th Street
Chicago, IL 60637
773-288-3688
• Transitional residence for homeless HIV-positive men and women. All residents required to have a case manager and/or be in a substance abuse program. Length of stay is assessed monthly. Also provides hospice housing. Free. English/Spanish.

Travelers and Immigrants Aid—San Miguel Apartments
907 West Argyle Avenue
Chicago, IL 60640
773-271-5800
773-271-5918—FAX
• Housing for men, women, and children with HIV/AIDS. English/Spanish.

Travelers & Immigrants Aid—Neon Street Center
4822 North Broadway,
2nd Floor
Chicago, IL 60640
773-271-6366
773-271-8810—FAX
• Multiservice drop-in center for homeless youth ages 13-21. Housing, food, counseling, education, and outreach. Free.

Travelers & Immigrants Aid—Rafael Center
4750 North Sheridan Road,
Suite 200
Chicago, IL 60640
773-989-0049
773-989-1935—FAX
• Residential housing for people with HIV/AIDS, residential recovery house, day and respite care, emergency shelters, and financial assistance for men, women and teens with HIV/AIDS. Free. English/Spanish.

Veterans Administration Medical Center—North Chicago
3001 Green Bay Road
North Chicago, IL 60064
847-688-1900, ext. 1551
847-578-3863—FAX
708-578-3841—Hearing-impaired TDD/TTY
• Services for eligible veterans including housing/shelter, day and respite care, and financial assistance.

Will County Center for Community Concerns
1 Doris Avenue
Joliet, IL 60433
815-722-0722
815-722-6344—FAX
• Emergency rent and mortgage assistance, utilities assistance, home rehabilitation, weatherization, low-income home energy assistance, and housing counseling. English/Spanish. Free.

Meals-On-Wheels and Other Food Programs

Call the following offices to determine your eligibility and meal prices.

Better Existence with HIV (BEHIV)
PO Box 5171
Evanston, IL 60204
847-475-2115
847-475-2820—FAX
• Food pantry. Serves northern Chicago and north/northwest suburbs. Free. English/Spanish.

Community Response
225 Harrison Street
Oak Park, IL 60304
708-386-3383
708-386-3551—FAX
• Food pantry serves the Austin area of Chicago and west suburban Cook County. Free. English/Spanish.

DuPage County Health Department AIDS Program
111 North County Farm Road
Wheaton, IL 60187
630-682-7979, ext. 7310
• Distributes non-perishable food to people living with HIV/AIDS in DuPage County. Free. English/Spanish.

Evanston Meals-at-Home
1350 Ashland Avenue
Wilmette, IL 60091
847-251-6827
• Meals delivered to homebound individuals 5 days a week. Special diets accepted. Sliding scale fees.

Groceryland
3902 North Sheridan
Chicago, IL 60613
773-244-0088
773-665-1000—Rogers Park/Edgewater, Chicago
773-486-0200—Humboldt Park, Chicago
773-224-1444—South Side, Chicago
• Open Hand grocery centers provide weekly food for people with HIV and AIDS. Referrals through HIV case managers. Free.

The HIV Coalition (HIVCO)
1471 Business Center Drive,
Suite 500
Mount Prospect, IL 60056
847-391-9803
847-391-9839—Hand-to-Hand
Food Line
847-391-9826—FAX
• Distributes non-perishable food to people with HIV/AIDS living in suburban Cook, Lake, McHenry, and Kane Counties. Free. English/Spanish.

Madison County AIDS Program (MADCAP)
2016 Madison Avenue
Granite City, IL 62040
618-877-5110
618-876-4952—FAX
• Home-delivered meals for people with HIV. English/Spanish.

Meals on Wheels— Riverside Medical Center
350 North Wall
Kankakee, IL 60901
815-935-7871
815-936-6559—FAX
• Meal services based on physician orders for residents of Kankakee, Bradley, and Bourbonnais.

Open Hand Chicago
1648 West Howard Street
Chicago, IL 60626
773-665-1000
773-665-0044—FAX
• Home-delivered meals program includes two meals (one hot, one cold box lunch) delivered by volunteers Monday-Friday, 5 p.m.-8 p.m. Modified meals available. Clients may also pick up food in four grocery centers throughout Chicago. Free. English/Spanish.

Transportation

Call your local public transportation system, township, or village to ask about special services for people with disabilities, including people with HIV/AIDS. In the Chicago metropolitan area, contact:

Regional Transit Authority (RTA)
ADA Paratransit Program
181 West Madison
Chicago, IL 60602
312-917-4357—Application forms
312-917-1339—FAX
312-917-1338—Hearing-impaired TTY/TDD
• Provides transportation discounts and services for people with disabilities, including persons with HIV/AIDS. Also offers door-to-door services to people who, as a result of their disability, are unable to use the main bus and rail system. Transportation provided by PACE and CTA. You must preregister for this service and be within the PACE/CTA service area. Applications available in English and Spanish.

FISH of Park Ridge
PO Box 86
Park Ridge, IL 60068
847-698-3478—24-hour answering service
• Transportation assistance to the doctor, hospital, shopping, and other places. Free of charge for people in the Park Ridge area.

Other Help with Basic and Emergency Needs

Actors' Fund of America
203 North Wabash, Suite 2104
Chicago, IL 60601
312-372-0989
312-372-0272—FAX
• Financial assistance, social services, case management, and community referrals for those who have made a living in the entertainment industries.

Association House of Chicago
2150 West North Avenue
Chicago, IL 60647
773-276-0084
773-276-7395—FAX
• Emergency food, shelter, and clothing. Shelter for women. Legal services and foster care. Residential and addiction recovery programs for the economically, mentally, and/or physically disabled. English/Spanish.

Austin People's Action Center
5931 West Corcoran Place
Chicago, IL 60644
773-921-2121
773-626-4911—FAX
• Emergency food pantry, advocacy and referrals, medical transportation. Free.

Catholic Charities
126 North Desplaines Street
Chicago, IL 60661
312-655-7715
312-263-4290—FAX

Catholic Charities— Southwest Suburban
10661 South Roberts Road
Palos Hills, IL 60465
708-430-0428
708-430-0502—FAX

**Catholic Charities—
West Suburban**
1400 South Austin Boulevard
Cicero, IL 60804
708-209-1110
708-209-1124—FAX
• Emergency assistance with basic needs, including food, clothing, and shelter. Information and referrals. English/Spanish.

**Catholic Charities—
Lake County**
671 South Lewis Avenue
Waukegan, IL 60085
847-249-3500
847-623-6750—FAX
• Emergency financial assistance for housing, food, and transportation. Free. English/Spanish.

Chase House—North, South, and West locations:
1133 North LaSalle
Chicago, IL 60610
312-751-8887
312-751-3904—FAX

2555 East 73rd Street
Chicago, IL 60649
773-374-0422
773-374-0370—FAX

1657 North Karlov
Chicago, IL 60639
773-486-9479
773-486-1240—FAX
• Family support services for HIV-impacted families. Food distribution, transportation, mental health referrals, family and youth/teen counseling, and day and respite care.

**Connection Crisis
Intervention and
Referral Services**
PO Box 906
Libertyville, IL 60048
847-362-3381
847-367-1080—24-hour crisis and referral service
800-310-1234—Teen Line
847-362-8783—FAX
• The best "one stop shop" if you need referrals to assistance programs, general social services, and mental health agencies in the Chicago metropolitan area. Trained crisis workers can help with a wide range of emergency and basic needs beyond HIV, such as domestic violence, shelter, and food. Provides telephone support and referrals for depression/suicidal thoughts. Free.

Direct AID
3439 North Halsted, Basement
Chicago, IL 60657
773-528-9448
• Financial assistance with rent, utilities, and food for people with and AIDS diagnosis in the Chicago metropolitan area.

Firman Community Services
144 West 47th Street
Chicago, IL 60609
733-373-3400
773-373-3602—FAX
• Emergency food distribution and clothing, child care for children age 3-13, and foster care services. Most services free except day care.

Genesis House
911 West Addison Street
Chicago, IL 60613
773-281-3917
773-281-0961—FAX
• Provides food, clothing, counseling, case management, and risk reduction education to women who have been or are involved in prostitution.

**Genesis House—
West Side Satellite**
743 South Sacramento
Chicago, IL 60612
773-533-8701
773-533-8705—FAX
• Provides food, clothing, counseling, case management, detox and treatment, and risk reduction education to women who have been or are involved in prostitution. Free medical care and HIV testing.

Illinois AIDS Hotline
800-243-2437—Hotline staffed 8 a.m.-11 p.m., 7 days/week
800-782-0423—Hearing-impaired TTY/TDD
• Referrals to health services, HIV case management, and general social services throughout Illinois. English/Spanish.

Illinois Department of Rehabilitation Services (DORS)
6200 North Hiawatha Street, Suite 300
Chicago, IL 60646
773-794-4800
773-794-4830—FAX
773-794-4826—Hearing-impaired TTY/TDD
• Home services accessible through case management. Program includes personal assistants, homemakers, home health program, home-delivered meals, respite care, and minor home remodeling to accomplish daily activities. Referrals to other offices in the Chicago metropolitan area. English/Spanish.

Marillac House
2822 West Jackson
Chicago, IL 60612
773-722-5157
773-722-1469—FAX
• Emergency food and clothing for persons in need.

NIA Comprehensive Center
1808 South State Street
Chicago, IL 60616-1611
312-949-1808
312-949-9415—FAX
• Respite care with light housekeeping up to 180 hours per year, family improvement counseling, case management, speech therapy, parenting classes. "Focus Program" for people with developmental disabilities. "SAFIT Program" for high-risk moms. Free.

People's Resource Center—Wheaton
1506 East Roosevelt Road
Wheaton, IL 60187
630-682-3844
630-682-3868—FAX
• Food pantry, clothing, medical, and dental assistance for low-income DuPage County residents.

Travelers & Immigrants Aid—Rafael Center
4750 North Sheridan Road, Suite 200
Chicago, IL 60640
773-989-0049
773-989-1935—FAX
• Comprehensive HIV/AIDS services including financial assistance, emergency shelters/housing, meals, day and respite care, and mental health services. Free. English/Spanish.

3. FINANCIAL PLANNING

Financial security can be difficult to achieve with or without HIV. However, living with a serious illness creates a special set of financial worries. Gaps in insurance coverage, the possibility of losing or having to leave a job, having to live on a fixed income, providing for your children's future—all these and more are enough to keep a person awake nights.

The best way to avoid this kind of worry and stress is to:

1) *Plan ahead.* Start putting together your financial "battle plan" as soon as possible. Saving money can bring great peace of mind. If you are still working and/or have other resources you can draw on, consider talking with an HIV-sensitive certified financial planner, investment counselor, or attorney skilled in asset management. (You can often locate such individuals through HIV/AIDS service organizations, where they give seminars on financial and legal matters.)

   If you don't have substantial financial resources, your case manager can refer you to agencies and individuals who can help you make the most of what you do have. These advisors can also show you how to protect yourself and your family in case of hardship.

   If you're concerned about not being able to meet your credit card payments after leaving your job or going on disability, ask your lenders if they offer credit protection plans for disability or unemployment. These plans generally charge a small premium each month, then cover all or a portion of your unpaid balance should you leave your job or become disabled. If you're not in the habit of paying off your cards each month, this kind of insurance can be a great help. While credit protection plans don't typically require medical screening, they must be applied for well *before* the need to make a claim arises.

2) *Know your rights.* If you become disabled or find yourself in financial peril as a result of your illness, you may be entitled to special consideration from creditors. That doesn't mean you can just ignore your obligations, however. If you have debts you cannot pay, it may be wise to write a letter to the creditor explaining that you are ill and need to arrange an alternative schedule for repayment. Many companies will be glad to work with you once they learn of your situation (and receive some reassurance that you want to pay your bill).

   Other creditors may not be so understanding—but that doesn't mean you should allow them or their collection agencies to harass you. If this happens, seek help from an attorney.

Work as long as you can and start looking into financial assistance programs <u>early</u>. Don't let your pride deny your stomach! My priorities are food, clothing, and shelter, but also entertainment. If I can't enjoy life, I tend to fall into a "what's the point?" attitude. I need a reason to take my meds, see my doctor, and take care of myself.

SANDI

I owed VISA a lot of money. I made a deal with them; I told them I was terminally ill, and we were able to come to an agreement. It was a big relief not to have them breathing down my neck.

"SAM"

3) *Try not to panic if the unforeseen happens.* Many people immediately think "bankruptcy" when faced with serious financial problems. However, declaring bankruptcy is not an option to enter into without careful consideration and legal consultation. Bankruptcy is usually a lengthy, hassle-ridden process that does years of damage to your credit rating. While filing will place an automatic stay on litigation against you, bankruptcy does *not* relieve you of all your debts. You are still responsible for taxes, school loans, child support, and alimony obligations.

There often are alternatives short of bankruptcy that will bring relief. But if you have sizable debts you cannot pay, explore your options with an attorney.

4) *Don't transfer assets unadvisedly.* Some people mistakenly believe they have a better chance of preserving their assets or qualifying for public assistance if they sell or give away their assets to someone else. Unless you're very careful, or are only dealing with very small amounts, the government is bound to find out about it. This may lead them to deny or reduce assistance benefits on the basis of fraud. There may also be financial repercussions for the person(s) acquiring your assets. Before making any decisions of this nature, talk to an attorney.

4. YOUR LEGAL RIGHTS

The stigma surrounding HIV disease has frequently led to discrimination against HIV-infected individuals. You may be concerned that employers, insurers, landlords, and others might try to deprive you of your rights. Unfortunately, that concern is justified.

The most important thing to realize is that HIV-related discrimination is illegal. Many courts have ruled that HIV is a handicap. As an HIV-infected person, you are protected from discrimination solely on the basis of your handicap. If you are deprived of your rights on account of your illness, you can fight back in court.

Just because you have HIV or AIDS, you *cannot* legally be:

- fired, reassigned, isolated, demoted, or denied full-time employment, unless the position requires the handling of food or demands medically invasive, exposure-prone procedures;
- evicted from your dwelling or refused housing or a mortgage.
- removed from school or day care;
- denied medical or dental treatment or treated improperly in a medical setting;
- forced to surrender custody or give up visiting your children;
- denied access to public schools, accommodations (such as retail shops, restaurants, or hotels), or transportation;
- deprived of your personal property;

I think people are in a bind, especially if they went into debt. A lot of our clients assumed they were going to die, and said, "I've got these credit cards, why don't I live it up now? I'm going to travel and find my guru in Tibet." Some people went on these spiritual quests, which aren't cheap. They incurred debt they didn't think they'd have to worry about—and then the new drugs came along. Now they're having to figure that stuff out, the dollars-and-cents dilemmas, as well as emotionally adjusting their expectations of their lives.

That may not sound like a stressful process, but it is. If you've been assuming that you're going to die and all of a sudden you have to be prepared to live, everything changes. We're all taught to plan for the worst-case scenario—so you can see the paradox.

DEBORAH STEINKOPF
EXECUTIVE DIRECTOR, BEHIV—
BETTER EXISTENCE WITH HIV

I want to emphasize how important it is to seek competent legal counsel around complicated things, especially if you own assets or are in a partnership. I'm significantly younger than my partner, Fred. Everything Fred and I own, we own jointly. We needed to structure our assets in such a way that if I had to go on Medicaid, we could lay a paper trail to make it look as though I have no assets without arousing any suspicions. That way, there'd be no danger of compromising Fred's "twilight years," so to speak, or losing everything we'd spent the last fifteen years building up. Fred will be retiring soon, so this was a big issue for us.

One option was to transfer everything to Fred's name—which I was unwilling to do. That was going too far for me. So our attorney put everything in a "life estate." It doesn't completely protect us, but it creates a situation where outsiders will have a very difficult time figuring out what belongs to whom, and whether I actually own anything. Like it or not, that's the kind of thing you have to do to protect yourself.

"RALPH"

- harassed by others; or
- improperly denied coverage under an existing insurance policy (dropped or denied benefits for no good reason).

If any of the above happen to you—or if someone discloses your HIV status to others without your consent—you may have grounds for a lawsuit. People who can prove they became infected via contaminated blood products after 1985, or those whose doctors were grossly incompetent in their failure to diagnose HIV infection in time for effective treatment may also want to consider legal action.

However, the Equal Employment Opportunity Commission (EEOC) now treats HIV discrimination claims on a "fast-track" basis. You also are not required to have legal representation to file a charge against your employer. Lawsuits can be major undertakings; many drag on for years. As the plaintiff, you'll have the burden of proving the other party guilty of unlawful discrimination, malice, or ill will. Unless you are backed up by excellent witnesses and documentation, proving your case can be extremely difficult. Still, you'll want to at least discuss your options with a private attorney, or an organization like the AIDS Legal Council of Chicago or the American Civil Liberties Union (ACLU). Usually a reasonable settlement can be reached through negotiation, without actually going through the lawsuit stage.

Finding and Working with an Attorney
By Emily P. Berendt, Attorney-at-Law

Emily Berendt is a sole practitioner who concentrates her practice in estate planning. She is the former Executive Director of Positive Approach to Health (PATH). Emily believes good communication is the single most important aspect of working with any attorney.

It is very likely that at some point during your tenure with HIV, you will find yourself in need of a good lawyer.

Discrimination based on HIV status or the perception of HIV status is still very much alive, in spite of the volumes of material that have been written on the subject. You are protected against discrimination by many federal and state laws, including the Federal Rehabilitation Act, the Illinois Human Rights Act, the Chicago Human Rights Ordinance (in Chicago only), the Cook County Human Rights Ordinance, and the Americans With Disabilities Act. There are other laws that may protect you depending on your circumstances, including Housing Ordinances and local Human Rights Ordinances in communities outside Chicago. Remember, you don't need an attorney to file charges with the Illinois Department of Human Rights, the Equal Employment Opportunity Commission (EEOC), or the Chicago Human Rights Committee.

Existence of these laws doesn't mean you will prevail without going to court, however. Unless your lawyer can negotiate favorably with the discriminating party, you will have to decide whether you can deal with the stress and expense of a lawsuit. In many cases, it may not be feasible.

When to Call a Lawyer

Besides asserting your rights when you have suffered discriminatory treatment, your lawyer can advise you on ways to avoid future problems when you do things like change jobs or purchase insurance. She or he can also help you with financial planning for the course of your illness and/or help you achieve goals in your estate plan.

Just a few examples of the many circumstances in which you may need a lawyer are:

- You are demoted, denied promotion, or terminated from your job while you are still able to perform all essential functions of the job.
- You are faced with HIV-specific questions on an application for a job or health insurance.
- You are denied payment of benefits by your health insurance carrier.
- Your dentist refuses to treat you.
- Your landlord, for no justifiable reason, asks you to move or refuses to renew your lease.
- Your landlord refuses to allow you to install a support rail beside your bathtub.
- Your children are singled out for different treatment in their school.
- You decide that, in order to avoid impoverishing your spouse with the cost of your illness, you want a divorce.
- You want your life partner and not your parent(s) to have control over your finances and health care if you become incompetent.
- You want to leave your property to your life partner instead of your family.
- You want to arrange for care and guardianship of your children.

Finding the *Right* Lawyer

Lawyers, like doctors, frequently concentrate or limit their practice to specific areas. This allows the lawyer to develop more expertise and facility in that area of the law. For example, your lawyer might handle employment discrimination claims, but not estate planning; or, be well prepared to do the closing on the sale of your home, but not your divorce or bankruptcy petition. Therefore, you may need more than one lawyer for different purposes.

It is very important to find a lawyer who understands HIV, is comfortable working with you, and makes you feel comfortable in turn. Unfortunately, this is not a matter of looking in the Yellow Pages. While the legal community is becoming more and more attuned to the needs of HIV-positive persons, it is still a subset of the larger community where misunderstanding and fear of HIV prevail. Fortunately, you can turn to such public interest groups as the AIDS Legal Council of Chicago, the American Civil Liberties Union (ACLU), and the

---

One of the things I did that was really quite futile was to go and see a lawyer about a year and a half after I tested positive. The lawyer showed me a huge book, maybe three inches thick, of all the cases of people with AIDS trying to sue whoever gave it to them. You have to prove they knew what they were doing and were intentionally trying to inflict harm on you. There was no way I could prove that about the blood company where I got my factor VIII.

ADAM

Legal AID Bureau, among others. In addition, most local HIV/AIDS service organizations give referrals to private attorneys. An advantage to looking for a lawyer in this manner is that you probably will be able to find one who understands the expense of HIV and is doing this work for a reduced or waived fee.

Perhaps the best way to find a lawyer is to ask a friend or acquaintance in a support group. If they have been satisfied with the lawyer's work, chances are you will be too.

What you are looking for as an HIV-positive person is a lawyer who:

- understands HIV disease, its progression, and modes of transmission;
- understands the social implications of HIV and their impact on your situation legally;
- understands the immediacy of some legal needs of a person who is HIV-positive and is willing to act quickly to meet them;
- accepts both traditional and non-traditional lifestyles, and has the ability to relate to you as a person in a non-judgmental manner;
- is willing to spend whatever time is necessary to discuss your needs in detail in a relaxed, non-stressful atmosphere;
- keeps up-to-date on the latest developments in the law that affect or are affected by HIV issues;
- practices in your area of legal need;
- understands your financial situation and is willing to be flexible about payment; and
- understands your physical constraints and is willing to be flexible about scheduling appointments. Some attorneys are even willing to come to you if necessary, or arrange for telephone conferences when office visits are not practical.

Working with Your Chosen Lawyer

Establishing the right relationship with your attorney from the start will make working together a useful and rewarding experience for both of you.

Your relationship with your lawyer must be based on complete openness and trust on both sides. You must tell your lawyer everything in connection with your case. Don't screen out facts that you think are not important. Trust your lawyer to do that in the final analysis. Your lawyer cannot completely represent you if she or he does not have all the facts. In return, you are entitled to an honest evaluation of your case and clear explanation of your options in plain language. If an aspect of your case is outside the lawyer's realm of competency, she or he must honestly tell you that and ask your permission to seek advice from another attorney or refer you elsewhere.

Keep in mind that the information you give your lawyer is confidential. The attorney-client privilege is similar to that which exists between doctor and patient. Even a court cannot compel your lawyer to break your confidence as to privileged communications. The privilege extends to husbands and wives who visit the lawyer together and share information among the three of them. It does *not* extend to unmarried couples, however. Therefore, information would be accessible if an unmarried couple, traditional or non-traditional, later has a breakdown in the relationship that results in a lawsuit.

Your first visit to your chosen lawyer should accomplish three things. It should:

- set the tone of honest, open communication for the relationship;
- result in a clear understanding of what you want from your lawyer and what your lawyer can give you, including perhaps a written retainer agreement; and
- provide you with a clear understanding of how you will be charged for your lawyer's services.

How Lawyers Bill Their Clients

Lawyers' fees can vary greatly due to a number of different factors. You probably will be asked to place a deposit, called a retainer, with your attorney to retain his or her services.

Attorneys may bill by the hour or by the task. Hourly rates can range from $75 to $250 and up. If you are billed at an hourly rate, you will be billed only for the hours the attorney actually spends working on your case.

Some areas of legal practice lend themselves to flat fee arrangements. Real estate closings and wills are two examples. If you are quoted a flat fee, it probably will not include various filing fees and other costs. You may also be advised that any work necessary in connection with your case that is outside the realm of the ordinary for the flat fee will be billed on an hourly basis.

Don't hesitate to call several lawyers and compare fees before you choose. Also, be sure to get a clear understanding of the fees to expect, preferably in writing, at your first visit.

Legal Assistance

AIDS Legal Council of Chicago
220 South State Street,
Suite 1330
Chicago, IL 60604
312-427-8990
312-427-8419—FAX

Outreach program office at:
Cook County Hospital
1900 West Polk Street,
Room 634-635
Chicago IL 60612
312-733-8026
312-633-8651—FAX
• Information and counseling on all manner of legal issues provided free to people living with HIV/AIDS in the Chicago metropolitan area. The Council refers cases requiring more attention or representation to volunteer professional attorneys with specialized expertise. A nominal registration fee is requested, but may be waived for inability to pay. AIDS Legal Council puts out a quarterly newsletter, and publishes the "AIDS Legal Guide," a handbook focusing on Illinois law as it relates to the rights and concerns of HIV-infected state residents. English/Spanish.

American Civil Liberties Union of Illinois (ACLU)
203 North LaSalle Street,
Suite 1405
Chicago, IL 60601
312-201-9740
312-201-9760—FAX
• Free legal representation or referrals for HIV-affected individuals experiencing discrimination. Focus is on test cases that can establish precedents protecting the rights of all persons living with HIV/AIDS. The ACLU has a full-time legal staff available to represent HIV-affected clients throughout Illinois.

Chicago Lawyers' Committee for Civil Rights Under Law, Inc.
100 North LaSalle Street,
Suite 600
Chicago, IL 60602
312-630-9744
312-630-1127—FAX
312-630-9749—Hearing-impaired TTY/TDD
• Class action and law reform litigation focusing on discrimination and prosecution of hate crimes, including those against people with HIV/AIDS. Offers assistance with wills and powers of attorney. Free. English/Spanish.

Chicago Volunteer Legal Services Foundation
100 North LaSalle Street,
Suite 900
Chicago, IL 60602
312-332-1624
312-332-1460—FAX
• Provides free legal services to low-income residents in metropolitan Chicago. Representation for HIV-affected individuals in areas of wills, small estate planning, divorce, custody, visitation, and employment benefits.

Cook County HIV Primary Care Center
1835 West Harrison Street
CCSN 1268
Chicago, IL 60612
312-633-3005
312-633-3002—FAX
• Offers legal assistance through AIDS Legal Council's on-site project. Free. English/Spanish.

Cook County Legal Assistance Foundation, Inc.
828 Davis Street, Suite 201
Evanston, IL 60201
847-475-3703
847-475-3033—FAX
847-475-5580—Hearing-impaired TTY/TDD
• Free legal representation for those with HIV/AIDS in the areas of Public Aid, food stamps, Medicaid/Medicare, SSDI and overpayments, nursing home residents' rights, landlord/tenant disputes, consumer law, and unemployment benefits. Additional locations in Oak Park and Harvey. Free. English/Spanish.

Crusader Clinic
120 Tay Street
Rockford, IL 61102
815-968-0286
815-968-3881—FAX
• Legal assistance for people with HIV. English/Spanish.

DuPage Bar Legal Aid Service
126 South County Farm Road
Wheaton, IL 60187
630-653-6212
630-653-6317—FAX
• Provides legal assistance to low-income residents in family law and bankruptcy. Telephone screenings are conducted 9 a.m.-noon, Mon-Fri.

Horizons Community Services
961 West Montana
Chicago, IL 60614
773-472-6469
773-472-6643—FAX
773-929-4357—Lesbian/gay Helpline, 6-10 p.m. daily
773-871-8873—24-hour Anti-violence Crisis Hotline
773-327-4357—Hearing-impaired TTY/TDD hotline
• Horizons' Legal Services Program maintains a volunteer pool of professional attorneys experienced at serving lesbians and gay men, with special expertise in HIV-related legal matters. Legal Services clients receive a one-time free consultation with one of these lawyers. Referrals to qualified attorneys if further legal assistance is needed. Call the Helpline for details.

Illinois AIDS Hotline
800-243-2437—Hotline staffed 8 a.m.-11 p.m., 7 days/week
800-782-0423—Hearing-impaired TTY/TDD
• Referrals to AIDS legal assistance programs throughout Illinois. English/Spanish.

Illinois Department of Human Rights
100 West Randolph Street, Suite 10-100
Chicago, IL 60201
312-814-6200
312-814-6251—FAX
• Investigates charges of HIV discrimination in housing, employment, public accommodations, and access to credit. English/Spanish.

Lambda Legal Defense and Education Fund
11 East Adams Street, Suite 1008
Chicago, IL 60603
312-663-4413
312-663-4307—FAX
• National advocacy organization dedicated to protecting legal and civil rights of lesbians, gay men, and people living with HIV/AIDS. Free.

Legal Assistance Foundation of Chicago
343 South Dearborn Street, Suite 700
Chicago, IL 60604
312-341-1070
312-347-8311—HIV Housing Law Project
312-341-1041—FAX
312-431-1206—Hearing-impaired TTY/TDD
• Legal counseling and advocacy for low-income persons in civil matters regarding welfare, Social Security, consumer rights, employment, landlord/tenant disputes, and certain areas of immigration. Clients must meet financial need requirements and reside in Cook County. Free. English/Spanish.

Prairie State Legal Services
975 Main Street
Rockford, IL 61103
815-965-2902
815-965-1081—FAX
815-965-5114—Hearing-impaired TTY/TDD
8:30 a.m.-5 p.m. Mon-Fri
• Serves Northern Illinois. Nine field offices, including Carol Stream, Waukegan, and St. Charles. Assists low-income persons with civil matters, such as disability, family law, health insurance, housing discrimination, living wills, powers of attorney, and SSI. Call for eligibility requirements. English/Spanish.

Test Positive Aware Network
1258 West Belmont
Chicago, IL 60657
773-404-8726
773-472-7505—FAX
773-404-9716—Hearing-impaired TTY/TDD
• Free weekly legal clinic provided to members by appointment only. Call for the location.

Books and Publications

AIDS and the Law: A Basic Guide for the Nonlawyer
Terl, Allan H.
Hemisphere Publishing, 1992
• Written specifically for those interested in the legal aspects of AIDS but who have no professional legal training.

AIDS in the Workplace: Legal Questions and Practical Solutions
Banta, William
Lexington Books, 1992
• Provides both employers and employees with comprehensive information on the medical, legal, and ethical issues concerning AIDS in the workplace.

AIDS Law Today: A New Guide for the Public
Burris, Scott, Harlin Dalton and Judith Miller
New Haven: Yale University Press, 1992
• This publication of the Yale AIDS Law Project is an updated and completely revised edition

assessing the status of AIDS law. "Must reading" for anyone needing to grasp the legal dimensions of HIV disease.

"AIDS Legal Guide"
Produced by the AIDS Legal Council of Chicago, 1994
Mail order: AIDS Legal Council of Chicago, 312-427-8990
• Straightforward handbook focusing on Illinois law as it relates to the rights and concerns of HIV-infected state residents. Uses a Q&A format in easy-to-understand language, then provides an in-depth discussion of the issue for use by attorneys and other interested persons. Covers topics including HIV testing, workplace concerns, insurance and financial matters, Social Security and Public Aid, housing issues, family law, divorce and visitation rights, privacy and confidentiality, medical malpractice and experimental drug liability, transmission liability, wills, living wills, and powers of attorney, school law, travel and immigration law, and military law. Free.

Using a Computer and Modem

AIDS Legal Council of Chicago
http://www.thebody.com/alcc/alccpage.html
• The Council provides legal services to financially needy people in the Chicago area who are affected by HIV. Various legal information and forms are available at this site.

The Body: A Multimedia AIDS and HIV Resource
http://www.thebody.com/cgi-bin/body.cgi
• An excellent site offering HIV/AIDS information and support resources. Topics include Financial & Legal Issues, and more. Links to other sites.

The HIV InfoWeb
http://carebase2.jri.org/infoweb/
• Legal resources are among many HIV topics at this site. Includes a search engine and links to other sites.

Using a Fax

NAPWA Fax
National Association of People with AIDS
202-789-2222—FAX
• Many helpful legal publications available by fax, including employment rights under the Americans with Disabilities Act, legal questions and answers, and worksheets on preparing a will. Request the "Living with HIV" fax catalog of fax documents in English. A Spanish catalog is also available. You must be at a fax machine to use the NAPWA Fax service.

Video

"What about My Kids?"
Mail order: Gay Men's Health Crisis, 212-337-1950
• Guides parents through the process of arranging guardianship of their children. (Note: legal explanations from service providers are specific to New York State.)

PART 6

Prepared for Whatever Comes

- Life Planning with HIV or AIDS:
  Wills, Living Wills, and Powers of Attorney
- A Matter of Letting Go
- On Surrender
- A Taste of Heaven
- Hospice Care
  Hospice and Other Resources
- On Saying Goodbye
- Epilogue

This is the section no one wants to read, about the issues few of us care to think about. But death and dying, and their attendant legal and financial considerations, are matters that all of us must eventually think about and act upon—regardless of our HIV status.

Many people who are otherwise very organized and conscientious tend to procrastinate when it comes to "getting their affairs in order." Decisions on living wills, funeral arrangements, and guardians for our children can be difficult and unpleasant ones to make. Yet the urgency that surrounds them makes it impossible for us to push them aside forever. Most people who have faced these decisions and gotten the paperwork over with express a profound sense of relief and accomplishment. The peace of mind you'll feel from knowing these things are taken care of may be one of the best incentives for tackling them now.

There is another side to death and dying, of course…an emotional and spiritual side. Serious illness has a way of forcing people to examine their lives and belief systems. This can be a very stressful process—or one that can bring a tremendous sense of inner peace.

HIV is a relatively new phenomenon. We do not yet know whether everyone with AIDS will eventually die from the disease. We do know, however, that all human beings must eventually leave this existence as we know it. It may help to remember that as you work through your feelings and beliefs about dying. It's one more way in which "you are not alone."

> *I still don't have what it takes to actually sit down and make out a will. And I know I have to do that. I could die tomorrow—any of us could—and my son doesn't have a father.*
>
> "MARIE"

> *I think now I should have talked to a lawyer or made arrangements to see a living will before I actually went in to sign one. I remember the day I went into the doctor's office to do it. I was kind of freaked out at what I was looking at, because I didn't know what it all meant. The doctor said that you had to initial this box, this box, or this box, and I'm like—wait a minute! I have to think about that. I couldn't do it there; I had to take it home and read it over three or four times before I knew what to do.*
>
> "ELIZABETH"

I haven't done any of the legal work, if something happens to me and Louie. I will. My problem is, I'm not the perfect parent, but I'm looking for the perfect parent!

CHRISTINE

Life Planning with HIV or AIDS: Wills, Living Wills, and Powers of Attorney
by Emily P. Berendt, Attorney-at-Law

Emily Berendt is a sole practitioner who concentrates her practice in estate planning. She is the former Executive Director of Positive Approach to Health (PATH). Asked to relate the single most important message she'd like to emphasize here, Emily doesn't hesitate: "Do it *now!*"

Your test is positive. Or your diagnosis is AIDS. Among your many concerns may be the fear of losing control over your own life decisions. Decisions such as, "Who will take care of me when I'm sick? Do I want to be 'hooked up' to a respirator if I can't breathe on my own? How will I pay for this expensive illness? If death is at hand, do I want to die in a hospital or at home? Do I want to be buried or cremated? Who should come to my funeral or memorial? What will happen to the people I love and must leave behind?"

You knew you would have to deal with these questions sometime in your distant future. Suddenly, the virus has telescoped your life. The future is here, and you're not prepared.

There are ways to prepare. There are steps you can take and documents you can use with the help of your attorney (and sometimes, on your own) to take and keep control of your own life decisions. This article will focus on wills, living wills, and powers of attorney. These are the most useful documents available for the largest number of people. There are other documents and arrangements that may be useful to your own individual situation.

Last Will and Testament

Your will, carefully written, signed, and witnessed, can pass any property you own at your death to the person or persons of your choosing. You can include or specifically exclude your biological family if you wish and provide only for your life companion and friends. You can set up trusts for loved ones, provide for the care of your pets, make gifts to charity, and make special arrangements tailored to your situation and your wishes.

Naming an Executor

When you plan your will, you name an executor to carry out its provisions. Your executor must be a U.S. resident, at least eighteen years of age, of sound mind, not disabled, and not a convicted felon.

Your executor's duties include:
- arranging your funeral;
- filing your will with the probate court;
- petitioning the court for appointment as your executor;
- preserving your assets;
- paying your final bills;
- making the distributions you have designated; and
- filing your final income tax return.

Where probate is appropriate, your executor will also be accountable to the court throughout the probate process. This is not a job to be taken lightly. The person who accepts it must be reliable and diligent. Never name an executor without first discussing it with that person and obtaining his or her agreement to accept the responsibility.

By transferring some of your property during your lifetime, you can sometimes avoid formal probate proceedings. If you own no real estate at death and the value of your assets is under $50,000, your executor can use a Small Estate Affidavit as authority to collect and distribute your property. This procedure avoids public notice and the long delay associated with probate. Although it will not be appropriate in all situations, it is definitely worth considering and discussing with your lawyer.

I generally advise my gay and lesbian clients who are leaving substantially everything to their life partner to consider naming a trusted third person as executor. Your life partner will suffer enough trauma from your loss without having the additional stress of probating your will and perhaps meeting with hostility from your biological family. In some cases, however, the life partner will be the obvious best choice for the job.

Bequests and Final Details

Additionally, if you are leaving substantially everything to your life partner, your will should clearly say that is your intention. It's advisable to leave small gifts to each member of your biological family to show that you did not simply "forget" them—thus leaving your will open to challenge based on your mental capacity. If you intend to completely disinherit your biological family, your will must state that intention clearly, and must completely give all your property to another person or persons.

When you sign your will, it should be a formal, solemn occasion. You will be asked if you have read the will, and if it reflects your wishes. You may be asked to name your family members and give some basic information like address and place of employment to establish your mental capacity. In most cases, a life partner who is also primary beneficiary should not be present. That way, it cannot later be said that he or she influenced you to sign the will in his or her favor.

Your attorney may want to make an audio or video tape of the signing ceremony for proof of your intention and capacity in the event the will is challenged. If you are taking any medications that affect your mental state, you should go off them if you can, far enough ahead of the signing to clear them from your system.

Naming a Guardian for Your Children

An important function of your will may be to name a person you wish the court to appoint as permanent guardian for your minor child or children. After formal court appointment, the guardian will be the

---

I have made verbal arrangements for my son. I should do it on paper. He's going to go with my sister. She's like me.

Sometimes I think, "Oh, my God! I'm going to die!" But then I realize it happens to everybody. I live in a neighborhood where we hear gunshots every night, and I could be standing at the gate getting my key out and be shot. It's something that could happen to anyone, never mind AIDS. Still, dying is hard to think about and it gets me very emotional.

Just recently, someone I knew died. She had nine children and didn't make any arrangements. Now they're lost. They're being tugged on by two sides of the family. It's bad.

I don't want DCFS to get ahold of my son, even if it's for a day. I don't what him to have to go through that. So I know I'm going to have to get busy, put my decisions in writing.

WENDY

> *I wanted to know where my kids were going to be, and that they were going to be safe and taken care of. That I'm passing them on into the care of someone I know will fulfill what I have started. Because when I'm feeling really bad, knowing I'm protecting my kids helps me get through it. I'm able to feel really good about making the plans and getting things in place.*
>
> SANDI

> *My mom and I talked about what it will be like in the end before she does go, what possessions will be mine after she is gone, who will be my guardians. It made me feel a little better, because I'll be with people I've known for a while.*
>
> PATRICK (AGE 11)

person actually responsible for their custody and care. The test the court will apply is whether appointment of the person you have named is in the "best interests of the child." The court will usually honor your choice. Your choice of guardian, however, cannot take away the rights of the other biological parent who is fit and willing to take custody and care. Nor can your choice take away the rights of the state if your child is a ward of the state.

Include a written statement of your reasons for choosing someone as guardian. This will tell the court what you think is in the best interests of your child and can be a very important part of the court's consideration. Your reasons may be particularly important if you are naming a person who is not the biological parent, or who is your gay or lesbian life partner.

Guardianship nominations that take effect after your death can be made in a separate document without making a will. To be effective, the paperwork must be completed before you become ill to the point of incompetence. All of the above considerations would still apply, and your intended guardian would still have to go to court to petition for appointment.

Permanent guardianship can be effectively established during your lifetime, but not without relinquishing many parental rights. If your intended guardian is willing to be flexible about letting you continue parenting, designating a permanent guardian during your lifetime could greatly reduce the disruption to your child's life at the time of your death. This can give you great peace of mind.

Illinois law provides for the appointment of short-term and standby guardians. These procedures, however, are not available when the minor has another living parent who is willing and able to care for the minor and who does not consent to the appointment. Neither is it available when the minor already has a court-appointed guardian.

A short-term guardian is appointed without court involvement for up to 60 days by simply signing the form naming the guardian. The effective date of the guardianship can be tied into a date such as "when I am admitted to the hospital." The short-term guardianship can be renewed at the end of the 60 days, as long as you have legal capacity. This procedure gives you a way to transfer to another adult the necessary authority to care for your child during periods of your absence or incapacity. The short-term guardian would, for example, have authority to consent to medical treatment for your child.

Standby guardianship is a flexible and relatively simple arrangement that can serve the needs of parents with HIV. No longer do you have to wait until you are so sick that a guardianship hearing must be conducted on an emergency basis, placing additional stress on everyone involved. Nor do HIV-positive parents have to surrender custody of their children while they are healthy, a time when the need for family unity is particularly strong. Rather, parents can continue to care for their children, secure in the knowledge that their children's future care has been established.

The standby guardian is appointed by the court. The appearance in court happens during your lifetime, and your appearance in court is not mandatory. Once appointed, your guardian's power is inactive (on standby) until you can no longer care for your child. At that time, the guardian's power becomes effective immediately and is in force for 60 days. The standby guardian may petition the court for permanent appointment within that 60 days. In most cases, they will have no trouble obtaining permanent appointment. The standby guardianship, therefore, is better insurance against your permanent disability or incapacity.

In some cases, adoption may be a viable method of providing continuity of care for your child. An attorney can give you more information on adoption and issues of custody and care of children of divorced parents.

Living Will

A living will is generally a simple, one-page document that tells your doctor not to use extraordinary measures to prolong your life if your condition is terminal. It allows you to die naturally with only the administration of pain relief and comfort care. Procedures that can prolong the dying process may include the use of a respirator, blood transfusions, and intravenous feeding and medication. You can insert specific instructions about these and other procedures into the document. Your living will must be signed by you and two witnesses.

A living will has several limitations, however. First, the document reflects your wishes at the time of signing. A living will does not allow you to change your mind without completely revoking it. It does not permit anyone to use judgment in deciding what you would have wanted but must be followed as written. You should therefore review your living will frequently to make sure you still feel the same way about your medical care as you did when you originally signed it.

Second, in order for your living will to be effective, your physician must make and record a diagnosis that your condition is terminal. A "terminal condition" is defined as an incurable and irreversible condition such that death is imminent and the application of death-delaying procedures serves only to prolong the dying process. Therefore, a living will is only applicable near the very end of life.

Third, the Illinois Living Will Statute specifies that artificial nutrition and hydration may not be withheld or withdrawn if death would result from starvation or dehydration rather than the underlying terminal condition. If you have strong feelings about not having feeding tubes and IVs, a living will may not be able to accomplish this for you.

Being able to plan ahead helps you to have peace of mind, knowing that the person you choose will be the one to care for your children. Having those plans legalized ensures that your wishes will be carried out. We've seen situations where family members or others come in and fight over who'll care for the kids when there's not a clear plan left by the parent.

Planning also keeps your children from the further trauma of being left in legal limbo after you're gone. If you don't plan, even if there's a will (which is contestable), it may not be clear who has the authority as guardian to enroll the child in school or get medical care. The child may go into DCFS custody until the matter is cleared up. There's no guarantee that siblings will stay together or that the parent's wishes will be followed.

By planning, you can help your child get used to the idea of what will happen to them when you're gone. The biggest question children have is, "Who is going to take care of me?" If they're prepared for what's coming, they can cope better. It's the unknown that's frightening.

PHYLLIS CHARLES
FORMER SUPERVISOR, SECOND
FAMILY PROGRAM, LUTHERAN
SOCIAL SERVICES OF ILLINOIS

If you want to be sure your wishes will be followed when you are unable to state them and you are not diagnosed as terminally ill, you should consider the use of a health care power of attorney as an alternative to your living will.

Durable Power of Attorney for Health Care

A more flexible and useful document than the living will, the Durable Power of Attorney for Health Care does not require that you be diagnosed as terminally ill for the document to take effect. Instead, it can allow your agent (the person you name to take the power) to take over your care immediately or at a date you name. It is not restricted to what is written, but allows your agent to use judgment in making decisions. Your agent can consider prior discussions with you, what he or she knows about your overall life philosophy, as well as any written statements you have included in the document. Your agent can also consider advances in medical technology or changes in the law.

This power lasts through your incompetency and only terminates upon your death unless you specify that it will terminate at another time prior to your death.

Your agent will have priority in visitation rights, access to your medical records, and the right to make any necessary health care decisions. These decisions may include acceptance or refusal of death-delaying treatments or procedures, and the right to refuse food and fluids. Your agent can be given the right to carry out your wishes for disposition of your body and funeral arrangements upon your death. (In this case, the power lasts beyond your death to the extent necessary for your agent to carry out your wishes.) Your agent's right to do these things is greater authority than your biological family's right to do these things. (Thus, you can rule out a family member trying to challenge the validity of this document.)

Your agent's power does not have to be so broad, however. You can limit his or her authority to a specific situation, such as funeral arrangements or placement in a nursing home. The person you nominate is not obligated to accept the power and act on it. If the person does act, however, he or she is protected from liability as long as the action taken was not negligent. Your death due to withdrawal or withholding of life support under a Durable Power of Attorney for Health Care cannot be considered suicide or homicide. Nor can it impair your life insurance benefits in any way. Your agent is required to keep records of receipts, disbursements, and significant actions.

Doing Your Homework

Both the living will and health care power of attorney require some homework before and after signing. The health care power should be discussed with your intended agent to determine that person's ability and willingness to carry out your wishes. If that person is unable or unwilling to act on the document, you need to look for someone else.

Both documents should be discussed with your doctor. Consider your state of health and possible course of treatment. Any specific instruction you wish to make as a result of these discussions should be written into the document.

If your doctor is unable or unwilling to comply with your living will or health care power, now is the time to find this out so you can change doctors. If you are already hospitalized when you sign either document, and your doctor is unwilling to comply with it, he or she is required to help you transfer to another doctor who will comply.

After signing either document, give copies to your doctor, who is required to make that information a part of your medical records. Give the original Durable Power of Attorney for Health Care to your agent and distribute copies of both documents to your family and friends. Finding the documents in your bottom drawer after your funeral obviously does no good. Put a card in your wallet with the name and phone number of your agent and your doctor. State on the card that you have a living will and/or Durable Power of Attorney for Health Care in effect.

Illinois Health Care Surrogate Act

The Illinois Health Care Surrogate Act recognizes that all persons have a right to make decisions relating to their own medical treatment, including the right to forego life-sustaining treatment. Persons who are unable to make decisions to forego such treatment have a right to have someone make those decisions on their behalf.

The Health Care Surrogate Act only applies if you lack capacity to give informed consent to treatment yourself, have no valid living will or Health Care Power of Attorney, and have one of three qualifying conditions:

1) a terminal illness;

2) permanent unconsciousness;

3) an incurable or irreversible condition;

If the requirements of the Act are met, your doctor will look to others to make decisions in the following order of priority:

- a court-appointed guardian of the person;
- a spouse;
- an adult child;
- a parent;
- an adult sibling;
- an adult grandchild;
- a close friend;
- a court-appointed guardian of the state.

Since the Act only applies in the absence of a valid living will or health care power, part of your task with your attorney is to determine whether the priority of the list conflicts with your personal wishes.

For example, if you're an unmarried person estranged from your biological family, you may want your life partner (identified under the Act as "close friend") to make your decisions. Since "close friend" is only looked to in the absence of any family under the Act, you'll want to be certain that you have a valid Power of Attorney for Health Care in effect to give your "close friend" the power you want her or him to have. The Power of Attorney for Health Care will override your biological family's power under the Act.

Or, as another example, if you are a person with no living relatives and a court-appointed guardian, you might want to override the authority of that guardian to make life-sustaining decisions by signing a living will. As long as the living will is valid, it controls.

Durable Power of Attorney for Property

A Durable Power of Attorney for Property is useful in allowing another person to conduct your personal business during your illness. The person you name as your agent in this document can have very broad powers to sell your property, manage your business, trade your stock, or fund your living trust, among others. Or, you can limit the power to only specific functions such as the power to collect and cash your paycheck or Social Security disability payment and pay your bills. This power also lasts through your incompetency and only terminates upon your death unless you name an earlier termination date.

As under a Durable Power of Attorney for Health Care, the person you name as your agent in a Durable Power of Attorney for Property is not obligated to accept and act on the power. However, if your appointed agent does act, he or she will be protected from liability as long as the action taken is not negligent. Your agent's actions also cannot be invalidated simply because your agent happens to have an interest in or benefit from the property managed. Your agent must keep a record of receipts, disbursements, and significant actions.

Any power of attorney or living will can be revoked at any time during your competency. Any oral command from you during your competency will override either document. Therefore, you are not giving up anything by getting these documents in place. You're only enhancing your own control and protection.

Doing It Yourself

Powers of attorney for health or property, and sometimes living wills, are available in many libraries and stationery stores that sell legal supplies. If you have access to a computer and modem, legal forms are also available from:

AIDS Legal Council of Chicago
http://www.thebody.com/alcc/alccpage.html

You can use these ready-made forms to create a binding legal document. This is both good and bad. The Illinois Statutory Power of Attorney forms have instructions written right into the form. If you are sure of your wishes and able to clearly state them in writing, you can fill out the forms yourself and save some money on attorney's fees. If you do not understand something though, or are not clear about the proper use of the forms, you can do more harm than good. Write down your questions and call an attorney. You may get enough information by phone to answer your questions—or, you may conclude you need an attorney to prepare the document for you. If you're the least bit uncertain, it will be worth the fee to be sure that you have a correctly executed form.

A Note on Early Planning

Wills, living wills, and powers of attorney are open to challenge by any person who would have it other than you have planned. This is especially true if you are an unmarried traditional or non-traditional couple because of potential or real conflicts with your biological family.

Even if your family is one where understanding, love, and support are unconditional, it may be best not to rely on them to carry out your wishes for major life decisions without putting those wishes down in legally binding documents. Even in the closest family, the combination of grief, shock, fear, guilt, and misunderstanding can cause one or more members to react unpredictably.

Something important to consider is timing. When I speak on life planning with HIV, I emphasize, "Do it now" as a theme of my presentation. Time is something you cannot waste with HIV. Early planning is the best planning. In the ideal situation, you will have your life plan in place before you test positive. Failing that, you should get things underway as soon as possible after a positive test or confirmed diagnosis of AIDS. The healthier you are when you sign any document, the less likely that any challenge will be made or will succeed if made. A healthy person isn't likely to be unduly influenced. Do it now.

That person who would have it otherwise—let's abbreviate that to PWHO—can also use the possibility of dementia to challenge and overturn your plans. HIV can cause central nervous system damage in varying degrees. AIDS Dementia Complex (ADC) shows up in a range of ways from mild confusion and short-term memory loss to severe social impairment and lack of ability to care for oneself. General public perception of dementia, however, is of the severe kind.

Therefore, the PWHO in your life is likely to claim that you were suffering from dementia when you signed your will or power of attorney. In fact, he or she could claim you were suffering from dementia whether you truly were or not, simply because of dementia being associated in the public mind with HIV. Again, the healthier you are when you make and document any decisions, the less likely a challenge based on ADC will be brought or will succeed if brought. Do it now.

Another note on dementia: if you do develop it, your capacity to sign documents will be questionable, not only to your PWHO but to your own attorney. Your attorney may be ethically obligated to refuse to draft documents for you. Adult guardianship proceedings may be the only way to then appoint someone to care for you or your property. By then, you may have lost control over who is appointed. Do it now.

Whatever your life plan includes, getting it down on paper is the most important thing you can do for yourself. Take action to recover some of the control that HIV has taken away from you. You will find that you can spend less time worrying about what the future will bring and more time on caring for your health and well-being in the present.

Do it now.

An earlier version of this article appeared in the January, 1991 issue of "Positively Aware." (Parts of this version have been substantially rewritten.)

A Matter of Letting Go
Contributed by Charlie Cox

Part of my strategy for living with AIDS has been learning to let go. I don't subscribe to the theory of, "I'm gonna fight this thing to my last ounce of breath!" There comes a time when you've got to face the fact that your life is going to end, and that it may end sooner and differently than you'd originally anticipated. When you reach this point, you sort of know you're not going to step in front of a truck or have a heart attack. You sort of know you're going to be sick and die in a hospital or at home. So you have a scenario, at least, that you can prepare for—unless, of course, they come up with a cure in the next few years.

A lot of people out there can't face death, can't talk about it. I can understand that. In my pre-HIV life, I had a habit of ignoring things that were coming up that I thought would be awful or horrible. But one of the lessons I've learned is that it's easier if you just face them and prepare for them. Get a real picture of what's in store and what options are available. I'm not saying we should dwell on death—but I also don't think it does any good to shy away from it.

The biggest thing that changed my feelings about all of this was being with Paul when he died. Paul was the most important person in my life, and I was really determined to be right there with him, by his side—partly, for selfish reasons. I wanted to see what death is, what happens. I wanted this to be a *known* thing. At the very least, I wanted to have one example of what goes on so it's not this big mystery. So I wouldn't have to lie in bed at night going, "Oh God, what's it gonna be like?!"

I came out of that experience so relieved; I felt blessed. Part of that is just being very close to someone at the most important moment of their life. But I was amazed—I thought, "This is not the horrible thing people make it out to be. This is actually kind of beautiful! Now I know one way it can be."

You always wonder. You see death on TV, and it's either they just drop because somebody shot them, or there's a lot of choking and clutching. Paul just kind of drifted away; he ran down like a clock. At a certain point, that next tick just didn't come. It was quite different than what I expected. It was really very peaceful.

On the other hand, I realized later that Paul was spared a lot of the indignities other people go through. He was in complete control of his mind and his speech until he fell asleep, five hours before he died. He was conscious, he was in charge—he held court with his family. It was an entertaining afternoon. It made me believe this is something that can be handled. I also know it's possible for it to be real ugly and hard. At least now, I have a sense of the range of possibility.

I learned a long time ago—in the dentist's chair, actually—that the worst way to manage pain is to tense up. Because you will feel that needle then, every inch of the way. If you just take some deep breaths and relax, the whole experience is much more tolerable.

I use that same psychology with thoughts of dying. Especially since Paul's death, it makes sense to me to just relax. Relax and move through it. It'll come whatever way it's gonna come. If I don't get all freaked and uptight about it, maybe it won't be so awful.

For me, the real fear was not so much death, but the process of dying with AIDS. I'm not afraid of death in the sense of my life ending. What I'm apprehensive about are all the messy, painful things that can go on before then. That's why Paul's death was such a relief for me. It's at least possible for it to be dignified.

This experience wasn't the only one that helped me learn to accept what's coming. Part of it has to do with the changes that have occurred in my body and my mind. Paul's death coincided with my first HIV-related symptoms. I had seven different skin things going on all at once. Up until then, I'd done a lot of stuff in my mind to try and deny it would ever happen. I'd think things like, "Maybe they got the test results mixed up. Or maybe I'm going to keep this at bay for a long time. I'm doing all the right things, I may never get sick from this." I remember being puzzled: where is it, how come it's not hitting?

All through 1988, I had never in my whole life been so healthy, physically or mentally. But by the spring of '89, I wrote in my journal, "This is not going to pass me by. It may not kill me, but I'm surely going to get sick." So by that year, with Paul gone and my own illness beginning to surface, I went through that first step: okay, I'm gonna have to pay some dues for this.

I sometimes think about— I'm probably not going to live to see my daughter get married, and what would I want to say to her? So I have these two books I write in for my kids...things I would want my daughter to know some day, things I'd like my son to know some day... and when I think about those things, I write them down. On my bad days, it's really scary to do. On good days, it's like, "God, I would have loved to have had a book like that from my mother." I think it has helped the relationships to be more real.

My whole family has a really good sense of humor. I buy something new, and Jenny will say, "Do I get that when you die?" And we kind of laugh about it. It's better to be open and honest and prepared than for it to be a big secret.

SANDI

PREPARED FOR WHATEVER COMES 253

Later, I took another step toward acceptance when I finally realized my health had gotten out of control. This isn't just weight loss anymore—this definitely is wasting. The diarrhea was getting a lot worse. And then, the KS appeared. That realization that I'd lost control was a major turning point, but my reaction was to try and stop all this as fast as possible, get back in control—survive all this as best I could.

Recently, within the past month or so, I've reached yet another point: realizing that I'm not always going to be able to control AIDS. I've finally realized, yeah—in all probability, this is going to kill me. At this point, it's not such a jarring thought. I'm used to it. I'd gone through all these other stages: maybe I don't have it; okay, I have it, but I might never get sick from it; okay, I'll get sick from it, but I just might survive it. And then, no—no I won't. This is real.

So now, I've entered a different phase. It's a kind of acceptance, as I said. My illness is not reversible, but I can manage it—for now. If I do things right, I can sort of put it on hold for awhile. I can't control it totally or change the ultimate outcome, but I can steer it. Still, I can already see the next point coming up on the horizon: the day when I find I can't steer any longer.

To some extent, I think that's happening to me already. One of the major letting-go points comes when you begin to run out of treatment alternatives—when you have to face the fact that the antiviral medications you've been taking aren't doing you any good anymore. Or maybe they're beginning to do you harm—the side effects are getting worse, toxicities are building. What I'm doing at the moment seems to be working; we'll see. But I feel as though my options are sort of drifting away from me.

Coming to grips with your mortality isn't just a physical or emotional process. There are also a lot of practical considerations involved. Everybody thinks it's going to be depressing to talk about wills and disability and stuff. But you have to talk about it, you have to face it, because if you don't then you won't be prepared. You'll find yourself surprised and caught in the lurch, with no resources in place.

There are people who won't come to TPA on nights where there's going to be a discussion of funerals or wills. I think that's stupid. You need to know about things like that, so if you care about the person who's going to be handling it later, you can help them out. Find out what's the cheapest way to do this, or what all the paperwork is.

So many people in the last month of their life wind up saying, "Oh, I should've done a health care power of attorney, I should've done a living will." But it's too late now, they're too sick. They really can't cope with it—and it may not even be legally binding at that point, because what kind of shape are they in? For me, all that's out of the way. It's done. I don't have to think about it anymore. It's just a load off my shoulders.

I approached a good friend three years ago and asked if she'd be willing to be my agent in my health care power of attorney. She agreed, but I've pressed her on it a number of times since then. I ask her, "Are you sure? We don't know what this is going to be like. I might be in hospitals for months, and your family life could suffer. You might have to spend a lot of time signing things and making decisions. I might be incapable of that."

But she's still willing to do this for me, so I know that's in place, I know it's there. I have a person I trust who knows my views who can make decisions pretty much the same way I would. It means I don't have to be frightened that someone's going to do stuff to me I don't really want done. The idea of being unable to communicate is extremely frightening to me. I've seen people in that position. They're conscious, in the sense that they know something's going on, but they're out of control. I've seen the fear in their eyes. It looks like an awful place to be in.

But if you know that being out of communication in that context doesn't totally deprive you of your rights and your wishes and your preferences—that there's someone who's going to take care of things for you—it helps. It relieves some of the anxiety. Because I don't have a lover to do that for me, I had to go out and find someone else who would.

The memorial service—that's another thing I've thought about. Actually having organized one and about to do another one, I've come to the conclusion that I don't want to leave a lot of detailed instructions. I just told the person I've lined up to handle those things, "You do whatever you feel you want to do. This is for you, it's for dealing with grief and parting. It's not going to do anything for me. Memorials are for the living, not the dead. I don't want any religious trappings or aspects, but other than that, anything goes. Do pizza and beer, be serious and ceremonial, or sit around and tell jokes—whatever the hell you want."

I really do believe that once you're dead, you're dead, and it's really none of your business what goes on. You've lost total control when you die—you don't have any more say! So it really makes no difference to me what they do at my memorial. Again, it's a matter of letting go.

On Surrender
By Juan Alegria, M.Div.

Many of us impose a tyranny of hope on ourselves. There's an undercurrent that says we can only live with this disease if we are filled with optimism, a positive attitude, and hopefulness. That in itself can be another burden, where you are not only angry and sad, but now you are expected to feel hopeful if you want to live.

The day before my daughter died, she told her sister she'd be going away. She said she'd been seeing a white hand reaching toward her. We asked if she was afraid of it, but she said no...so we told her to go ahead and reach out for it. The next morning she got up briefly, then shut down her body. She died within eight hours. I believe to this day she chose to do that.

ROSA

This is just another version of the idea that AIDS is punishment, that if we are sick it's our fault, and if we are going to be well we have to "earn" it. Our society has a picture of medicine as savior, disease as enemy, and we assume that all things have to move from chaos to order. But that's incredibly arrogant, and actually the opposite of what's true. Bodies break down, bones become dust to create other forms of life. There's not necessarily a "lesson" in AIDS, and there's not necessarily something to speak about in regretful tones if we surrender to it. AIDS is a condition that is part of our communal planetary experience, and we have to find more mature responses to it.

Whatever we feel, think, or do about AIDS should be based on truth and honesty—even when it goes against our assumptions of "how things should be." If you refuse to accept HIV or if you feel bitter, and just hate it with all your guts, and don't want to move beyond it, that doesn't mean you have a deficit. Surrender may be the ultimate courageous statement of our essence. There are as many ways of responding to AIDS as there are people and circumstances. We are a part of complex, mysterious, and sometimes conflicting energies moving around us, and we don't have to struggle to develop a reverent or positive sense about HIV. A legitimate response for the community is one that recognizes that those who choose not to fight represent an important piece of the human response to this horror. The people who take that route are heroes and "she-roes" in a different way.

A Taste of Heaven
by John Fortunato

John Fortunato has been a pastoral psychotherapist in private practice for over twenty years. He also has served as a spiritual director and retreat leader. John is the author of many articles and two books: <u>Embracing the Exile: Healing Journeys of Gay Christians</u> and <u>AIDS: The Spiritual Dilemma</u>, both published by HarperCollins.

HIV will probably be the most powerful spiritual force you ever encounter. It begins by raising the biggest question of life, "What is the meaning of death?" In the process of dealing with that issue, you will also be likely to face that other major human question, "What is the meaning of life?" If you take this process seriously, you may well be able to use HIV to make your life richer than it ever could have been without it.

My hope is that, in the next few pages, I can offer you some ways to think about this part of your spiritual journey that will help you work through your feelings and thoughts about the meaning of your life with HIV...and your eventual death with HIV.

"I am going to die."

That's almost always the biggest thing that hits people when they first learn they're infected. They often become obsessed, overwhelmed, and immobilized by the thought. You may be, too. For most of us, dying is a terrifying idea—and if that's where you are, you should give yourself permission to go ahead and be overwhelmed for now.

As you read this, you may be one step past that perfectly normal state of panic—or if not, you soon will be. Really. And when you are ready to hear it, you'll get a lot of good advice from counselors and doctors and nurses and support groups and books NOT to focus on dying from AIDS, but on living with HIV.

That is very good advice. Until you die, no matter what from, you have to deal with life. It is a major part of your spiritual journey. But I want to encourage you not to let well-meaning people bamboozle you out of thinking about death if that's what you need to do.

Sometimes people close to you will attempt to jostle you out of thinking or talking about dying. They probably are trying to be supportive, but they may also be too scared themselves to talk about death. Don't let them harass you. If you need to talk with somebody about what death means to you, find someone who will hang in with you. Because the reality is, most of the time HIV infection leads to AIDS, which is a fatal illness. That's real. You'd be loony if the thought of dying weren't on your mind a lot right now.

What about an Afterlife?

People who have a fatal illness need to find some answer to the question, "What happens to me when I die?" You will need to work that one out for yourself. Don't be surprised if some of your old answers aren't convincing anymore.

For instance, the answer you may have been taught when you were young was, "We die and go to heaven to be with God." That still may be just what your intuition and head and heart tell you. If so, meditation on heaven and earth and being with God will probably be very comforting to you. But you alternatively may find that the traditional Judeo-Christian idea of what happens at death no longer seems real.

People believe all sorts of things about what happens at death. Many believe that we simply return to the earth and our lives are over. Some believe that we are reincarnated and return to earth again, perhaps thousands and thousands of times. Still others believe we go through a period of cleansing or purifying, and then go to heaven to be with God. Certain Christians believe that after we are buried we remain, in a sense, dormant until Jesus returns at the end of time and resurrects us. And some of us believe that our spirits immediately enter a different state of being which we might call "heaven."

People also have many notions of what heaven is or might be like, ranging from something like an earthly paradise to a cosmic state of being that we as earthly creatures cannot possibly grasp. Most people who believe in an afterlife envision it as a place that is peaceful, happy, and joyous. Someone once described his view of heaven as "a dimension

---

When Sarah died, I had an out-of-body experience. I went with her, up from the couch to the picture window. I stopped at the window, and she went on through it. That was my not wanting to let go. I actually went with her when her spirit left. I am sure today that there is something after this life. I know it; I believe it. Something left Sarah's body. It was so real! There was a sensation of movement. I got to the window and I couldn't go any further. She left and I came back.

When I came back and realized what had happened, I screamed her name, stood up, and held her, and screamed, "I can't believe she did it. She really did it!" I kept asking my sister if it was really true. For the first time in months, we took all the tubes out of Sarah.

JULIE

For me, the most painful part of thinking about dying is thinking about my children. I don't ever want to lose them and I don't ever want them to lose me. But I know that in reality, there is nothing I can do to stop God's perfect plan for each one of us. And so trusting in that I'm doing the one thing that I know being a mother is all about, I'm trying to teach my children about the world we live in and how we can make it a better place.

In all that I do right now, today and tomorrow, whenever I talk about AIDS and that which surrounds it, I have the peace of knowing that whatever happens to me, my words and my love and my hope will live on. I think that is the greatest gift I could ever give my children; they will know how to love and how to hope. And they will survive.

SHARI

of being which is the answer to the question mark of life," the response to all of life's yearning and strife and uneasiness and pain.

You will need to spend some time thinking about what you believe happens when you die. It will probably come and go as a theme in your spiritual journey as you begin living with HIV. My guess is that it will come up for you a lot when you don't feel well and recede some when you are feeling better. That's fine.

Remember one thing: there aren't any right or wrong answers. Just trust your guts. They will tell you. The right answer for you about what happens when you die will be the one that helps untangle the knot in your stomach that appears when you get scared about dying.

The Other Half of the Journey

Then, there's living. Once you know you have this disease that in all probability is eventually going to be fatal, life just isn't the same anymore. If you never thought about "the meaning of life" before, you will now. Gold is only valuable because it is scarce. And days, too, become much more valuable to people once they realize they only have a limited number of them.

Of course, we all have a limited number of days. But it seems to be very human that only when people are forced to look dying in the face do they really "get" how short and valuable life is. This will probably happen to you, too.

Over time, you will find that your values are going to change a lot. You may well discover that things you used to think were important are really dumb, and some things you basically ignored before are suddenly very critical. Maybe you will find that friendships are much more valuable to you now, and that your collection of leaded crystal has lost its sparkle. Or maybe your appreciation of the beauty of nature is greatly heightened, or of human-made things like architecture or theater or art.

You probably will also find that the balance between your time alone and your time with others will change. Some HIV-infected people find they want to spend more time alone, quietly contemplating things. Others find they want to be with people more now than ever before.

My advice is that you be very attentive to yourself about all of this. Try to make time each day to reflect on how your life is going, what you see changing, and what you need to do to get your spiritual needs met. Because that's what all of this is about. By making sure that the set-up of your life helps take care of the things you find valuable, you will be tending to your spiritual journey. Taking time to smell the roses (if you like smelling roses) is every bit as much of a prayer for some people as getting down on their knees and talking to God is for others. What I want you to do is take excellent care of your soul as you learn to live with this disease.

An Unexpected Gift

Almost everyone I have known with HIV at some point says, "I didn't learn how to live until I got this virus." They often add, sadly, "I wish I had learned sooner. Now that I know what's important to me, I don't want to die." Those are very valid and important feelings. You're entitled to have them and don't let anybody talk you out of them. What they mean mostly is that you have learned how to make your life very meaningful and rich, and that you have learned to love it.

There is bad news and good news about your newfound zest for life. The bad news is, once you've had a taste of life that is lived richly and fully, it's sort of like chocolate and me. I just can't stop. I want all the chocolate in the universe. You want to live forever now that you love it. So it's sad that you will probably live a shorter life than you might have without HIV.

The good news is that most people die without ever getting to taste life the way you have. That is a sad commentary on our times. Most of us today don't know how to live. We civilized folks basically operate in a "make-it-through" mode, spending most of our lives doing things that make our souls shrivel up and die. What a waste! So you may have gotten a gift along with HIV: an appreciation for human life as it was intended to be lived. Maybe that will help you glimpse a vision of what happens to you at the end of life. Maybe life lived fully and richly is "a taste of heaven."

Taking the First Steps

If you've been part of a religious tradition in the past that still appeals to you, or if you're currently a member of a church that nourishes you, I would suggest that you take the ideas presented above and see what your tradition says about them. You'll need to find the right words and images to help support and comfort you through your journey with HIV, whether those words are "eternal life in Jesus Christ," or "resting in the bosom of Abraham," or "being transformed into everlasting glory," or "returning to Mother Earth." You may want to find books or scriptures that you find comforting, whether they are the Bible or the Book of Mormon or a volume of poetry. Trust yourself as you explore the right things to surround yourself with at this time.

A final piece of advice: people who are especially committed to being conscious about their spiritual journeys—like monks and religious sisters—spend their entire lives trying to make sense of life and death. You are not going to figure this all out for yourself in a few weeks! Be patient as you try to make spiritual sense of your life with HIV. Just take one day at a time. You don't need to figure out the meaning of everything today. You only need to try to understand today *today*. The best way to avoid being spiritually overwhelmed as you deal with this is to be very hard on yourself about not putting too much on your plate. If you find yourself doing that, be ruthless and take something off. It will be there tomorrow. Really.

Turn it over to God. You've got to turn it to someone higher than yourself. You know all those foxhole prayers: "Get me out of this, Lord, and I'll do whatever you want"? This ain't one we'll get an answer to quickly.

Go ahead and scream. Do it, because God forgives us for whatever we've done. When the body's gone there's nothing left but the spirit. Say it how you feel. Somebody has to understand, there's gotta be <u>some</u>body who can hear it.

AIDS isn't the only bad thing that's happened to me. I've lost a hand, I never had a mother, lots of stuff. A lot of things have happened to me in my life, but somehow I came through okay. Someone loves me. You've got to trust God and let Him take care of you, and it will be easier. Be around people who believe in God. Don't hang around negative people.

KAREN

Survivor guilt. That's a big one. Some of our clients who are long-term survivors have lost a lot of friends and lovers to AIDS. They, themselves, have been able to benefit from the new treatments; they're doing really well. Still, the impact that's had on them emotionally is really heavy—especially if they were caregivers themselves, already having buried so many people they loved, and having prepared themselves for death. Now all of a sudden, they're going to be around! They're having expectations of living out a normal life span, or close to it…and they're looking around, and so many people they used to know and hang out with and party with are gone. Chicago's become a ghost town for many gay men, at least the big core community that used to be there. Those left behind often feel incredibly isolated and guilt-ridden—that somehow, <u>they</u> made the cut-off to be able to take advantage of the new drugs, while their loved ones didn't.

DEBORAH
STEINKOPF
EXECUTIVE DIRECTOR, BEHIV—
BETTER EXISTENCE WITH HIV

Hospice Care

Hospice provides a supportive environment for terminally ill patients. The emphasis is on death with dignity, and on keeping patients as comfortable and pain-free as possible.

In most hospice programs, care is provided in-home by a specially trained team of doctors, nurses, therapists, social workers, and clergy. Their role is to meet the physical, emotional, social, and spiritual needs of the patient in his or her last months of life. Hospice team members also support the patient's primary caregiver(s), family members and extended family, helping to guide and comfort them to maximize their involvement and minimize burnout. Help is available 24 hours a day, 7 days a week.

A few hospice programs offer group residential facilities for patients who are alone or whose home situation cannot accommodate their needs. Inpatient hospice staffs include highly skilled pain management specialists. Every effort is made to create a home-like, loving environment.

For the most part, though, hospice is not a place so much as it is a philosophy. Life quality is given priority over life quantity. Patients generally choose hospice having made the decision that aggressive tests and treatments are no longer effective or desirable. Patients find it comforting to know that while in hospice, they will not be put on machines, stuck with needles, or forced into the usual barrage of diagnostic invasions typical of a hospital setting.

Hospice gives patients the opportunity to find a sense of peace and self-awareness—focusing on whatever has given them the most meaning in their lives. Dr. Robert Hirschtick, writing in "Positively Aware," has this to say on what hospice can offer:

> *This approach is sometimes derided as "giving up." But it's okay to give up. It's okay to give up on medications that cause nausea and fatigue when their benefits have long since ebbed. It's okay to give up on painful biopsies and endoscopies that increasingly yield "non-diagnostic" results. This type of giving up offers tremendous freedom. Freedom to be selfish and be cared for. Freedom to cry. Freedom to express fear and discuss death. Freedom to mend relationships. Freedom to say goodbye. The energy that had been channeled toward staying alive is freed up to be refocused on feeling and living well….*
>
> *Hospice is not only for people on their "death bed," although such people have benefited from hospice. Hospice is not euthanasia. The philosophy does not condone active hastening of death. The decision to join hospice is not irrevocable. An individual may leave the program and resume aggressive care at any time….*

Hospice has been described in TIME magazine as a way of "bargaining away pain and isolation in return for peace and acceptance." It affords an opportunity to work through anger and fear en route to a higher level of serenity. Those who have opted to go this way have given up what the disease would have taken anyway and have gained an otherwise unobtainable tranquillity. Not a bad bargain.

From "Hospice: A Philosophy of Living," in "Positively Aware," the newsletter of Test Positive Aware Network, December, 1991. Reprinted with permission.

Hospice and Other Resources

Listed below are many hospice and support programs. Most communities have hospice programs, which you can find in the Yellow Pages under "Hospices." Or call the Illinois AIDS Hotline (800-243-2437) for referrals throughout Illinois.

Keep in mind that your hospice choices may be determined by your insurance coverage, hospital, and physician. Some hospice programs are Ryan White funded, have sliding scale fees, or are free to eligible people. Check your options with your insurance company, health care provider, or case manager.

Advocate Health Care
2311 West 22nd Street, Suite 300
Oak Brook, IL 60521
800-564-2025
• 24-hour private duty care including RNs, LPNs, and homemakers. Home health visits include RNs, physical, occupational, and speech therapists, and home health aides. At-home hospice care, home health continuous care, and infusion services. Public Aid accepted. English/Spanish.

Advocate Home Health Services
8950 Gross Point Road, Suite E
Skokie, IL 60077
847-966-8700
847-966-8743—FAX
• Provides home care, homemaker services, and physical, occupational, and speech therapy. Day care is also available. Public Aid accepted.

Advocate Hospice
1441 Branding Street, Suite 240
Downers Grove, IL 60515
630-963-6800
708-386-9191—Ryan White Hospice Network
630-963-6877—FAX
• Hospice services include medical care for pain control and symptom management, social services, pastoral and bereavement counseling. Ryan White CARE Act Hospice Network provides hospice care to medically indigent PWAs in the greater Chicago/Suburban area. Public Aid accepted. English/Spanish.

Apria Healthcare Group
565 Lamont Road
Elmhurst, IL 60126
630-941-6440
630-941-6409—FAX
• Infusion therapy, nutrition, nursing, pharmacy, and social services. Women's health program.

Care-Med Chicago
322 South Green Street
Chicago, IL 60607
312-738-8622
312-738-9753—FAX
312-738-5299—Hearing-impaired TTY/TDD
• Comprehensive home care including RN visits, social services and mental health care, pastoral care, IV, and physical, respiratory, speech, and occupational therapies. Home health aides, medical equipment, and hospice. Public Aid accepted. English/Spanish.

Coram Healthcare
1471 Business Center Drive, Suite 500
Mount Prospect, IL 60056
847-803-9600
847-803-8635—FAX
• Infusion therapy, skilled clinical nursing, pharmacy, nutrition, and social work services. Multidisciplinary care team dedicated to HIV services.

Center for New Beginnings
10300 West 131st Street
Palos Park, IL 60464
708-923-1116
708-923-6524—FAX
• Individual and group support for bereavement and for persons affected by HIV/AIDS. Serves Chicago metropolitan area. Free.

Columbia Home Care
550 West Webster Avenue
Chicago, IL 60614
773-883-0016
773-883-9415—FAX
• Comprehensive home health services, case management, psychiatric home health, and hospice. Public Aid accepted. Call for south Chicago location information. English, Spanish, American Sign Language.

Community Nursing Service—West
1041 West Madison
Oak Park, IL 60302
708-386-4443
708-386-7453—FAX
• Hospice care in Chicago's west suburbs. Sliding scale fees. Public Aid accepted. English/Spanish.

DeKalb County Hospice
213 East Locust
DeKalb, IL 60115
815-756-3000
815-758-0962—FAX
• Support services for the terminally ill and their families. Information, referrals, and respite and bereavement support. Free. English/Spanish.

Fox Valley Hospice
200 Whitfield Drive
Geneva, IL 60134
630-232-2233
630-232-0023—FAX
• Hospice care provided in Chicago's far west and northwest suburbs. Free

Harbor Light Hospice
800 Roosevelt Road,
Building C, Suite 206
Glen Ellyn, IL 60137
630-942-0100
630-942-0118—FAX
• Hospice and bereavement services and support in west suburban Chicago.

Home Care Resources—Hospice of West Suburban Hospital
1000 West Lake Street
Oak Park, IL 60301
708-383-4663
708-383-9429—FAX
• General hospice care providing services to develop a supportive, caring environment working with the patient and family. Offers RN/LPN, HHA services, various therapies, and pastoral and bereavement support.

Home Health Plus
175 East Hawthorn Parkway
Vernon Hills, IL 60061
888-733-3750
847-362-3295—FAX
• Five locations throughout the Chicagoland area. In-home and residential hospice and home health services. Nursing, nutritional counseling, spiritual counseling, bereavement support, volunteers, medical social workers, and home health aides. Traditional home care services, including therapies, infusion therapy, and private duty service. English, Spanish, Russian, French, Haitian, Polish, and Asian languages (including Taiwanese and Korean). Public Aid and Medicare accepted.

Horizon Hospice
833 West Chicago Avenue
Chicago, IL 60622
312-733-8900
312-733-8952—FAX
• Provides in-home and residential hospice and support services to terminally ill people, including persons with HIV/AIDS and their families and caregivers. Bereavement support group. Serves the Chicago area. Public Aid accepted. English/Spanish.

Hospice House of Alexian Brothers
800 West Beisterfield Road
Elk Grove Village, IL 60007
847-981-5574
847-981-5914—FAX
• Inpatient or in-home care for persons with AIDS. Bereavement care. Support services for the terminally ill and their families.

Hospice of DuPage
690 East North Avenue
Carol Stream, IL 60188
630-690-9000
630-690-9064—FAX
• Services for the terminally ill, including pain and symptom control, nursing, CNA visits, social worker visits, and bereavement and chaplain support. 24-hour on-call availability. Sliding scale fees. Public Aid accepted.

Hospice of the Great Lakes
3130 Commercial Avenue
Northbrook, IL 60062
847-559-8999
847-559-9005—FAX
• Hospice care to residential and nursing home patients and their caregivers and families.

Hospice of Highland Park Hospital
718 Glenview Avenue
Highland Park, IL 60035
847-480-3858
847-480-3941—FAX
• Hospice and home health services. Offers nursing and social work visits, as well as bereavement support and counseling.

Hospice of Kankakee Valley
1015 North 5th Avenue, Suite 5
Kankakee, IL 60901
815-939-4141
815-939-1501—FAX
• Home-centered hospice care, management of pain and symptoms, and bereavement counseling. Arrangements for in-home medical equipment, medications, and medical services. 24-hour on-call nurses and counselors. Sliding scale fees. Public Aid accepted. English/Spanish.

Hospice of the North Shore
2821 Central Street
Evanston, IL 60201
847-467-7423
847-866-6023—FAX
800-526-0844—Hearing-impaired TTY/TDD
• Full range of hospice care support services, including medical management, nursing visits, social services, support, and volunteer assistance. Services provided in-home and at extended care facilities. English/Spanish.

Hospice of Northeastern Illinois
410 South Hager Avenue
Barrington, IL 60010
800-425-4444
847-381-5599
847-381-5713—FAX
• Full-service hospice with nursing visits, CNA, social worker, chaplain, and bereavement support. Medicare-certified; Public Aid accepted. English/Spanish.

In-Home Health Care
2000 Glenwood Avenue, Suite 103
Joliet, IL 60435
815-725-8400
815-725-8473—FAX
• Comprehensive home health care, hospice, and long-term care services. Offices in Joliet, Morris, Worth, Chicago, Schaumburg, and Oakbrook Terrace. Medicare accepted. English/Spanish.

Joliet Area Community Hospice
335 West Jefferson
Joliet, IL 60435
800-360-1817
815-740-4107—FAX
• Multidisciplinary hospice and home health services, including social workers, pastoral care, and volunteer services. Public Aid accepted. English/Spanish.

Lake Forest Hospice
660 North Westmoreland
Lake Forest, IL 60045
847-234-5600
847-234-9365—FAX
• Full service hospice services, psychosocial and spiritual support. English/Spanish.

Northwestern Memorial Hospice
303 East Superior Street, Passavant 9E
Chicago, IL 60611
312-908-7476
312-908-4070—FAX
• Inpatient and home hospice care for terminally ill patients. Home care offers a full range of services including nurses visits and home infusion. Bereavement support for the terminally ill and their families. Medicare accepted.

Olsten Kimberly Quality Care
220 Remington Boulevard, Suite 127
Bolingbrook, IL 60440
800-908-3388
630-378-9721—FAX
• Home care services, includes visiting RNs, therapists, infusion therapists, homemakers, and companions trained in care of AIDS patients. Public Aid accepted. Multilingual.

Rainbow Hospice, Inc.
1550 North Northwest Highway, Suite 220
Park Ridge, IL 60068
847-699-2000
847-699-2047—FAX
• Home-based hospice care and support services for the terminally ill. Sliding scale fees.

Rush Hospice Partners
1035 Madison Street
Oak Park, IL 60302
708-386-9191
708-386-9933—FAX
708-681-6233—Hearing-impaired TTY/TDD
• In-home, residential, and inpatient hospice services in Cook, Lake, and DuPage Counties. Emotional, spiritual, and bereavement support for the terminally ill, their families, caregivers, and others. Ryan White CARE Act Hospice Network provides hospice care to medically indigent PWAs in the greater Chicago/Suburban area. English/Spanish.

St. Thomas Hospice
7 Salt Creek Lane
Hinsdale, IL 60521
630-850-3990
630-850-3953—FAX
• Multidisciplinary at home or inpatient hospice services for the terminally ill and their families. Sliding scale fees. Public Aid accepted.

STAR Hospice
2615 West Washington Boulevard
Waukegan, IL 60085
847-360-2220
847-360-2185—FAX
• Hospice care, support services, and home health care. Medicare accepted.

Unity Hospice
439 East 31st Street
Chicago, IL 60616
312-949-1188
312-949-0158—FAX
• Home-based and inpatient care for patients with terminal illnesses. Counseling and support services for individuals and families. Medicare accepted.

VNA North Hospice
5215 Old Orchard Road, Suite 700
Skokie, IL 60077
847-581-1717
847-581-1919—FAX
• Full-range home care for the terminally ill, including case management, skilled nursing, aides, social work counseling, and psychological, spiritual and emotional support for patients and families. Public Aid accepted. English/Spanish.

Vitas Corporation
7301 North Lincoln Avenue, Suite 201
Lincolnwood, IL 60646
800-762-5444
847-568-9009—FAX
• Hospice and home-based support services in Cook, Lake, and DuPage Counties. Public Aid accepted. English/Spanish.

Vitas Innovative Hospice
580 Watersedge Drive
Lombard, IL 60148
630-495-8484
630-495-1598—FAX
• Full-service home care, "Patients without Primary Caregiver" program. Nursing home care, inpatient and contract hospice beds available, bereavement support.

West Towns Visiting Nursing Service
6438 West 34th Street
Berwyn, IL 60402
708-749-7171
708-749-7185—FAX
• Offers home-based hospice, bereavement, and spiritual support to the terminally ill in west/southwest Cook and southeast DuPage Counties. Public Aid accepted. English/Spanish.

Long-Term Care Facilities

Many local hospitals offer or can help you arrange long-term care. Discuss your options with your health care provider, case manager, or insurance provider.

AIDS Care
315 West Barry
Chicago, IL 60657
773-935-4663
773-935-4662—FAX
• Long-term housing with continuum of care through personal physicians and outside agencies. Residents are provided with case management, food, and basic necessities, as well as pastoral care and counseling. Public Aid accepted.

Alden Nursing Center—Lakeland
820 West Lawrence Avenue
Chicago, IL 60640
773-769-2570
773-769-1551—FAX
• Comprehensive long-term care for those with HIV/AIDS. Public Aid accepted. Multilingual.

Bonaventure House
PO Box 148187
Chicago, IL 60614
773-327-9921
773-327-9113
• Residential service for PWAs offering case management, residential health care and hospice services, support groups, pastoral care, and transportation to doctor appointments.

Chicago House and Social Service Agency
PO Box 14728
Chicago, IL 60614
773-248-5200
773-248-5019—FAX
• Operates three facilities and scattered site apartments, each geared toward a different stage of HIV disease. Eligibility based on diagnosis, need, ability to live in a group setting, and willingness to abide by rules banning drug/alcohol use. Provides case management to clients in residences and to the community. Sliding scale fees. English/Spanish.

Glen Oaks Nursing Center
270 Skokie Boulevard
Northbrook, IL 60062
847-498-9320
847-498-2990—FAX
• Provides long-term care for people with HIV/AIDS. Grace Pavilion HIV/AIDS nursing care unit provides tube feeding, IV and oxygen therapies, and hyperalimentation. Physical and occupational therapy, art and music therapy, and rehabilitation, as well as support groups, pastoral care. Public Aid accepted. English/Spanish.

Oak Forest Hospital
15900 South Cicero Avenue
Oak Forest, IL 60452
708-633-3731
708-687-7979—FAX
• Long-term inpatient care in an HIV/AIDS unit, as well as psychological and spiritual support. Public Aid accepted. English, Spanish, Polish, and French.

Snow Valley Nursing and Rehabilitation Center
5000 Lincoln Avenue
Lisle, IL 60532
630-852-5100
630-852-9747—FAX
• Medicare-certified skilled nursing and rehabilitation center for long- and short-term stays. Hospice-affiliated.

Foster Care for Children

Association House of Chicago
2150 West North Avenue
Chicago, IL 60647
773-276-0084
773-276-7395—FAX
• Foster care and legal services. Residential and addiction recovery programs for the economically, mentally, and/or physically disabled. Shelter for women. English/Spanish.

Casa Central
1401 North California
Chicago, IL 60622
773-276-1902
773-276-0465—FAX
• Transitional housing for families, adult day care, foster care, and day care. Sliding scale fees. English/Spanish.

The Children's Place
3059 West Augusta Boulevard
Chicago, IL 60622
773-826-1230
773-826-0705—FAX
• Temporary residential home for children from birth-5 years. Services available to natural or foster parents and siblings. English/Spanish.

Firman Community Services
144 West 47th Street
Chicago, IL 60609
733-373-3400
773-373-3602—FAX
• Foster care services, child care for children age 3 to 13 years. Most services free except day care.

Illinois Department of Children and Family Services (DCFS)
750 West Montrose Avenue
Chicago, IL 60613
773-989-5884
773-989-3478—FAX
• Support services for HIV-affected families, children, and youth. Group home for HIV-positive adolescents age 13-18 who are wards of the state. Referrals and help in accessing foster care, child day care, and respite care. Permanency Planning program helps HIV-positive parents plan for the care of their children. Provides family presentations, counseling, legal services, homemaker, and early intervention services. Free. English/Spanish.

Kaleidoscope—Star Program
1279 North Milwaukee Avenue, Suite 250
Chicago, IL 60622
312-278-7200
312-278-5663—FAX
• Child welfare agency providing services to HIV-affected children and their families. Foster care, independent living programs for adolescents age 18-21, and in-home services for families in need. Support groups for foster parents of HIV-positive children. English/Spanish.

Lutheran Social Services of Illinois
1144 West Lake Street
Oak Park, IL 60301
708-445-8341
708-445-8351—FAX
• "Second Family" program assists HIV-positive parents in making long-term plans for their children. Prospective adoptive "second families" trained and licensed. Support group for gay/lesbian parents affected by HIV, and case management for parents. "Positive Care" program places state wards with HIV/AIDS, and works with families in reuniting children with their parents. The program also offers medical care, parenting classes, and support groups. English/Spanish. Free.

Funeral Arrangements

Department of Veterans Affairs—Veterans Service Division
800-827-1000
8 a.m.-4:00 p.m., Mon-Fri (except federal holidays)
• Provides financial assistance to cover transportation and cemetery plot costs. Deceased must have been a veteran on pension or died in a VA hospital.

**Illinois Department
of Public Aid**
624 South Michigan Avenue
Chicago, IL 60605
800-252-8635
8:30 a.m.-4:45 p.m. Mon-Fri
• Information and eligibility requirements for financial assistance for funeral arrangements. English/Spanish.

Social Security Administration (Illinois)
800-772-1213—English/Spanish
7 a.m.-7 p.m., Mon-Fri
• Social Security may provide a one-time payment to cover burial costs. Payable to the surviving spouse or child.

Books and Publications

After You Say Goodbye: When Someone You Love Dies of AIDS
Froman, Paul Kent
Chronicle Books, 1992
• Presents a very personal approach to grief, fear, discrimination, and the outrage that frequently accompanies the death of a loved one from AIDS. Offers practical, individual strategies and solutions to the emotional problems encountered by those dealing with their loss.

AIDS and the Hospice Movement
Ament, Madalon O. and Claire Tehan
Harrington Park, 1991
• Discusses all aspects of AIDS and hospice care, including eligibility criteria and variations in the normal grieving process.

American Cancer Society, Inc.
800-227-2345
• Request their booklet, "Questions and Answers about Pain Control." It explains the physiology of pain and how to relieve it with and without medication.

Among Friends: Hospice Care for the Person with AIDS
Buckingham, Robert W.
Prometheus, 1992
• Indispensable resource for PWAs and loved ones who are concerned about appropriate care.

On Death and Dying
Kubler-Ross, Elizabeth
Macmillan Publishing, 1991

Videos

"Living with Loss: Children with HIV"
Mail order: Child Welfare League of America, 800-407-6273
• Explores positive ways to cope with loss for families and others caring for children with HIV/AIDS.

"Thinking About Death"
Mail order: Lambda Rising Books, 800-621-6969
• People with HIV and their loved ones talk about mortality, mourning, and loss from different spiritual perspectives.

"What About My Kids?"
Mail order: Gay Men's Health Crisis, 212-337-1950
• Guides parents through the process of arranging guardianship of their children. Legal explanations from service providers are specific to New York.

On Saying Goodbye
by C. J. Hawking, M.Div.

C. J. Hawking is a former Hospice Chaplain at Illinois Masonic Medical Center. She wrote this essay in 1992 based on her experiences there and in San Francisco during her chaplain residency year.

There are as many ways to die as there are people. Each person's death experience is unique, and, when you think about it, usually reflects their personality. I also believe that each person's death experience is sacred.

We have been taught by our society that death is failure, defeat, an unhappy ending. Having spent time with people who are dying with AIDS (after they have lived with AIDS for up to seven years), I am convinced that the dying process can be life-affirming, joyful, and healing.

I once served as a hospice chaplain to seven AIDS patients who lived together in a community setting. When one patient died, the effect rippled through the household. One 33-year-old patient, having experienced multiple deaths in this community, turned to me one day and asked, "Do you think a person can prepare for death?"

I found great wisdom and maturity in his asking that question. We explored it together at length. Let me share a few of our discoveries.

Goodbye to Work

To cease breathing is not the first death an AIDS patient encounters. The first death often comes when you leave your job. In our culture, saying goodbye to your job means saying goodbye to status, community standing, financial security—and to your identity, in a very real way. We live in a time in which society too often values you more for what you can do than for who you are.

Some people living with AIDS are fortunate enough to be able to plan when to leave their workplace. Others become ill very suddenly and unexpectedly. For them, there are no handshakes, no "retirement" parties, or fond farewells. In a situation like this, where there was no closure, it can be very difficult to accept the fact that this part of your life is over.

If you have already left your job and it's not feasible or desirable to return to say your goodbyes, I would suggest that you say them by using your imagination. Picture yourself going into the building one last time…greeting the security guard, pressing the elevator button, clocking in, and so on. Now imagine yourself at your desk or locker, on your last day…your belongings packed and ready to go. Imagine yourself going around to say goodbye to everyone. What would you say? What has working here meant to you? Who would you avoid? Hug? Exchange phone numbers with?

As you go through this exercise, be aware that this is a part of your past. You will not be returning. You may want to do this while sitting in a car outside the building. Say goodbye to the building, the street, the coffee shop on the corner. Be aware of what you have gained from the work experience and the loss you now feel.

Goodbye to Home

Having to move out of your own house or apartment is often the next big loss to be faced. Some of the patients I've known have become ill so quickly that family and friends had to perform the actual moving job. If this was the case for you, and you never had a chance to say a proper goodbye to "your place," use your imagination to go back and move out personally. Picture each room as it was when you last saw it. Sort through your artwork, clothes, furniture, dishes, books and so on. Which ones were your favorites? What did each piece mean to you? Whom would you like to pass these things along to?

Go from room to room in your mind. What memories are held within each one? Relive the good times, the struggles, the life you had there. This has been your space. What is special about it? Think back. Laugh. Cry. Live it!

As I write this, two of our hospice patients are sorting through their treasured belongings and giving gifts and keepsakes to their loved ones. This is the greatest testimony to life I have ever witnessed: these people using their last weeks to make gifts for others.

Goodbye to Loved Ones

Saying goodbye to your loved ones is usually the most challenging, as well as the richest experience a dying person goes through. Think about the important people in your life. Focus on each one. What are the characteristics you have valued in them? What have they taught or shown you? What have you given them? Reflect on your most special times together. Envision a conversation in which you share your thoughts and memories.

When the time comes to actually meet with some or all of these special people, let this sharing process be mutual. Be prepared to let them be vulnerable with you. Also, be prepared that they may not respond in exactly the way you would like them to. Give them the space to be comfortable with what they want to say, and how they want to remember you and be remembered by you.

Goodbyes on Top of Goodbyes

Goodbye to your job, your co-workers, your belongings, your home, your friends, your family, your breadth of independence—how will you be able to stand all this loss? I can't answer that question for you because I haven't gone through it myself. But I can tell you what I have seen work for others.

Life is a paradox. The more you have to say goodbye to, the more fullness and richness you have had in your life. The deeper the pain, the deeper the joy you have felt. As you wave your hand to say goodbye to the beauty of life, raise your voice to give thanks for all that you've been privileged to be a part of.

I'm artistic. I draw, sew, do photography. I want my daughter to be photographed a lot—and me, my husband, all of us as a family unit—so she can see us together when I'm gone.

I've thought about do I want to draw something for her, do a diary or something. On the flip side, and it may be denial, I'll think, "I'll be here forever." Some days, I look at her and wonder if I'll be able to see her go to school. The hard thing for me to accept is that I'm in this position.

HIV has made me respect life. It's made me a better person, more well-rounded. I'm looking at things deeper. I'm trying to learn about other cultures. I'm also a more feeling person now. I look at my child who doesn't have HIV, and I think about what a miracle it all is.

EVIE

Two other things I would suggest: try to maintain your sense of humor, and remember that you needn't be alone as you go through the final stages.

There is a saying that we come into this world alone, and we leave it alone. That is not entirely true. While others can't go with you, they can be with you. You won't be alone if you don't want to be alone. Stay open to the possibilities. I've made friends with patients five days before they died. Don't close yourself off from the potential for love in your life while your life is still ongoing.

Saying Goodbye with AIDS

Most of the insights I've shared so far are more or less universal, no matter what the cause of death. However, I believe there are some aspects unique to AIDS as a cause of death that deserve special note.

As unjust as it is, there still exists a stigma surrounding AIDS and the people dying from it. It would be a terrible waste to spend your last days on earth worrying about this or letting it affect the way you fashion your goodbyes.

After the stigma, what strikes me most is that we are all too young to be burying our friends, lovers, brothers, sisters, sons, daughters, neighbors, and so forth. For some of us, we are burying our friends before we bury our grandfathers. This feels unnatural. It is unnatural! Let's just acknowledge that upfront.

If at all possible, don't waste your energy pretending. Energy and time are too precious now to pretend you don't have AIDS, that you're not gay or an IV drug user, or that you're not dying and scared as hell about it. As one of my favorite patients would say (and I quote him often), "I don't have time for this!"

You do have time, however, for many other things: to reflect, laugh, cry, remember, give, take, love, sigh, enjoy, bitch, and raise your voice in thanks and your hand to wave goodbye…knowing that you are cherished and will be missed.

Epilogue
By Joseph Zendell
Former HIVCO President

It's tough writing an epilogue to this book. I feel almost as if I'm writing an epilogue to my life, and that's pretty depressing. What comes to mind now, as I sit here with 7 T cells and this damned virus in my body, is fear. Oh, not fear of death. Death will either be a release, an eternal sleep, or a great adventure.

No. What I fear is dying…badly. I fear the pain and the lingering, wasting away of what I once was. I am desperately afraid of losing my dignity, becoming a burden and a helpless invalid.

I remember the months before my beloved Michael died. How much he needed me as he became weaker and unable to lift his head. How heart wrenching it was to care for him, knowing that the end was at hand. And yet I was proud to be able to be with him those last months, and pleased that I could help him through the process of dying. There was never any fear in his eyes, just strength and courage.

Each day now I struggle between trying to accept the inevitable, death, and the need to fight on—to try new and encouraging alternative techniques. To hope that somehow, I'll beat the odds.

What an incredibly illogical, human thing this is, this thing called "hope." It is often the only thing we have that keeps us from going absolutely nuts. I hope for a cure. I hope for new and useful treatments. I hope that I can outlast this disease and continue what has been a wonderful life.

That "there is hope" is perhaps the only way we can really deal with this dreaded and cruel plague. It isn't rational. It isn't, perhaps, terribly productive. But the alternative is to give up, and that I will never do. Michael never did.

Neither should you.

APPENDICES

APPENDIX A

Needs Assessment Form

Make a list of what I need in terms of:

1. Health care and emotional support:

_____

_____

_____

_____

_____

_____

2. Financial and legal assistance:

_____

_____

_____

_____

_____

3. Housing, food, and day-to-day living:

_____

_____

_____

_____

_____

_____

APPENDIX B

Appointment Form

Copy this form and use it to keep track of appointments with doctors, therapists, case managers, and other health care and social service providers.

Record of Visit with Health Care or Social Service Provider

Date:_____   Provider:_____

Reason for visit:
_____

My health since last visit:
_____
_____
_____

Questions and things to discuss:
_____
_____
_____

New test results:
_____
_____
_____

Notes from discussion/referrals/next steps:
_____
_____
_____

Next appointment date:_____

APPENDIX C

More important than any single T cell or viral load test is how your results look over time and in relation to each other. Copy this form and use it to help track your test results.

Health Record

Date	T Cells	Viral Load	Other Tests	Treatments	Health	Notes
Example: 4/1	300	4,000	positive parasite screen	AZT/3TC	diarrhea	start Flagyle for parasite; continue AZT/3TC; retest 4/14 for parasite

APPENDICES 275

APPENDIX D

Record of Contacts Related to HIV

Copy this form and use it to keep track of interactions with case workers, entitlement or insurance agencies, attorneys, or others.

Date	Person/Agency	Call or Visit	Topic	Notes	Next Steps	Completed
Example: 4/1	*John Smith at counseling center*	*phone call*	*SSDI application*	*I need to call Ms. Johnson to verify information*	*call SSDI office by 3/5*	*called 3/2*

RESOURCES INDEX

Resource	Phone	Page
A		
Access Living	312-226-5900	225
ACLU Foundation—National Prison Project	202-234-4830	179
Actors' Fund of America	312-372-0989	229
Adams County Health Dept.	217-222-8440	15
ADD—Residence for Women	773-271-3418	22
Advocate Health Care	800-564-2025	262
Advocate Home Health Services	847-966-8700	262
Advocate Hospice	630-963-6800	262
Advocate Hospice—Ryan White Hospice Network	708-386-9191	262
AIDS Alternative Health Project	773-561-2800	101
AIDS Care	773-935-4663	225, 265
AIDS Care Network	815-968-5181	31, 146, 207
AIDS Clinical Trials Information Service (ACTIS)	800-TRIALS-A	91
AIDS Foundation of Chicago	312-922-2322	9, 15, 66, 207
AIDS Legal Council of Chicago	312-427-8990	13, 225, 238, 240, 251
AIDS Ministry of Illinois	815-723-1548	153, 207, 225
AIDS Pastoral Care Network	773-334-5333	29, 153
AIDS in Prison Project—The Osborne Association	212-673-6633	179
AIDS Research Alliance Chicago	773-244-5800	91
AIDS Support Coalition	815-459-1985	31, 146
AIDS Treatment Data Network	800-734-7104	13, 105
AIDS Treatment News	800-873-2812	98, 104, 105
Alcoholics Anonymous AIDS Awareness of New Town Alano Club	773-271-6822	171
Alcoholism and Drug Dependence Program (ADD)—Lutheran Social Services	773-282-7693	171
Alden Nursing Center—Lakeland	773-769-2570	265
Alexian Brothers Medical Center	888-394-9400	66
American Cancer Society	800-227-2345	266

American Civil Liberties Union of Illinois (ACLU)	312-201-9740	179
American Dietetic Association	312-899-0040	130
American Dietetic Association—Consumer Hotline	800-366-1655	133
American Foundation for AIDS Research (AMFAR)	800-39AMFAR	91, 104
American Indian Health Service	773-883-9100	29
American Red Cross—Mid-America Chapter	312-440-2000	21, 160
Apria Healthcare Group	630-941-6440	262
Ascension Respite Care Center	312-751-8887	25, 146, 207
Asian American AIDS Foundation	773-989-7220	29, 225
Association for Individual Development	630-859-1291	225
Association House of Chicago	773-276-0084	29, 171, 225 229, 266
Aunt Martha's Youth Services	708-747-2701	28
Austin People's Action Center	773-921-2121	225, 229

B

Bethany Ministries	847-945-1678	31, 153
Better Existence with HIV (BEHIV)	847-475-2115	20, 146, 207 225, 228
Bishop's Task Force on AIDS of the Greek Orthodox Diocese of Chicago	312-337-4130	153
Body Positive	212-566-7333	104
Bonaventure House	773-327-9921	225, 265
Branden House	800-244-0996	171
Brass Foundation	773-994-2708	171
Bridge House	312-266-0404	171
Brother-to-Brother—Mt. Sinai Family Health Ctrs.	773-288-6900	30, 146

C

Camp Getaway	773-334-5333	25
Care-Med Chicago	312-738-8622	262
Casa Central	773-276-1902	226, 266

Catholic Charities	312-655-7715	153, 207 226, 229
Catholic Charities—Lake County	847-249-3500	153, 208 226, 230
Catholic Charities—Southwest Suburban	708-430-0428	207, 226, 229
Catholic Charities—West Suburban	708-209-1110	208, 226, 230
CAVDA—Citizens AIDS Project	847-398-3378	21
CDC National AIDS Clearinghouse	800-458-5231	8, 13, 19, 26 32, 33, 91, 114 136, 160, 162
CDC National AIDS Hotline (English)	800-342-2437	8, 16, 169, 207
CDC National AIDS Hotline (Spanish)	800-344-7432	8, 16, 168, 207
Center for Addictive Problems	312-266-0404	172
Center for Natural and Traditional Medicines	202-234-9632	101
Center for New Beginnings	708-923-1116	31, 146, 262
Champaign-Urbana Public Health District	217-352-7961	15
Chase House—North	312-751-8887	27, 230
Chase House—South	773-374-0422	27, 230
Chase House—West	773-486-9479	27, 230
Chicago Adolescent HIV Network (CAHN)	312-633-7438	27
Chicago Dental Society	312-836-7300	77
Chicago Dept. of Public Health	312-744-8500	66
Chicago Dept. of Public Health—HIV/AIDS Services	312-747-2437	66
Chicago Dept. of Public Health—Englewood Clinic	312-747-5278	66
Chicago Dept. of Public Health—Lakeview Clinic	312-744-2572	66
Chicago Dept. of Public Health—Roseland Neighborhood Health Center	312-747-9500	66
Chicago Dept. of Public Health—South Side Clinic	312-747-0120	66

Organization	Phone	Pages
Chicago Dept. of Public Health—Uptown Clinic	312-744-1935	66
Chicago Dept. of Public Health—West Town Clinic	312-744-5470	66
Chicago Health Outreach	773-275-2060	169
Chicago House and Social Service Agency	773-248-5200	208, 226, 265
Chicago Lawyers' Committee for Civil Rights Under Law	312-630-9744	238
Chicago Medical Society	312-670-2550	66
Chicago Medical Society 24-Hour Tel-Med Line	312-670-3670	66
Chicago Recovery Alliance	773-471-0999	168
Chicago Volunteer Legal Services Foundation	312-332-1624	238
Chicago Women's AIDS Project	773-271-2242	22, 146, 160, 208
Child Welfare League of America	800-407-6273	26
Children's Home and Aid Society of Illinois—Viva Family Center	773-252-6313	25, 30, 32
Children's Memorial Hospital	773-880-3718	22, 25, 66-67
Children's Memorial Hospital—Hemophilia Treatment Center	773-880-4620	67
Children's Place	773-826-1230	25, 226, 266
Circle Family Care	773-921-8100	153, 208
Circle of Hope	815-334-9116	21, 146
Clean Start—Illinois Masonic Center for Addiction Medicine	773-477-2000	172
Coach House Drop-In Center—Woodlawn Organization	773-288-4088	101
Coalition for Positive Sexuality	773-604-1654	160
Columbia Home Care	773-883-0016	262
Columbia Michael Reese Hospital & Medical Center	312-791-3455	67
Community Counseling Centers of Chicago	773-769-0205	208
Community Economic Development Association (CEDA)	312-207-5444	226
Community Nursing Service—West	708-386-4443	262

Community Response	708-386-3383	20, 146, 208 226, 228
Community Supportive Living Systems	773-239-0501	226
Comprension y Apoyo a Latinos en Oposicion al Retrovirus (CALOR)	773-235-3161	30, 146, 208
Connection Crisis Intervention & Referral Services	847-367-1080	11, 230
Connection Crisis Intervention Teen Line	800-310-1234	11, 230
Cook County Dept. of Public Health	708-445-2530	101, 208
Cook County Hospital— HIV Primary Care Center	312-633-3005	20, 67, 101 146, 172 208, 238
Cook County Hospital— Women and Children's HIV Program	312-633-5080	20, 22, 25 67, 172
Cook County Legal Assistance Foundation	847-475-3703	238
Coram Healthcare	847-803-9600	262
Cornerstone Services	815-774-3660	226
Critical Path AIDS Project	215-545-2212	13, 91, 102, 104
Crusader Clinic	815-968-0286	67, 209, 238

D

Daniel Hale Williams Center	773-538-6700	67
DeKalb County Hospice	815-756-3000	263
Dept. of Health and Human Services	800-654-8595	176, 226
Dept. of Veterans Affairs— Veterans Service Division	800-827-1000	201, 266
Direct AID	773-528-9448	230
Duane Dean Recovery Project	815-939-0125	172
DuPage Bar Legal Aid Service	630-653-6212	238
DuPage County Health Dept. AIDS Program	630-682-7979	146, 209 227, 228
DuPage County Medical Society	312-670-9630	66

E

El Rincon Community Clinic	773-276-0200	30, 147, 172
Erie Family Health Center	312-666-3488	30, 67, 209
Evanston Meals-at-Home	847-251-6827	228

F

Family AIDS Support Network	773-404-1038	32
Family Guidance Center	312-943-6545	172
Family Service and Mental Health Center	708-383-7500	147
Firman Community Services	733-373-3400	230, 266
FISH of Park Ridge	847-698-3478	229
Fox River Valley Center for Independent Living	847-695-5818	147, 209, 227
Fox Valley Hospice	630-232-2233	263

G

Garfield Counseling Center	773-533-0433	172, 209
Gateway Foundation—Northwest	773-862-2279	172
Gateway Foundation—South	773-476-0622	22, 172
Gay and Lesbian Physicians of Chicago	312-670-9630	33, 66, 77
Gay Men's Health Crisis	212-807-6655	8, 13, 19 28, 32, 160
Gay Men's Health Crisis—Publications	212-337-1950	13, 161
Genesis House	773-281-3917	23, 227, 230
Genesis House—West Side Satellite	773-533-8701	23, 227, 230
Gerber Hart Gay & Lesbian Library and Archives	773-883-3003	17
Glen Oaks Nursing Center	847-498-9320	265
Greater Community AIDS Project	217-351-2437	227
Groceryland—Humboldt Park	773-486-0200	228
Groceryland—North Side, Chicago	773-244-0088	228
Groceryland—Rogers Park/Edgewater	773-665-1000	228
Groceryland—South Side, Chicago	773-224-1444	228

H

Harbor Light Alcoholism and Drug Dependence Service	312-733-0500	172
Harbor Light Hospice	630-942-0100	263
Harm Reduction Outreach	815-961-1269	169
Haymarket House	312-226-7984	23, 172, 209
Healthcare Alternative Systems—North	773-252-3100	173
Healthcare Alternative Systems—South	773-254-5141	173
Healthcare Alternative Systems—West	773-252-2666	173
Heartland Human Services	217-342-7058	15
Hemophilia Foundation of Illinois	312-427-1495	20, 25, 209
Hemophilia Foundation—National Info Line	800-42-HANDI	20
HIV Coalition (HIVCO)	847-391-9803	13, 22, 147, 229
HIV Coalition Hand-to-Hand Food Line	847-391-9839	22, 229
HIV Positive Action Coalition	773-871-0130	21
HIV Services Consumer Access Line	312-747-9650	204
HIV Talk Radio Project	312-541-TALK	20
Holy Family Hospital	847-297-1800	67
Home Care Resources—Hospice of West Suburban Hospital	708-383-4663	263
Horizon Hospice	312-733-8900	147, 263
Horizons Community Services	773-472-6469	28, 147, 239
Horizons Community Services Lesbian/Gay Hotline	773-929-HELP	28, 147, 239
Horizons Anti-Violence Crisis Hotline	773-871-8873	28, 147, 239
Hospice House of Alexian Brothers	847-981-5574	263
Hospice of DuPage	630-690-9000	263
Hospice of the Great Lakes	847-559-8999	263
Hospice of Highland Park Hospital	847-480-3858	263
Hospice of Kankakee Valley	815-939-4141	263
Hospice of Northeastern Illinois	800-425-4444	264
Hospice of the North Shore	847-467-7423	264

Howard Area Community Center	773-262-6622	209
Howard Brown Health Center	773-871-5777	21, 23, 28 67, 134, 147 173, 209

I

Illinois AIDS Hotline	800-243-2437	9, 17, 77, 147 160, 168, 207 230, 239
Illinois Alcoholism & Drug Dependence Assn.	800-252-6301	171
Illinois Dept. of Alcoholism and Substance Abuse (DASA)	312-814-3840	173
Illinois Dept. of Children and Family Services (DCFS)	773-989-5884	25, 27, 266
Illinois Dept. of Human Rights	312-814-6200	239
Illinois Dept. of Public Aid	800-252-8635	202
Illinois Dept. of Public Aid—Comprehensive Health Insurance Plan (CHIP)	800-367-6410	197, 202
CHIP Board of Directors	800-962-8384	197
Illinois Dept. of Public Health—AIDS Drug Assistance Program	800-825-3518	92
Illinois Dept. of Public Health HIV/AIDS Section Chicago Springfield	312-814-4846 217-524-5983	21, 27, 93, 202 21, 27, 93, 202
Illinois Dept. of Public Health—Continuation of Health Insurance Coverage (CHIC) Program	800-825-3518	194, 202
Illinois Dept. of Rehabilitation Services (DORS) Chicago Springfield Illinois Director of Insurance	773-794-4800 217-782-2093 217-782-4515	223, 231 223 201, 202
Illinois Insurance Information Service	800-444-3338	202
Illinois Masonic Medical Ctr. "Strong Spirit" Program	773-296-8400	101
Illinois Masonic Medical Ctr. Triad Clinic	773-296-8400	67
Illinois State Dental Society	217-525-1406	77
Illinois State Medical Society	312-782-1654	33, 63

ImpactAIDS, Inc.	505-995-0722	19, 32, 33
In-Home Health Care	815-725-8400	264
Institute for Advanced Study of Human Sexuality	415-928-1133	161
Interventions	312-633-4990	173, 209
Interventions—Central Intake	312-850-9411	171
Interventions—Crossroads	773-239-1400	173
Interventions—Wauconda	847-526-0404	173

J

Jackson County Health Dept.	618-684-3143	16
Jewish AIDS Network Chicago	773-463-7251	153
Jewish Children's Bureau of Chicago	847-568-5100	26
Joliet Area Community Hospice	800-360-1817	264
Joshua Ministries Support Group	847-618-4255	32, 148

K

Kaleidoscope—"Star" Program	312-278-7200	26
Kelzer Care Center	773-268-8438	227
Komed Health Center	773-268-7600	68

L

Lake County Alcoholism Treatment Center	847-360-6540	173
Lake County Health Dept.	847-360-6891	147
Lake Forest Hospice	847-234-5600	264
Lambda Legal Defense and Education Fund	312-663-4413	239
Lawndale Christian Health Center	773-521-5006	153, 209
Legal Assistance Foundation of Chicago	312-341-1070	239
Legal Assistance Foundation of Chicago—HIV Housing Law Project	312-347-8311	227
LesBiGay Radio	773-973-3999	20
Love & Action Midwest, Inc.	708-392-3123	153, 210
Loyola University Medical Center—HIV/AIDS Clinic	708-216-5024	68
Lutheran Family Mission	773-287-2921	26

Lutheran General Hospital Addiction Treatment Program	847-696-6050	173
Lutheran General Hospital—Nesset HIV Center	847-318-9320	68
Lutheran Social Services of Illinois	708-445-8341	23, 26, 147, 210, 266

M

Madison County AIDS Program (MADCAP)	618-877-5110	210, 229
Make-A-Wish Foundation	312-943-8956	26
Marillac House	773-722-5157	231
Meals on Wheels—Riverside Medical Center	815-935-7871	229
Medicare Hotline	800-638-6833	220
Men's Network—Heart of Illinois HIV/AIDS Center	309-671-8418	28
Midwest AIDS Training and Education Center (MATEC)	312-996-1373	33
Minority Outreach Intervention Project (MOIP)	773-276-5990	30, 147, 210
Mt. Sinai Hospital	773-257-6547	68

N

National Association of People with AIDS (NAPWA)	202-898-0414	9, 21-22, 97
National Drug and Alcohol Treatment Referral Routing Service	800-662-HELP	171
National HIV Telephone Consultation Service Warmline	800-933-3413	33
National Hotline for Gay and Lesbian Youth	800-347-TEEN	29
National Minority AIDS Council	202-483-6622	33
National Native American AIDS Hotline	800-283-2437	8
National Pediatric HIV Resource Center (NPHRC)	800-362-0071	26, 33
National Runaway Switchboard	800-621-3230	11
National STD Hotline	800-227-8922	8
Near North Health Service Corporation	312-337-1073	173
New City Health Center	773-737-5400	68

New Phoenix Assistance Center	773-978-6322	227
NIA Comprehensive Center	312-949-1808	231
Night Ministry	773-935-8300	27, 153
Northern Illinois AIDS Resource Center	815-633-1660	227
Northern Illinois Council on Alcohol and Substance Abuse—Women and Children's Center	847-785-8660	173
Northwest Community Hospital	847-618-4255	32, 148
Northwestern Hemophilia Treatment Center	312-908-9660	68
Northwestern Memorial Hospice	312-908-7476	264
Northwestern Memorial Hospital—HIV Center	312-908-8358	68

O

Oak Forest Hospital	708-633-3731	68, 266
Olsten Kimberly Quality Care	800-908-3388	264
Omni, Incorporated Initiative	773-278-6106	174, 227
Open Door Clinic	847-695-1093	68, 210
Open Hand Chicago	773-665-1000	229
OUTpost	217-239-4688	29

P

Parents, Families, Friends of Lesbians & Gays (P-FLAG)—		
Chicago Area	773-472-3079	32
National	202-995-8585	32
Parental Stress Services—24-Hour Hotline	312-3PARENT	11, 148
Pastoral Counseling Center of Lutheran General Hospital	847-518-1800	154
Peer Services	847-492-1778	174
People with AIDS Coalition—Hotline	800-828-3280	8, 30, 97
People's Resource Center—Wheaton	630-682-3844	231
Peoria City/County Health Dept.	309-679-6013	16
Pets Are Wonderful Support (PAWS)	415-241-1460	185

Pilsen Little Village Community Mental Health Center	312-226-5864	210
Planned Parenthood—Chicago Area	312-427-2276	23, 160
Planned Parenthood—Chicago-Area Hotline	312-427-2275	23, 160
Positive Approach to Health (PATH)	847-618-4255	148, 234, 244
Prairie State Legal Services	815-965-2902	239
Pride Youth—LINKS North Shore Youth Health Service	847-441-9880	29
Prism Youth Network—Oak Park Area Lesbian and Gay Association	708-FUN-FIND	29
Project Inform	415-558-8669	8
Project Inform—Hotline	800-822-7422	8
Project VIDA	773-522-4570	28, 30, 101
Prologue	800-DOCTORS	66
Provident Hospital	312-572-2724	68
Public Action to Deliver Shelter (PADS)		
DuPage PADS	630-682-3846	227
Hesed House (Aurora)	630-897-2165	227
Northwest Suburban (Cook County)	847-622-5476	227
PADS Place (Lake County)	847-249-0737	227
South Suburban PADS (Cook County)	708-754-4357	227
Southwest Chicago	773-737-7070	227
Tri-Village PADS (Maywood)	708-681-5517	227
PWA Coalition	212-647-1415	104, 180
PWA Health Group	212-255-0520	104, 180

R

Rainbow Hospice	847-699-2000	264
Ravenswood Community Mental Health Center Crisis Line	773-769-6200	11
Regional Transit Authority (RTA)—ADA Paratransit Program	312-917-4357	229
Reimer Foundation	773-935-SAFE	160
Renz Addiction Center	847-742-3545	174
Review	630-629-6946	29

RFMH/HIV Center	212-740-0046	24
Rock Island County Health Dept.	309-793-1955	16
Roseland Christian Health Ministries	773-291-6050	69, 101
Roseland Community Hospital HIV Clinic	773-995-3469	69, 101
Rush Hospice Partners	708-386-9191	264
Rush Presbyterian—St. Luke's Medical Center	312-942-5865	69

S

San Francisco AIDS Foundation—Subscriptions	800-959-1059	104
Serenity House	630-620-6616	174
Share Program	847-882-4181	174
Snow Valley Nursing and Rehabilitation Center	630-852-5100	266
Social Security Administration—Illinois	800-772-1213	217, 220, 267
South Suburban Council on Alcoholism and Substance Abuse	708-957-2854	174
Southern Illinois University School of Medicine	217-782-0181	16, 69, 210
Southern Illinois University School of Medicine—HIV Care Consortia	217-782-7683	16
St. Catherine's of Genoa Catholic Worker	773-288-3688	174, 228
St. Clair County Health Dept.	618-233-7703	16
St. Francis Hospital of Evanston	847-316-2775	69
St. Joseph Hospital	888-712-CARE	69, 101
St. Thomas Hospice	630-850-3990	264
STAR Hospice	847-360-2220	264
Starlight Foundation	312-251-7827	26
Stop AIDS	773-871-5777	22
African-American Program	773-752-7867	22, 30, 161
Latino/a Program	773-235-2586	161
North Side	773-871-3300	160
Sulzer Regional Library	312-744-7616	17

T

Take-A-Hike	708-366-5713	137
Talkline Help Lines		
Adults	847-228-6400	11
Kids	847-228-5437	11
Teens	847-228-8336	11
Teen Living Programs	773-883-0025	28
Teens Tap AIDS Hotline	800-234-TEEN	9
Test Positive Aware Network	773-404-8726	17, 19, 21, 22 29, 30, 31, 91 102, 137, 148 207, 239
Travelers & Immigrants Aid	312-629-4500	31
Travelers & Immigrants Aid—Chicago Health Outreach	773-275-2586	69
Travelers & Immigrants Aid—Neon Street Center	773-271-6366	28, 228
Travelers & Immigrants Aid—Rafael Center	773-989-0049	174, 210 228, 231
Travelers & Immigrants Aid—San Miguel Apartments	773-271-5800	228
Treatment Action Group	212-260-0300	104
Treatment Alternatives for Safer Communities (TASC)	312-787-0208	210
TASC Health Services	312-738-8933	210
Trinity United Church of Christ HIV/AIDS Support Ministry	312-409-AIDS	148, 154

U

UIC Community Outreach Intervention Project		
Austin	773-379-1137	174, 211
North	773-561-3177	174, 211
South	773-536-4509	174, 211
West	773-252-4422	174, 211
Unity Hospice	312-949-1188	265
University of Chicago Hospitals	773-702-1000	69
University of Illinois at Chicago	773-561-3177	69, 211
University of Illinois at Chicago Community Health Project	773-536-4509	70

University of Illinois at Chicago Hospital HIV/AIDS Project— Family Center for Immune Deficiency	312-996-8337	25, 69

V

Veterans Administration Medical Center— North Chicago	847-688-1900	70, 175, 228
Veterans Affairs Dept.— Hines V.A. Hospital	708-343-7200	70, 175
Veterans Affairs Medical Center— West Side	312-666-6500	70
VIDA/SIDA	773-278-6737	17, 31, 102
Vitas Corporation	800-762-5444	265
Vitas Innovative Hospice	630-495-8484	265
VNA North Hospice	847-581-1717	265

W

WATCH Program	773-702-4317	23
Way Back Inn	708-345-8422	174
Weiss Memorial Hospital	773-564-5333	70, 102
West Town Visiting Nursing Service	708-749-7171	211, 265
Western Clinical Health Services	312-251-5020	175
Westside Association for Community Action	773-277-4400	211
Will County Center for Community Concerns	815-722-0722	228
Will County Health Dept.	815-727-8670	16, 211
Will County Health Dept.— HIV/AIDS Care Consortia	815-727-5062	16, 211
Windy City Rainbow Alliance of the Deaf— Voice	773-275-1715	29
TTY/TDD	312-738-9755	29
Winfield Moody Community Health Center	312-337-1073	70
Winnebago County Health Dept.	815-962-5092	16
Women Alive	213-965-1564	14, 24
Women Alive—Hotline	800-554-4876	24

Women and Infants Transmission Study (WITS)	312-996-7479	23
Women's Information Service and Exchange	800-326-3861	24
Woodlawn Organization Substance Abuse Services	773-493-6116	175
WORLD (Women Organized to Respond to Life-Threatening Diseases)	510-658-6930	24
Wyler Children's Hospital of the University of Chicago	773-702-3853	70

Web sites

Access Project: Patient Assistance Programs http://www.aidsnyc.org/network/access/pa.html	97
Act Up: Real Treatments for Real People http://www.aidsnyc.org/rtrp/index.html	12, 134
AIDS Daily Summary http://www.cdcnac.org/summary/html	12
AIDS Education Global Information Service (AEGIS) http://www.aegis.com/	12
AIDS Hotlines and Service Organizations http://www.thebody.com/hotlines.html	12
AIDS Legal Council of Chicago http://www.thebody.com/alcc/alccpage.html	251
AIDS Research Information Center (ARIC) http://www.critpath.org/aric/aricinc.htm	13
American Civil Liberties Union (ACLU)– National Prison Project (NPP) http://www.aclu.org/index.html	179
The Body: A Multimedia AIDS and HIV Resource http://www.thebody.com/cgi-bin/body.cgi	13, 105, 134, 148, 240
CDC National AIDS Clearinghouse http://www.cdcnac.org	13
Closing the Gap http:www.omhrc.gov/ctg/ctg-aids.htm	13, 31
Critical Path AIDS Project http://www.critpath.org/	102
The Food & Drug Administration (FDA) HIV and AIDS Page http://www.fda.gov/oashi/aids/hiv.html	13, 91, 105
Gay Men's Health Crisis (GMHC) On the Web http://www.gmhc.org/	13, 161

The HIV/AIDS Treatment Information Service (ATIS) http://www.hivatis.org/	13, 31, 105
The HIV InfoWeb http://carebase2.jri.org/infoweb/	14, 91, 105, 240
The Journal of the American Medical Association (JAMA) HIV/AIDS Site http://www.ama-assn.org/special/hiv/hivhome.htm	14, 105
"The Kite," http://www.silcom.com/~chc	179
Marty Howard's HIV/AIDS Home Page http://www.smartlink.net/~martinjh/	14, 202
National AIDS Treatment Information Project http://www.kff.org	105
National Institute of Allergy and Infectious Disease (NIAID) Gopher Site gopher://odie.niaid.nih.gov/11/aids	14
National Library of Medicine (NLM) AIDS Information Gopher Resource, gopher://gopher.nlm.nih/gov/11/aids	14, 91, 106
National Women's Law Center http://essential.org/afi/nwlc.html	179
NOAH: New York Online Access to Health AIDS Information Page http://www.noah.cuny.edu/aids/aids.html	14, 133
Osborne Association–AIDS in Prison Project http://www.aidsnyc.org/aip/links.html	179
POZ Magazine http://www.POZ.com	148
Safer SexPage http://www.cmpharm.ucsf.edu~troyer/safesex.html	161
Test Positive Aware Network http://www.tpan.com/alternat/index.htm	102, 148
Yahoo AIDS/HIV Search Site http://www.yahoo.com/Health/Diseases_and_Conditions/AIDS_HIV/	14

INDEX

A

AABD (Aid to the Aged, Blind or Disabled), 220-21, 222
abdominal pain
   as drug side effect, 79, 83
   as symptom, 88, 135
abortion
   and clinical drug trials, 90
   decisions on, 162, 164
abstinence from sexual activities, 155, 157, 159
abusive relationships, 53. *See also* domestic violence
   HIV infection from, 119
acceptance, 110, 254
Access Living, 225
Access Project: Patient Assistance Programs (Web site), 97
ACLU. *See* American Civil Liberties Union
Acquired Immune Deficiency Syndrome. *See* AIDS
activated lymphocytes, as immunomodulators, 84
"Active Duty: Lending Support to PWAs" (video), 18
Actor's Fund of America, 229
Act Up: Real Treatments for Real People (Web site), 12, 134
acupuncture, 61, 98, 101
ADA (Americans with Disabilities Act), 111-12, 234
Adam, stories and opinions, x, 56, 165, 168, 213-16, 235
   on case managers, 206
   on sexual activities, 157
   on support, 141-42
   on telling others, 120
Adams County Health Department, 15
addiction treatment. *See* substance abuse programs/treatment
ADD–Residence for Women, 22
adoption
   as option for care of child, 247
   by people living with HIV/AIDS, 164
advocacy, 49
   organizations, 21-22
Advocate Health Care, 262
Advocate Home Health Service, 262
Advocate Hospice, 262
   Ryan White Hospice Network, 262
AFDC (Aid to Families with Dependent Children), 220, 222, 223
African Americans, 57-60. *See also* people of color
   resources for, 29-30, 146, 148, 161, 173, 210
afterlife, 256-58
After You Say Goodbye: When Someone You Love Dies of AIDS (Froman), 267
agents for powers of attorney. *See* Durable Power of Attorney
AIDS (Acquired Immune Deficiency Syndrome), 2-3, 5-6. *See also* HIV; people living with HIV/AIDS
   on health insurance forms, 190
   seen as punishment, responses to, 149-50, 256
AIDS, God and Faith: Continuing the Dialogue on Constructing Gay Theology (Long and Clark), 154
"AIDS, Medicine, & Miracles" conference (April 1996, in Denver), 46
AIDS, people with. *See* people living with HIV/AIDS
AIDS Alternative Health Project, 101
"AIDS and Addiction" (video), 175
AIDS and the Healer Within (Bamforth), 154
AIDS and the Hospice Movement (Ament and Tehan), 267
AIDS and the Law: A Basic Guide for the Nonlawyer (Terl), 239
AIDS Benefits Handbook, The, 202
AIDS Care, 225, 265
AIDS Care At Home: A Guide for Caregivers, Loved Ones, and People with AIDS (Greif and Golden), 32
AIDS Caregiver's Handbook, The (Eidson, editor), 134
AIDS Care Network, 31, 146, 207
AIDS Clinical Trials Information Service (ACTIS), 91
AIDS Confidentiality Act, Illinois, 111
AIDS Daily Summary (Web site), 12
AIDS-defining illnesses (CDC list), 3, 6. *See also* illness; *individual diseases and symptoms*
AIDS Dementia Complex (ADC), 79, 251-52
AIDS Drug Assistance Program, 92-93, 219
AIDS Education Global Information Service (AEGIS) (Web site), 12
AIDS Foundation of Chicago
   HIV Care Consortia, 15, 207
   Information Line, 9, 66
"AIDS/HIV Treatment Directory," 104
AIDS Hotlines and Service Organizations (Web site), 12
AIDS in the Workplace: Legal Questions and Practical Solutions (Banta), 239

AIDS Law Today: A New Guide for the Public (Burris, Dalton, and Miller), 239
AIDS Legal Council of Chicago, 111, 192, 225, 235-36, 238
    Web site, 13, 240, 251
AIDS Legal Guide, 240
AIDS Ministry of Illinois, 153, 207, 225
AIDS Pastoral Care Network/ Equipo de Cuidado Pastoral Contra el SIDA, 29, 153
AIDS-Related Complex (ARC), on health insurance forms, 190
AIDS Research Alliance Chicago, 91
AIDS Research Information Center (ARIC) (Web site), 13
AIDS Support Coalition, 31, 146
AIDS Treatment Data Network, 13, 105
AIDS Treatment News, 98, 104, 105
Aid to Families with Dependent Children (AFDC), 220, 222, 223
Aid to the Aged, Blind or Disable (AABD), 220-21, 222
"Al," personal story, 124
Alcoholics Anonymous (AA), 22, 171, 227
Alcoholics Anonymous AIDS Awareness of New Town Alano Club, 171
Alcoholism and Drug Dependence Program (ADD), 171
alcohol use, 129, 143, 166-67, 170
    abuse, 40, 43, 129 (*see also* substance abuse; substance abuse programs/treatment)
    discussing with doctor, 73, 76
    interaction with medications, 79, 83
    and safer sex, 156

Alden Nursing Center–Lakeland, 265
Alegria, Juan, on surrender, 255-56
Alexian Brothers Medical Center, 66
"Alive and Kicking" (newsletter), 180
All Care, Inc., 179
alternative treatments. *See* supplemental treatments
Alyna, personal story, 144
Amazon.com Books, 17
American Cancer Society, Inc., 266
American Civil Liberties Union (ACLU)–National Prison Project (NPP), 179
American Civil Liberties Union of Illinois (ACLU), 238
American Dietetic Association, 130
    Consumer Hotline, 133
American Indian Health Service, 29
American Red Cross/Mid-America Chapter, 21, 160
American Sign Language, 21, 160, 225, 262
Americans with Disabilities Act (ADA), 111-12, 234
America Online AIDS and HIV Research Center, 12
Among Friends: Hospice Care for the Person with AIDS (Buckingham), 267
anal intercourse, 1, 156, 157
anemia, 79, 163
anger, 36, 56, 137, 138, 141, 187, 255
anonymity, and HIV testing, 126
anorexia (loss of appetite), 6, 132
antibiotics, table 94-96
antibodies
    as immunomodulators, 84
    in infant's blood, 162

anti-tumor agents, as immunomodulators, 84
antivirals (antiretrovirals), 4, 78-83, 86, 155, 254, *table* 94-96. *See also individual drugs by name*
anxiety, 37, 141
AOL (America Online), 12
appetite, 130-31
    loss of, 6, 132
Apria Health Care Group, 262
ARC (AIDS-Related Complex), on health insurance forms, 190
artifical nutrition, 133, 247, 248
artificial insemination, 164
art therapy, 141
Ascension Respite Care Center, 25, 146, 207
Asian American AIDS Foundation, 29, 225
Asian Americans, 29, 58, 69-70, 225, 263. *See also* multilingual services; people of color
Bo Gyung, 131, 152
assertiveness. *See also* proactivity
    in working with a doctor, 72, 73
assets, financial, 218
    legal arrangements concerning, 234, 244-45
Association for Individual Development, 225
Association House of Chicago, 29, 171, 225, 229, 266
"attacker" (CD8) cells, 2, 4. *See also* T-cell count(s)
attitude, 38-39
    of long-term survivors, 48-49
attorneys. *See* lawyers; legal services
Aunt Martha's Youth Services, 28
Austin People's Action Center, 225, 229

AZT (Retrovir; ZDV; zidovudine), 4, 78-79, 83, 136
　use during pregnancy and childbirth, 7, 162

B

bacteria in foods, harmful effects, 135
bankruptcy, 233
baptismal certificate, as documentation, 212
baseline exams, 72-73
bDNA test, viral loads measured by, 74
Beatty, Nora, 141
Be Good to Yourself: A Resource Guide for Inmates Living with HIV, 180
BEHIV (Better Existence with HIV), 20, 84-85, 146, 170, 205, 207, 225, 228
bereavement support services, 146, 147, 153, 211, 262-65
Berendt, Emily P., 234-35, 244-50
"BETA" (Bulletin of Experimental Treatments for AIDS), 104
Betadine™ solution, 183, 184
Bethany Ministries, 31, 153
Better Existence with HIV (BEHIV), 20, 84-85, 146, 170, 205, 207, 225, 228
bilingual (Spanish/English) services, 20-22, 28-33, 162, 204, 207-11, 229-31. See also Hispanic-Americans
　dental services, 77
　food programs, 228-29
　on food safety, 136
　for homeless people, 176
　hospice care, 262-65
　at hospitals and clinics, 66-70
　housing assistance, 225-28
　information on safer sex resources, 160-61
　for legal assistance, 238-39
　long-term care facilities, 265-66
　for needle exchange programs, 168-69
　spiritual support resources, 153-54
　substance abuse treatment, 71-75
　support groups and mental health services, 146-48
　telephone hotlines, 8, 9-10, 16
　treatment options, 91, 101-2, 106
　Web sites, 14
　for women and children, 22-23, 25-27
birds, as pets, 183
birth certificate, as documentation, 212, 218
birth control, 90, 156. See also condoms
Bishop's Task Force on AIDS of the Greek Orthodox Diocese of Chicago, 153
blame, 38, 56
bleach, use for disinfection, 119, 168, 177, 181, 182
blood
　disorders, questions on health insurance forms, 190
　donation, 124-25, 181
　of newborns, antibodies in, 162
　presence in risky sexual practices, 133, 134
　rules for handling, 122, 123, 181
　tests, 195 (see also HIV tests)
　transfusions, 1, 247
blood products, HIV-infected, 1
Body, The: A Multimedia AIDS and HIV Resource (Web site), 13, 105, 134, 148, 240
body fluids, 1, 181
"Body Positive" (newsletter), 39, 104
body tissue donation, 125
body weight. See weight
Bo Gyung, personal story, 131, 152
Bonaventure House, 225, 265
bone marrow damage, as possible side effect of AZT, 79
books and publications, 17-18, 19, 33, 56, 97, 214-15
　for and about children, 26-27
　for and about women, 24
　on death and dying, 267
　for families, friends, and caregivers, 32
　on food and nutrition, 134
　on legal rights and assistance, 239-40
　on people living with HIV/AIDS in prisons, 180
　for people of color, 31
　on safer sex, 161
　on Social Security Administration programs, 218
　on spirituality, 154
　for teens, 28
　treatment information, 86, 102-3, 104-5
booksellers, 17-18. See also Lambda Rising Books
Branden House, 171
Brass Foundation, 171
breast feeding (nursing), 1, 90, 162, 223
Bridge House, 171
Brother to Brother–Mt. Sinai Family Health Center, 30, 146
Buddhism, spiritual support from, 151, 152
buyers' clubs, 97-98, 104

C

caffeine use, 73, 129, 166
Callen, Michael, 47-48
calories, 130
Camp Getaway, 25

INDEX **299**

cancer, 88-89
    anticancer drugs, *table* 94-96
    cervical, 6, 72, 89
    Kaposi's sarcoma, 6, 47, 88, 254
candidiasis, 87. *See also* yeast infections
carbohydrates, 130
care consortia, HIV, 15-16, 65
caregivers, 58, 140, 204, 260
    resources for, 31-32, 70, 134, 143-44, 163
Caregiver's Journey, The: When You Love Someone with AIDS (Pohl and Deniston), 32
Care-Med Chicago, 262
"Caring for Infants and Toddlers with HIV Infection" (video), 18, 164
"Caring for School Aged Children with HIV Infection" (video), 18, 164
Carmen, personal story, 141
Casa Central, 226, 266
case management, 20, 28, 65, 66-70, 187, 224-27
    advice on life insurance, 199
    aid in financial planning, 232
    government assistance programs, 203-11
    for homeless people, 176
    information on AIDS Confidentiality Act, 111
    information on applying for SSDI, 217
    for people of color, 29-30
    women's and children's services, 22-23, 25-26
Catholic Charities, 153, 207-8, 215, 226, 229-30
cats, 183
cat scratch disease, 183
CAVDA–Citizens AIDS Project, 21

CDC (Centers for Disease Control), 15, 19, 111
    AIDS-defining illnesses list, 3, 6
    definition of long-term survivor, 48
    evaluation of home tests for HIV, 126
    National AIDS Clearinghouse, 8, 19, 26-27, 32, 114, 162
        information on clinical trials, 91
        information on food safety, 136
        information on safer sex, 160
        resources for professionals, 33
        Web site, 13
    National AIDS Hotline, 8, 16, 168, 207
CD4 ("helper-T") cell counts, 2, 4, 74. *See also* T cell count(s)
CD8 ("attacker") cells, 2, 4. *See also* T-cell count(s)
celibacy, 155, 157, 159
Center for Addictive Problems, 172
Center for Natural and Traditional Medicines, 101
Center for New Beginnings, 31, 146, 262
Centers for Disease Control. *See* CDC
certified financial planners, 232
cervical cancer, 6, 72, 89
cervical caps, 156
cesarean section (C-section) for HIV-infected women, 165-66
Champaign-Urbana Public Health District, 15
Charles, Phyllis, 248
Charlie, stories and opinions, xi, 5, 51, 75, 130, 252-55
    on alternative treatments, 98
    on blood drives, 125
    on health insurance, 190

    on medications, 79
    on sexual activities, 157
    on spirituality, 151
    on support groups, 142
    on telling others, 107, 115-16
Chase House, 27, 230
chemotherapy, use in treatment of KS, 6
chest X-rays, 72
chewing problems, possible solutions, 132
CHIC (Continuation of Health Insurance Coverage), Illinois, 194, 202
Chicago Adolescent HIV Network (CAHN), 27
"Chicago Area HIV/AIDS Services Directory" (Bejlovec, editor), 97
Chicago Board of Education, policy on HIV-infected students, 114
Chicago Dental Society, 77
Chicago Department of Health, clinics and health centers, 66
Chicago Health Outreach, 169
Chicago House and Social Service Agency, 208, 226, 265
Chicago Lawyer's Committee for Civil Rights Under Law, Inc., 238
Chicago Medical Society, 66
    24-Hour Ted-Med Line, 66
Chicago Recovery Alliance, 168
Chicago Volunteer Legal Services Foundation, 238
Chicago Women's AIDS Project, 22, 146, 160, 208
childbirth, 1, 7, 162, 165-66
child care, 204, 230, 233
children, 53, 61, 65, 138, 142
    bookstores for, 17-18
    custody, 108, 233, 238, 246-47, 248
    eligibility for government programs, 218, 222, 223

foster care services, 266
guardians for, 19, 235, 240, 243, 245-47, 248
HIV infection in, 1, 3, 121-23, 152, 162-64, 165
medication for, 79
nutritional needs, 131
schools' treatment of, 112-14, 118, 235
services, 22, 25-26, 70
use of protease inhibitors, 82
videos concerning, 18, 19
viral load counts, 74, 82
publications for and about, 26-27
services for, 22, 25-27, 32, 140-41, 146, 208, 226, 228
at hospitals and clinics, 66-67, 70
stories and opinions, x, 113, 121, 141, 142, 246
telephone hotlines, 11
telling about HIV/AIDS, 108, 121-23
Children and the AIDS Virus (Hausherr), 27
Children's Home and Aid Society of Illinois–Viva Family Center, 25, 30, 32
Children's Memorial Hospital, 22, 25, 66-67
Hemophilia Treatment Center, 67
Children's Place, The, 25, 226, 266
Child Welfare League of America, 26
chills, as a drug side effect, 79
"Chinese Medicine and HIV," 102
CHIP (Comprehensive Health Insurance Plan), Illinois, 197, 202
chiropractics, 98
chlamydia, 87, 155, 156

Christine, stories and opinions, 79, 152, 203, 244
on children, 123, 164
churches, 58-59, 149-50, 153-54, 259. See also religion
Circle Family Care, 153, 208
Circle of Hope, 21, 146
Clean Start–Illinois Masonic Center for Addiction Medicine, 172
clinical research trials, 5, 23, 25, 64, 89-92, 214
at hospitals and clinics, 67-70
participation by people of color, 61-62
patient's right and responsibilities, 76
video on, 19
clinics, 66-70, 126, 157, 209, 210, 215
at Cook County Hospital, 213-14
prevention counseling, 160
specialized, 64, 65
strategic decisions on visits to, 55
use by people of color, 59-62
Closing the Gap (Web site), 13, 31
CMV (cytomegalovirus), 87
Coach House Drop-In Center–Woodlawn Organization, 101
Coalition for Positive Sexuality, 160
"COBRA Continuation Options: Questions and Answers," 202
COBRA (Consolidated Omnibus Budget Reconciliation Act) of 1986, 191, 193-95
cocaine, 170
colitis, as a form of CMV, 87
Columbia Home Care, 262
Columbia Michael Reese Hospital and Medical Center, 67

combination therapies ("cocktails"), 78-83
"Common Threads: Stories from the Quilt" (video), 18
communication, 72, 158, 255. See also telling others
between attorney and client, 236-37
between parents and children, 121-23
Community and Economic Development Association of Cook County (CEDA), 226
Community Counseling Centers of Chicago, 208
Community Nursing Service–West, 262
Community Response, 20, 146, 208, 226, 228
Community Supportive Living Systems, Inc., 226
complementary treatments. See supplemental treatments
Complete Guide to Safe Sex, The (book and video), 161
Comprehensive Health Insurance Plan (CHIP), Illinois, 197, 202
Comprension y Apoyo a Latinos en Oposicion el Retrovirus (CALOR), 30, 146, 208
computers, 11-12
use for information (see Internet; Web sites)
condoms, 1, 155, 156-57, 160
availability in jails and prisons, 177
female condoms, 157
Confide (mail-in kit for HIV testing), 125-26

confidentiality, 75, 120, 121, 234
 of attorney-client communications, 236-37
 of medical information, 64, 72, 73
  obtained by employer, 110-11
  obtained by insurance carrier, 191
  in prisons, 177
  in place of employment, 110-11
  in talking with case manager, 205
  and telling children, 121-23
Connection Crisis Intervention and Referral Services, 11, 230
 Teen Line, 11, 230
Consolidated Omnibus Budget Reconciliation Act (COBRA) of 1986, 191, 193-95
contestability clause, in health insurance policies, 196
Continuation of Health Insurance Coverage (CHIC), Illinois, 194, 202
Cook County Department of Public Health, 101, 208
Cook County Hospital
 AIDS clinic, 213-14
  HIV Primary Care Center, 20, 67, 101, 146, 172, 208, 238
  Outreach Program, 225, 238
  Women and Children's HIV Program, 20, 22, 25, 67, 172
Cook County Legal Assistance Foundation, Inc., 238
cookers, sharing as dangerous activity, 156
coping skills, 49, 57-60, 124-25, 129
 emotional support, 137-48
Coram Healthcare, 262
Cornerstone Services, Inc., 226
"Correct Care" (newsletter), 180

corticosteoids, *table* 94-96
cough, as symptom, 6, 88
counseling, 53, 56, 65, 224. *See also* case management; mental health, services; substance abuse programs/treatment
 at hospitals and clinics, 66-70
 on results of HIV tests, 126
Cox, Charlie, 252-55. *See also* Charlie
credit cards, 92, 232, 233
credit protection plans, 232
Critical Path AIDS Project, 13, 91, 102, 104
Crixivan (indinavir sulfate), 83, *table* 95
cross-training programs, 136
Crusader Clinic, 67, 209, 238
cryptococcal meningitis, 88
cryptococcosis, 88
cryptosporidiosis, 88
C-section (cesarean section) for HIV-infected women, 165-66
curriculum package, for use in high schools, 33, 114
custody of children, 108, 233, 238, 246-47, 248
cytomegalovirus (CMV), 87

D
Daniel Hale Williams Center, 67
DCFS (Illinois Department of Children and Family Services)
 custody of children after parent's death, 245, 248
ddC (HIVID; zalcitabine), 79, *table* 96
ddI (didanosine; Videx), 4, 79, *table* 94
death and dying, 149, 150-51, 243
 awareness of one's mortality, 37-38, 42
 denial of cause, 58
 fear of, 36-37, 45, 122, 145, 150
 high viral load count as risk

factor, 74
 hospice care (*see* hospice care)
 "letting go," 252-56
 preparation for, 243, 244-52, 254 (*see also* Durable Power of Attorney; living wills)
 saying goodbye, 269-71
 as a spiritual journey, 256-59
 survivor guilt, 268
DeKalb County Hospice, 263
delavirdine (Rescriptor), 80, *table* 94
delivery. *See* childbirth
dementia, 79, 251-52
denial, 37, 110, 121, 143, 269
 among people of color, 57-59
 as factor in substance abuse, 166-67
dental care, 25, 33, 67-70, 77, 107, 193
 discrimination in, 233, 235
dental dams, 156, 177
Department of Health and Human Services, 176, 226
Department of Veteran Affairs–Veterans Service Division, 201, 266
depression, 36, 56, 123, 137, 141, 143, 144-45
D4T (stavudine; Zerit), 4, 79, *table* 96
diapers, 181, 182
diaphragms (birth control devices), 156
diarrhea
 as a drug side effect, 79, 83, 99
 possible solutions, 131, 132
 as symptom, 6, 87, 135, 154, 163
didanosine (ddI; Videx), 4, 79, *table* 94
diet. *See* food and nutrition
dietitians, 130-31
dildoes, 155, 156
Direct AID, 230

disability, 111-12, 117, 198, 199, 216-17
   dealing with creditors, 232-33
   eligibility for MANG, 222
   health insurance coverage, 193
   insurance, 198 (*see also* Social Security Disability Insurance)
   life insurance coverage, 200
   talking about, 254
discrimination against people living with HIV/AIDS, 63, 75, 107
   in employment, 110-12
   on health insurance, 192
   legal rights, 233-35
disease. *See* illness
divorce, 235, 238
doctors, 33, 49, 55, 56, 62-76, 107. *See also* OB/GYN care
   advice on exercise, 136
   and health insurance claims, 192
   help in telling others, 109
   HIV specialists, 63-65
   infant's HIV status determined by, 162-63
   lawsuits, 234
   living wills and health care powers of attorney, 249
   nutritional information, 130
   physician referral services, 65, 66
   reporting HIV status of children and teens, 112-13
   role in applying Illinois Health Care Surrogate Act, 249
   role in treatment and treatment choices, 78, 81, 83, 85, 103
      consulting on supplemental treatments, 98-99, 103
   work with homeless people, 176
dogs, 183
domestic violence, 53. *See also* abusive relationships

programs, 226, 230
   shelters, 157, 176, 226
DORS (Illinois Department of Rehabilitation Services), 220, 223, 231
   agencies working with, 207, 208, 209
drugs, pharmaceutical/prescription. *See* medications
drug use, 39-40, 41, 108, 129, 143, 166-75. *See also* substance abuse; substance abuse programs/treatment
   discussing with doctor, 73, 76, 83
   firing or non-hiring on basis of, 112
   injection equipment, 125, 156, 170, 176
      guidelines for use and sterilizing, 168, 181
      needle exchange programs, 168-69
      transmission of HIV through shared, 1, 39, 44, 76, 170, 177
   interaction with antivirals, 79
   in jails and prisons, 177
   negative attitudes toward, 149-50
   and safer sex, 156
Duane Dean Recovery Project, 172
Dunning, Thomas, 170
DuPage Bar Legal Aid Service, 238
DuPage County Health Department AIDS Program, 146, 209, 227, 228
DuPage County Medical Society, 66
Durable Power of Attorney
   challenges to, 251-52
   for Health Care, 71-72, 205, 248-50, 254-55

   Illinois Health Care Surrogate Act in case of absence of, 249-50
   for Property, 250
dying. *See* death and dying

E

Early Care for HIV Disease (Baker, Moulton, and Tighe), 18
"Eating Defensively: Food Safety for Persons with AIDS" (video), 19
eating habits. *See* food and nutrition
Ebbert, Shelly, 158
education on HIV/AIDS, 20, 21-22, 46
   as help in telling others, 108-9
   need for among people of color, 57-59
   for prisoners, 177-80
   role in taking charge of one's life, 54, 56, 138
   for school personnel and students, 46, 113-14
EIA (ELISA) test for HIV, 125
elderly, the
   Medicare for, 219
   time between infection and diagnosis, 3
ELISA (EIA) test for HIV, 125
"Elizabeth," stories and opinions, x, 51, 65, 120, 137, 243
   on hope, 47
   on spirituality, 150-51
El Rincon Community Clinic, 30, 147, 172
emergency room doctors, seen by people of color, 60
emotions, 36-38, 53, 55-56, 157. *See also individual emotions*
   books on, 214
   involved in telling others, 108, 109
   support, 46, 137-48, 176, 203

personal perspectives on, 141-45
employee assistance/benefit programs, 167, 238
  health insurance, 189, 192
employment, 216, 268
  applying for, 112, 117
  blood drives, 124-25
  discrimination in, 233, 235
  group health insurance, 189-95
  leaving or switching, 269-70
    effect on health insurance coverage, 190-91, 193-95
  and revealing HIV status, 110-12, 116, 117
encephalitis, 87
enema equipment, sharing as dangerous activity, 156
enteral nutrition (EN), 133
entitlement agencies. *See* government assistance
enzymes, used by HIV to replicate itself, drugs inhibiting, 78-79
Epivir (lamivudine; 3TC), 79, 83, *table* 95
Epstein-Barr virus, 89
Equal Employment Opportunity Commission (EEOC), HIV discrimination claims, 234
Erie Family Health Center, 30, 67, 209
Essential HIV Treatment Fact Book (Douglas, Harding, and Pinsky), 18
ethnic differences, 60
Evanston Meals-at-Home, 228
Evie, stories and opinions, 120, 162, 269
exercise, 129, 136-37
extension of benefits provision, in group health insurance, 194

F

families, 41, 53, 55, 137, 235, 253. *See also* children; parents
  decision-making under Illinois Health Care Surrogate Act, 249-50
  denial, 58
  effects of wills, living wills, and powers of attorney, 245, 248, 251-52
  resources for, 31-32, 140-41
  telling, 107, 109-10, 115, 118, 121
Family AIDS Support Network, 32
Family and Medical Leave Act (FMLA), 195
Family Guidance Center, 172
Family Service and Mental Health Center, 147
fatigue
  as drug side effect, 79, 83
  possible solutions, 133
  as symptom, 6, 39, 87
fats, dietary, 130
FAX services for information and referrals, 8, 9, 11, 14-16, 20-22, 27-29, 31-33, 77, 98, 229-31
  case management, 207-11
  clinical drug trials information, 91
  food and nutrition, 134, 136
  hospice care, 262-65
  housing assistance, 225-28
  insurance, 194, 201, 202
  legal assistance, 238-39, 240
  long-term care facilities, 265-66
  needle exchange programs, 168-69
  patient assistance programs, 93, 97
  on physicians, hospitals, and clinics, 66-70
  safer sex resources, 160-61
  services for people of color, 29-31
  services for women and children, 22-26
  spiritual support, 153-54
  substance abuse treatment, 171-75
  support groups and mental health services, 146-48
  transportation, 229
  treatment, 86, 101-2, 106
FDA (Food and Drug Administration), 4, 13, 92
fear, 36-37, 55, 57, 138, 140, 145
feces, guidelines for handling, 181
feeding tubes, 133, 247
feline immunodeficiency virus (FIV), 183
feline leukemia virus (FeLV), 183
fever
  as a drug side effect, 79-80, 83
  as symptom, 6, 86-88, 135
Final Exit (Humphry), 71-72
finances, 61, 65, 108, 187, 232-33, 234. *See also* insurance
  assistance, 70 (*see also* Medicare; Public Aid; Social Security)
  covered in clinical drug trials, 89-90
  Durable Power of Attorney for Property, 250
  handled by the executor of a will, 244-45
  information needed for applying for public assistance, 212-13
  meeting costs of medications (*see* medications, meeting costs)
Firman Community Services, 230, 266
fish, as pets, 183
FISH of Park Ridge, 229
fisting, risk involved, 156

flexibility, of long-term survivors, 49
fluids, 83, 131
FMLA (Family and Medical Leave Act), 195
Food and Drug Administration (FDA), 4, 13, 92
    HIV and AIDS Page (Web site), 13, 91, 105
food and nutrition, 41, 73, 98, 129-36
    assessments, 68, 69, 210
    assistance, 22-23, 204, 207-8, 215, 224-25, 228-31
        food stamp program, 223
        for homeless people, 176
        WIC, 223
    books and publications on, 134
    food safety, 135-36
    hygiene measures concerning, 181
    possible solutions to symptoms and side effects, 132-33
    restrictions required by new drugs, 5
    right to withhold, 247, 248
    videos on, 19, 134
Food Stamps (FS), 220, 223, 238
For Those We Love: A Spiritual Perspective on AIDS, 32
Fortunato, John, 149-50, 256-59
foster care, 266
Fox River Valley Center for Independent Living, 147, 209, 227
Fox Valley Hospice, 263
fraud, in treatment options, 99-100, 101
friends, 31-32, 53, 55, 137
    telling, 107, 109-10, 118
FS (Food Stamps), 220, 223
funeral arrangements, 243, 244, 255, 266-67
    rights of the power of attorney agent, 248

fungal infections, 87-88, 163
    antifungals, *table* 94-95

G

GA (General Assistance), 218, 220, 221, 223
Gail, stories and opinions, 42-43, 119, 142
gammaglobulin, as immunomodulator, 84
Garfield Counseling Center, 172, 209
"Gary," stories and opinions, 52, 54, 129, 159
gas and bloating, 132, 135
Gateway Foundation, 22, 172
Gay and Lesbian Physicians of Chicago, 33, 66, 77
Gay and Lesbian Task Force, 215
"Gay Man's Guide to Safe Sex, The" (video), 161
gay men and youth, 13. *See also* homosexuality; partners
    resources for, 8, 23, 26, 28-29, 33, 139
        bookstores, 17-18
        support groups, 39, 139
    survivor guilt, 268
Gay Men's Health Crisis (GMHC), 8, 13, 19, 28, 32, 160
    publications, 13, 161
    On the Web, 13, 161
General Assistance (GA), 218, 220, 221, 223
Genesis House, 23, 227, 230
    West Side Satellite, 23, 227, 230
genital warts, 155
George, stories and opinions, xi, 6, 118, 131, 165, 169
    on making changes, 39-42
    on sexual activities, 156
    on 12-step programs, 167
Gerber Hart Gay & Lesbian Library and Archives, 17

"Getting It Right: A Young Gay Man's Guide to Safe Sex" (video), 161
Gina, stories and opinions, 53, 158
Glen Oaks Nursing Center, 265
gloves, wearing
    as a hygiene measure, 181-82, 184
    during sexual activities, 155, 156
gonorrhea, 87, 88
Good Vibrations Guide to Sex, The (Winks and Semans), 161
government (public) assistance, 187, 188, 203-31. *See also* Public Aid; Social Security Administration
Greater Community AIDS Project, 227
grief, 38
Groceryland, 228
group disability insurance, 198
group health insurance, 189-95, 197. *See also* health insurance continuation options, 190-91, 193-95
    filing for disability, effects of, 198
    HIV-related claims, 191-92
    renewal rates, raising, 190, 191
group life insurance, 195, 199. *See also* life insurance
    filing for disability, effects of, 198
group therapy. *See* support groups
Growing Up Positive: Stories from a Generation of Young People Affected by AIDS (Lucas), 28
growth factors, as immunomodulators, 84

guardianship, adult, 252
    decision-making under Illinois Health Care Surrogate Act, 249-50
guardianship of children, 235, 243, 245-47, 248
    video on, 19, 240
Guia Para Vivir Con La Infeccion VIH, La (Bartlett and Finkbeiner), 31
Guide to Living with HIV Infection (John, Bartlett, and Finkbeiner), 18
"Guide to Social Security and SSI Disability Benefits for People with HIV Infection," 218
guilt, feelings of, 36, 38, 53, 138, 144, 149-50, 152, 157, 268
gums, bleeding, and HIV transmission, 156, 182
gynecology. See OB-GYN care

H

hand washing, importance of, 181, 184
Harbor Light Alcoholism and Drug Dependence Service, 172
Harbor Lights Hospice, 263
Harm Reduction Outreach, 169
Hawking, C. J., 268-70
Haymarket House, 23, 172, 209
headaches
    as drug side effect, 79-80
    as symptom, 6, 87-88
health (medical) care, 33, 107, 112. See also clinics; doctors; hospitals; treatment
    Adam on obtaining, 213-16
    during clinical drug trials, 89, 214
    in jails, 119
    for people of color, 59-62
    for women, 22-23 (see also OB-GYN care)

Healthcare Alternative Systems, 173
    Residential Programs, 173
health departments, city and county, 16-17, 45, 65
    care consortia, 15-16
    clinics, 126, 157
    HIV status of children and teens reported to, 112-13
    prevention counseling, 160
health insurance, 40, 65, 71, 188-97, 214. See also Medicaid; Medicare
    COBRA, 190, 193-95
    coverage of mental health services, 139
    employers' attempt to limit, 111
    filing for disability, effects of, 198
    HIV-related claims, 190, 191-92
    legal rights, 234, 235
    prescription drug coverage, 5, 92
    substance abuse treatment coverage, 167
health journal, 73
Health Maintenance Organizations (HMOs), 71, 189, 191
    COBRA coverage, 193
"Healthy Start" program, 222
hearing impaired, services for, 21, 29, 160, 209, 225, 262. See also TTY/TDD
Heartland Human Services, 15
"helper-T" (CD4) cells, 2, 4, 74. See also T-cell count(s)
hemophiliacs, 1, 120, 141
    services for, 20, 25, 67, 68, 139, 209
Hemophilia Foundation–National Info Line, 20
Hemophilia Foundation of Illinois, 20, 25, 209

hepatitis, 125
herbal remedies, 62, 98
heroin, 39-40, 41, 170
herpes, 87, 88, 89, 155, 156
Hirschtick, Robert, 260-61
Hispanic-Americans, 58, 59-60, 146, 148, 209. See also bilingual services
    resources for, 29-31, 161, 173
histoplasmosis, 88
HIV (Human Immunodeficiency Virus), xi, 1-4. See also people living with HIV/AIDS
    in infants and children, 162-63 (see also children; infants)
    mutation into drug-resistant form, 81
    reinfection, 155, 177
    replication of, drugs inhibiting, 78-79, 80
    telling other about infection (see telling others)
    tests for (see HIV tests)
    transmission (see transmission)
"HIV/AIDS Clinical Trials: Knowing Your Options" (video), 19, 91
HIV/AIDS Treatment Information Service (ATIS) (Web site), 13, 31, 105
HIV Coalition (HIVCO), The, 13, 22, 147, 229
HIVID (ddC: Zalcitabine), 79, table 96
HIV InfoWeb, 14, 91, 105, 240
"HIV Nutrition Guidelines: Practical Steps for a Healthier Life" (Wong), 134
HIV-positive (HIV+; HIV-antibody positive), xi, 1-4. See also HIV; HIV tests; people living with HIV/AIDS
HIV Positive: Working the System (Rimer, Robert, and Connally), 18

HIV-Positive Action Coalition (HIVPAC), 21
HIV Services Consumer Access Line, 204
"HIV+ Survival Guide: Diet for Living in the Age of AIDS" (video), 134
HIV Talk Radio Project, 20
HIV tests, 16-17, 66-70, 112, 125, 198. *See also* T-cell count(s)
   and blood donating, 124-25
   ELISA, 125
   for infants, 162
   mail-in kits, 125-26
   needle-free, 127
   and requirements for health insurance, 189-90, 191, 195
   Western Blot, 125
HMOs (Health Maintenance Organizations), 71, 189, 191
   COBRA coverage, 193
holistic healing techniques. *See* supplemental treatments
Holistic Protocol for the Immune System, A (Gregory), 102
Holy Family Hospital, 67
Home Access (mail-in kit for HIV testing), 125-26
homebound teachers, 114
home care, 204, 223, 262-65
   coverage under health insurance, 92
   coverage under Medicare, 219
   hospice care, 260, 262-65
Home Care Resources–Hospice of West Suburban Hospital, 263
Home Health Plus, 263
homeless, the, 176, 223
   services for, 27-28, 207, 226, 227
homeopathy, 98

home testing for HIV, 125-26, 126
homosexuality, 45, 57-58, 108, 125, 149-50. *See also* gay men and youth; lesbians
Honest Herbal, The: Use of Herbs and Related Remedies (Tyler), 102
hope, 4, 34-49
HOPWA (Housing Opportunities for People with AIDS), 224
Horizon Hospice, 147, 263
Horizons Community Services, 28, 147, 239
hospice care, 69, 70, 147, 223, 228, 260-65
   coverage by Medicare, 219, 264-65
   patient right and responsibilities, 76
Hospice House of Alexian Brothers, 263
Hospice of DuPage, 263
Hospice of Highland Park Hospital, 263
Hospice of Kankakee Valley, 263
Hospice of Northeastern Illinois, 264
Hospice of the Great Lakes, 263
Hospice of the North Shore, 264
hospitals, 64, 66-70, 213-14, 215-16. *See also individual hospitals by name*
   Living Will and Durable Power of Attorney for Health Care lodged with, 71-72
   patient right and responsibilities, 76
   physician referral lines, 65
   use by people of color, 60
hotlines, 8-11, 138, 207
   on HIV tests, 126-27
   information on pharmacies and buyers' clubs, 97
   role in taking charge of one's life, 56

   for safer sex resources, 160
   on substance abuse treatment, 171
housing, 270
   discrimination in, 233, 234-35
housing and rent assistance, 15-16, 215, 220, 223-28, 229-31. *See also* shelters
   case management, 204, 208, 210
   for veterans, 70
   for women, 22-23
Housing Opportunities for People with AIDS (HOPWA), 224
Howard, personal story, 76
Howard Area Community Center, 209
Howard Brown Health Center, 21, 28, 67, 147, 173, 209
   pamphlets on nutrition, 134
   personal experience with, 139
   Women's Program, 23
hugs, 46
Human Immunodeficiency Virus. *See* HIV
human resources departments, in businesses, 111
humor, sense of, 159, 187, 271
Humphry, Derek, 71-72
hydration, artificial, withholding of, 247, 248
hygiene guidelines, 129, 181-82, 184

I

I Know the Time Is Now: A Journey Living with AIDS (Kavanaugh), 154
Illinois, state of, care consortia funded by, 15-16
Illinois AIDS Hotline, 9, 17, 77, 147, 160, 168, 207, 230, 239
Illinois Alcoholism & Drug Dependence Association, 171

Illinois Department of
Alcoholism and Substance
Abuse (DASA), 173
Illinois Department of Children
and Family Services
(DCFS), 25, 27, 266
custody of children after
parent's death, 245, 248
Illinois Department of Human
Rights, 239
Illinois Department of Insurance,
202
Illinois Department of Public
Aid. See Public Aid
Illinois Department of Public
Health, 21
CHIC Program, 194, 202
HIV/AIDS Section, 27, 93,
194, 202
Ryan White AIDS Drug
Assistance Program, 92-93
Illinois Department of
Rehabilitation Services
(DORS), 220, 223, 231
agencies working with, 207,
208, 209
Illinois Director of Insurance,
201, 202
Illinois Health Care Surrogate
Act, 249-50
Illinois HIV Health Fraud
Information Network, 101
Illinois Human Rights
Commission, on dental
treatment, 77
Illinois Insurance Information
Service, 202
Illinois law
AIDS Confidentiality Act, 111
Illinois Health Care Surrogate
Act, 249-50
Living Will Statute, 247
on revealing names of sexual
partners or needle sharers,
76
on short-term and stand-by
guardians, 246-47
Illinois Masonic Medical
Center–Triad Clinic, 67
"Strong Spirit Program," 101
Illinois State Dental Society, 77
Illinois State Medical Society,
33, 63
illness (disease), 2-6, 74
caused by food poisoning, 135
dangers to HIV-infected
children, 114, 163
fear of, 36-37, 122
opportunistic infections, 4, 6,
48, 73, 86-89
Immune Power: A
Comprehensive Treatment
Program for HIV (Kaiser),
18, 102
immune system, 4, 73-74, 129,
137. See also T-cell count(s)
alternative therapies, 99, 130
of cats, 183
food poisoning effects, 135
immunomodulators effects, 84
of infants and children, 114, 162
pregnancy effects, 164
reinfection effects, 155
immunization. See vaccination
immunoglobulins, 84, table 95
immunomodulators, 84,
table 94-96
Impact AIDS, Inc., 19, 32, 33
implants (birth control devices),
156
incest, compared with HIV
infection, 143
income tax, federal. See Internal
Revenue Service
incompetence, legal arrangements
made prior to point of, 246
indinavir sulfate (Crixivan), 83,
table 95
individual health insurance, 188
infants, 23, 182
eligibility for WIC program,
223
HIV infection in, 18, 82,
162-64
viral load counts in, 74
infections. See opportunistic
infections
in-home care. See home care
In-Home Health Care, 264
insomnia, as a drug side effect,
79, 83
Institute for Advanced Study of
Human Sexuality, 161
insurance, 187, 188-202, 215. See
also health insurance; life
insurance
disability, 198 (see also Social
Security Disability
Insurance)
intake interview, with case
manager, 203
interferons, 84, table 95
Interim General Assistance, 219
interleukins, as
immunomodulators, 84
Internal Revenue Service
executor's filing of final
return, 244
return as documentation for
assistance, 212
International Aids Conference,
VII, Katoff's speech, 48
Internet, 9, 17, 24, 86. See also
Web sites
Interventions, 173, 209
Interventions Central Intake, 171
Interventions Crossroads, 173
Interventions Wauconda, 173
In the Lap of the Buddha
(Harrison), 154
intimacy, 157
intravenous feeding and
medication, 92, 133, 247
investment counselors, 232
Invirase (saquinavir), 83, table 96
isolation, 38, 59, 116, 139, 145
"It's Like This..." (video), 24

J

Jackson County Health Department, 16
jail. *See* prisons and jails
Jenny, stories and opinions, 121
Jewish AIDS Network Chicago, U.A.H.C., 153
Jewish Children's Bureau of Chicago "Take Five" Programs, 26
Jim, stories and opinions, 54, 71, 98, 121, 137, 139
   on pets, 183
   on spirituality, 152
jobs. *See* employment
Joe, stories and opinions, 76, 98, 137, 190, 206
Johnson, Daniel, 82
Johnson, Magic, 57-58
Joliet Area Community Hospice, 264
Joshua Ministries Support Group/ Northwest Community Hospital, 32, 148
Journal of the American Medical Association (JAMA) HIV/AIDS Site, 14, 105
Julie, personal story, 257

K

Kaleidoscope-Star Program, 26
Kaposi's sarcoma (KS), 6, 47, 88, 254
Karen, stories and opinions, 168, 259
Karissa, personal story, 113
Katoff, Lew, 48
"Keeper's Voice, The" (periodical), 180
Kelzer Care Center, 227
kidney ailments,
   as drug side effect, 83
kissing, 155-56, 181
"Kite, The" (Web site), 179
Komed Health Center, 68
KS (Kaposi's sarcoma), 6, 47, 88, 254

L

Lake County Alcoholism Treatment Center, 173
Lake County Health Department, 147
Lake Forest Hospice, 264
Lambda Legal Defense and Education Fund, 239
Lambda Rising Books, 17, 18, 27, 28, 31, 32, 102, 134, 202
   videos available from, 19, 102, 134, 154, 267
Lamivudine (Epivir; 3TC), 79, 83, *table* 95
"LAP Notes" (newsletter), 24
Latinas/os. *See* bilingual services; Hispanic-Americans
Lawndale Christian Health Center, 153, 209
lawyers (attorneys), 187, 234-37. *See also* legal services
   billing methods, 237
   services related to telling others, 108, 110, 117
leave of absence, medical, 195
legal alien status, as qualification for SSI, 218
Legal Assistance Foundation of Chicago, 239
   HIV Housing Law Project, 227
legal services. *See also* lawyers
   advice on health insurance, 192
   assistance, 67, 203, 204, 215, 225, 227, 233-40 (*see also* AIDS Legal Council of Chicago)
   for preparation for death, 243, 244-45, 249-50 (*see also* Durable Power of Attorney; living wills; wills)
   relating to financial arrangements, 232-33, 234
lesbians, 23, 26, 149. *See also* homosexuality
   resources for, 17-18, 28-29, 33, 139, 160
   newsletter, 24
   support groups, 39, 139
<u>Lesbian Sex Book, The</u> (Caster), 161
LesBiGay Radio, 20
"letting go," 252-55
Lewis, Jim, 35-39
libraries, 17, 214-15
life
   orientation to of long-term survivors, 48
   quality of, 41
      as a hospice care concern, 260
   as a spiritual journey, 256-59
   taking control of, 40-44, 52-62
"life estate," putting assets into, 234
life expectancy, 5-6
   for HIV-infected infants, 163
life insurance, 195, 199-201, 248
   employers' attempt to limit, 111
   filing for disability, effects of, 198
   "living" or "accelerated" benefits, 200
   for veterans, 201
   viatical settlements, 200-201
life partners. *See* partners
lifestyle, changes in, 37-38, 39-42, 62, 129, 136-37
   food and nutrition, 130-36
life support/life-sustaining treatment
   under Durable Power of Attorney for Health Care, 248
   under Health Care Surrogate Act, 249
   and hospice care, 260
   under a living will, 247
   physician's respect for patient's wishes, 65
lifetime health insurance benefit caps, 192
litter boxes, emptying, 184
liver damage, as drug side effect, 79, 83

"Living Proof" (video), 19
"Living Well with HIV/AIDS: A" (Davis, Newman, and Salomon), 134
living wills, 71-72, 108, 205, 243, 247-49, 254
   challenges to, 251-52
   Illinois Health Care Surrogate Act in case of absence of, 249-50
   physician's respect for, 65
Living with AIDS: A Guide to Resources in New York City, 213
   information on insurance, 192-93, 195, 196, 198, 200
"Living with Loss: Children with HIV" (video), 19, 267
long-term care facilities, 265-66
long-term survivors, 3, 47-49
   survivor guilt, 268
Losing Uncle Tom (Jordan), 27
loss, feelings of, 37
Love and Action Midwest, Inc., 153, 210
Loyola Medical Center–HIV/AIDS Clinic, 68
"Luis," stories and opinions, xi, 6, 35, 51, 73
Lutheran Family Mission, 26
Lutheran General Hospital
   Addiction Treatment Program, 173
   Nesset HIV Center, 68
   Pastoral Counseling Service, 154
Lutheran Social Services of Illinois, 23, 26, 147, 210, 266
lymphoma, 47

M

MAC (MAI; mycobacterium avium complex; mycobacterium intracellulare), 86, 87, 183
Madison County AIDS Program (MADCAP), 210, 229
magazines. See books and publications
mail order booksellers, 17-18. See also Lambda Rising Books
Make-A-Wish Foundation, 26
Making It: A Woman's Guide to Sex in the Age of AIDS (Patton and Kelly), 161
managed care, 85
   HMOs, 71, 189, 191, 193
MANG (Medical Assistance No Grant), 220, 222
"Marie," stories and opinions, xi, 98, 142, 151, 155, 203
   on making a will, 243
   on telling others, 117, 122
marijuana use, 168, 170
Marillac House, 231
Martelli, personal story, 4
Martin, Annie, 119, 123
Marty Howard's HIV/AIDS Home Page (Web site), 14, 202
Mascaro, Michelle, 191, 204-5, 212
massage, 62, 98, 101, 155
masturbating, 155, 156
material misrepresentation, on health insurance claims, 196
Meals on Wheels–Riverside Medical Center, 229
measles
   avoidance of people with, 181
   danger to HIV-infected children, 114, 163
Medicaid, 65, 71, 188, 218, 238
   eligibility for, 194, 197, 218
   medication coverage, 85, 92
   MediPlan, 220, 221-22
   qualification for DORS, 223
Medical Assistance No Grant (MANG), 220, 222
medical benefits. See health insurance
medical care. See clinics; doctors; health care; hospitals
medical history, 72, 112. See also medical records
   health insurance requirements, 190, 196
Medical Information Bureau, 195
medically disabled. See disability
Medical Management of AIDS, The (Sande and Volberding, eds.), 33
medical records
   access to of the power of attorney agent, 248
   confidentiality (see confidentiality)
   group health insurance requirements, 192, 196
   living wills and health care powers of attorney included in, 249
   provision of for viatical settlement, 200
medical treatment. See doctors; medications; treatment
Medicare, 139, 215, 219-20, 238
   acceptance for hospice care, 264-65
   for SSDI recipients, 219
Medicare Hotline, 220
medications (pharmaceutical drugs), 4-5, 35, 41, 56, 78-85, 103. See also individual drugs and drug types by name
   clinical trials (see clinical research trials)
   combination therapies ("cocktails"), 78-83
   effect on nutritional needs, 131
   information on as part of medical history, 72
   meeting costs, 5, 67, 70, 85, 92-98, 213-16
   coverage under COBRA, 193
   Medicaid and Federal AIDS Drug Assistance Program, 219

pharmaceutical companies programs, 85, 93-98
non-FDA approved, 92
patient's rights and responsibilities concerning, 75-76
prophylactic treatments, 6, 86-89
recording in health journal, 73
reducing risk of HIV transmission, prisoners' possible need for, 177
resistance to, development of, 80, 81, 82, 83
side effects (*see* side effects)
use by homeless people, 176
MediPlan. *See* Medicaid
meditation, 98, 150, 257
memorial service, 255. *See also* funeral arrangements
meningitis, as symptom, 40
Men's Network–Heart of Illinois HIV/AIDS Center, 28
menstrual period, intercourse during, 1
mental health, 36-38. *See also* emotions
services, 41, 67-68, 70, 138-41, 146-48, 158 (*see also* counseling; 12-step programs)
Midwest AIDS Training and Education Center (MATEC), 33
mind-body connection, role in long-term surviving, 47
Minority Outreach Intervention Project (MOIP), 30, 147, 210
Monk, Elizabeth, 140
mothers. *See* parents; women
motor skills, slow development of, in infants and children, 163
mouth(s)
reasons for dentists' reluctance, 77
risks in sexual activities, 156
symptoms found in, 6, 39, 163

Mt. Sinai Hospital, 68
multilingual services, 9, 11, 22, 29, 225, 265-66. *See also* bilingual services
for hospice care, 263-64
at hospitals and clinics, 67, 69-70, 101
mumps/measles/rubella (MMR) immunization, 163
muscle aches, as drug side effect, 79, 99
mutation, of HIV into drug-resistant form, 81
My Brother Has AIDS (Davis), 27
mycobacterium avium complex (MAC; MAL; mycobacterium intracellulare), 86, 87, 183
My Dad Has HIV (Alexander, Rudin, and Sejkora), 27
"My Suggestions for Those Diagnosed with AIDS" (Sherman), 55-56

N
Nance, Brent, 188
NAPWA Fax. *See* National Association of People with Aids
Narcotics Anonymous (NA), 68, 167, 227
NASBA test, viral loads measured by, 74
National AIDS Treatment Information Project
FAX service, 15
Web site, 105
National Association of People with AIDS (NAPWA), 9, 21-22, 97
NAPWA Fax, 15, 97, 98, 106, 185, 218
information on clinical trials, 91
legal publications, 240
publications on food and nutrition, 134, 136

publications on women's issues, 24
resources for people of color, 31
viatical settlements, 202
National Drug and Alcohol Treatment Referral Routing Service, 171
National Hemophilia and AIDS/HIV Network for the Dissemination of Information, 20
National Hemophilia Foundation, 215
National HIV Telephone Consultation Service Warmline, 33
National Hotline for Gay and Lesbian Youth, 29
National Institute of Allergy and Infectious Disease (NIAID) Gopher Site, 14
National Library of Medicine (NLM) AIDS Information Gopher Resource (Web site), 14, 91, 106
National Minority AIDS Council, 33
National Native American AIDS Hotline, 8
National Organization for the Reform of Marijuana Laws, 169
National Pediatric HIV Resource Center (NPHRC), 26, 33
"National Prison Project Journal, The" (periodical), 180
National Runaway Switchboard, 11
National STD Hotline, 8
National Women's Law Center, Web site, 179
Native Americans, 8, 29. *See also* people of color

nausea and vomiting
    as drug side effect, 79-80, 83, 99
    possible solutions, 133
        antinausea drugs, *table* 95-96
    as symptom, 88, 131, 135
Near North Health Service Corporation, 173
need-based programs
    Public Aid, 220-23
    SSDI not a, 216-17
    SSI as a, 218-19
needles (syringes), IV, 125, 156, 170, 176
    exchange programs, 168-69
    guidelines for use and sterilizing, 168, 181
    transmission of HIV through shared, 1, 39, 44, 76, 170, 177
nelfinavir (Viracept), 83, *table* 95
neurological problems, as symptom in infants and children, 163
neuropathy, 79
    antineuropathy drugs, *table* 95
neutropenia, as a drug side effect, 79
nevirapine (Viramune), 79-80, *table* 95
newborns. *See* infants
New City Health Center, 68
New Joy of Gay Sex, The (Silverstein and Picano), 161
New Phoenix Assistance Center, 227
newsletters. *See* books and publications
NIA Comprehensive Center, 231
Night Ministry, 27, 153
night sweats, as symptom, 6, 87
NOAH: New York Online Access to Health AIDS Information Page (Web site), 14, 133

non-employed people, individual health insurance, 189
non-Hodgkin's lymphoma, 89
non-nucleoside reverse transcriptase inhibitors (NNRTIs), 4, 79-80
"non-progressors," 3, 47-49, 298. *See also* people living with HIV/AIDS
Northern Illinois AIDS Resource Center, 227
Northern Illinois Council on Alcohol and Substance Abuse (NICASA)–Women and Children's Center, 173
Northwest Community Hospital, 32, 148
Northwestern Hemophilia Treatment Center, 68
Northwestern Hospital–HIV Center, 68
Northwestern Memorial Hospice, 264
Norvir (ritonavir), 83, *table* 96
"Notes from the Underground" (publication), 104
No Time to Wait: A Complete Guide to Treating, Managing, and Living with HIV (Siano), 18
nucleoside analogues (NRTIs; nucleoside reverse transcriptase inhibitors; RTIs), 78-79
    protease inhibitors used in conjunction with, 80, 83
numbness, emotional, 36, 137
nursing (breast feeding), 1, 90, 162, 223
nutrition. *See* food and nutrition
"Nutrition and HIV" (video), 19, 134
Nutrition and HIV: A New Model for Treatment (Romeyn), 134

O

Oak Forest Hospital, 68, 266
OB/GYN (obstetrics-gynecology) care, 1, 7, 22, 23, 66-67, 68, 70
    pregnancy and delivery decisions, 162, 165-66
Olsten Kimberly Quality Care, 264
Omni, Incorporated Initiative, 174, 227
On Death and Dying (Kubler-Ross), 267
Open Door Clinic, 68, 210
Open Hand Chicago, 229
opportunistic infections, AIDS-related, 4, 6, 48, 73, 86-89. *See also* illness
optimism, of long-term survivors, 49
oral sex, 57, 156, 157
    transmission of HIV through, 1
Orasure, as needle-free HIV test, 127
organs, enlarged, in infants, 163
organ transplants, 1, 125, 181
Osborne Association–AIDS in Prison Project, 179
OUTpost, 29
Outreach Program, Cook County Hospital, 225, 238

P

PADS. *See* Public Action to Deliver Shelter
PADS (Public Action to Deliver Shelter), 227
pain management
    complementary therapies' benefits in, 99
    drugs, *table* 95
    with hospice care, 260
    under a living will, 247
Palmer, Joan, 204

pancreatitis, as a drug side effect, 79
panic, 137
Pap smear, 72
Parental Stress Services, 11, 148
parenteral nutrition (PN), 133
parents, 11, 23, 39, 82, 138, 144. *See also* women
   custody, 108, 233, 238, 246-47, 248 (*see also* guardianship)
   telling, 109, 121
   telling children, 121-23
Parents, Families, Friends of Lesbians & Gays (P-FLAG), 32
partners, 53, 71, 235, 268. *See also* sexual partners
   life partners
      arrangements for bequest in will, 245
      legal rights, 234, 235, 250
      naming as guardians, 246
part-time workers, health insurance, 189
passport, as documentation, 212
pastoral care, 67, 69-70, 153-54, 209, 225
Pastoral Counseling Center of Lutheran General Hospital, 154
PATH–Positive Approach to HIV, 42-43
Patrick, stories and opinions, x, 142, 246
"Paul," stories and opinions, 51, 72, 139
PCP (Pneumocystis carinii pneumonia), 6, 40, 74, 86
PCR (polymerase chain reaction), viral loads measured by, 74
Peer Services, Inc., 174
pelvic inflammatory disease (PID), 6, 72, 87
penetration, sexual, 156-57, 158.

See also anal intercourse; vaginal intercourse
pentamidine, 79, *table* 96
People Like Us Books, 17
people living with HIV/AIDS, xi, 1-7, 35-49, 129
   diagnosis, xi, 35-47, 107
   discrimination against (*see* discrimination)
   financial aspects (*see* finances; government assistance; insurance)
   finding and working with a doctor, 63-76 (*see also* doctors)
   food and nutrition (*see* food and nutrition)
   homelessness, 176, 223
   insurance (*see* disability; health insurance; life insurance)
   legal aspects (*see* lawyers; legal services)
   long-term survivors, 3, 47-49, 268
   medical care (*see* dental care; health care; treatment)
   patient rights and responsibilities, 75-76
   in prisons and jails, 44-46, 177-80
   sexual activities, 155-61
   support (*see* support; support groups)
   taking charge of their lives, 51, 52-62
   telling others, 51, 55-56, 107-27
people of color, 57-60. *See also* African-Americans
   Refugee and Repatriation Assistance, 221
   resources for, 8, 29-31, 139, 210
   support groups for, 39, 146, 148

People's Resource Center–Wheaton, 231
People with AIDS Coalition, Inc., 8, 30, 97
Peoria City/County Health Department, 16
peripheral neuropathy, as a drug side effect, 79
pets, 182-85
Pets Are Wonderful Support (PAWS), 182, 185
P-FLAG (Parents, Families, Friends of Lesbians & Gays), 32
pharmaceutical drug companies, patient assistance programs, 85, 93-97
pharmaceutical drugs. *See* medications
pharmacies, 92, 97-98
phone sex, 155
physical therapist, advice on exercise, 136
physicians. *See* doctors
Pilsen Little Village Community Mental Health Center, 210
"PI Perspective" (publication), 104
Planned Parenthood, Chicago Area, 23, 160
   Hotline, 23, 160
plasma donation, 125, 181
platelet count, 163
PN (parenteral nutrition), 133
pneumonia, 163
   pneumocystis carinii (PCP), 6, 40, 74, 86
Polymerase Chain Reaction (PCR) test, 74, 162
poppers (amyl nitrate; butyl nitrate), 156
Positive Cooking, 134
"Positive Faith" (video), 154
"Positively Aware" (publication), 104, 188, 260-61
pot smoking, 168, 170

power of attorney. *See* Durable Power of Attorney
"POZ" (publication), 104
   Web site, 148
PPO (Preferred Physician) plan, 191
Prairie State Legal Services, 239
pre-existing conditions, health insurance clauses on, 189, 190, 191, 192, 194, 196
pregnancy, 138, 162, 164-66
   clinical trials during, 90
   combination therapies used during, 82
   conceiving with HIV-positive father, 164
   effects of megadoses of vitamins, 130
   and eligibility for Medicaid, 222
   eligibility for Special Pregnant Women and Children Program, 222
   infection of fetus during, 1, 7, 162
   prenatal care, 68, 70
   and viral load counts, 74-75
Presumptive Supplemental Security Income, 219
prevention. *See* sexual activities; transmission
Pride Agenda (bookstore), 17
Pride Youth–LINKS North Shore Youth Health Service, 29
Prism Youth Network–Oak Park Area Lesbian and Gay Association, 29
prisons and jails, 210
   advocacy groups, 177, 179-80
   treatment of HIV-positive inmates, 44-46, 119, 177-80
proactivity, 48-49, 51, 52-62, 72, 111
probate process, 244-45
Project Inform, 8

Project VIDA, 28, 30, 101
Prologue, 66
property
   Durable Power of Attorney for, 250
   limitations on for SSI, 218
   SSDI not limited by amount of, 216
   transfer of during lifetime, 245
prophylactic (preventive) treatments, 4, 6, 86-89, 163
prostitution, services for women involved in, 227, 230
protease inhibitors, 4-5, 80-83, 84, *table* 95-96
   use in conjunction with other medications, 79-80, 83
   use in infants and children, 82
proteins, 130
protocols, 78, 81. *See also* clinical research trials
Provident Hospital, 68
psychotherapy. *See* mental health, services
Public Action to Deliver Shelter (PADS), 227
Public Aid, Illinois Department of, 157, 188, 218-19, 220-23, 238, 267
   appeals process, 203
   CHIP program, 197, 202
   Medicaid (*see* Medicaid)
   programs accepting payment from, 23, 30, 102, 209, 211
   hospice care, 262-65
   hospitals and clinics, 67-70, 101-2
   housing assistance, 225, 226
   long-term care facilities, 265-66
   substance abuse treatment, 171-74
public assistance. *See* government assistance; Public Aid
publications. *See* books and publications; *individual publications*
public health departments. *See* health departments, city and county
PWA Coalition Newsline, 104, 180
PWAs. *See* people living with HIV/AIDS

Q

Que es un Virus? Un Libro para Ninos Sobre el SIDA (Fassler and McQueen), 27
"Questions and Answers about Pain Control" (American Cancer Society), 267

R

radiation, use in treatment of KS, 6
Rainbow Hospice, Inc., 264
"Ralph," stories and opinions, 116, 129, 144, 234
   on health insurance, 190, 192
   on treatment, 81, 99
"rapid-progressors," 3. *See also* people living with HIV/AIDS
Ravenswood Community Mental Health Center Crisis Line, 11
Reader's Guide to Alternative Health Methods (Zivicky), 102
Refugee and Repatriate Assistance (RPA), 220, 221
Regional Transit Authority (RTA), 229
Reimer Foundation, 160
reincarnation, belief in, 257
relatives. *See* families
religion. *See also* churches; spiritual support
   support from, 46-47, 149-54, 259
rent. *See* housing and rent assistance
Renz Addiction Center, 174

Rescriptor (delavirdine), 80, *table* 94
respite services, 204, 223
rest and relaxation, 137
retinitis, as a form of CMV, 87
Retrovir. *See* AZT
retrovirus, 4. *See also* HIV
Review, 29
rights
   legal, 232-37
   as a patient, 75-76
rimming, risk involved, 156
ritonavir (Norvir), 83, *table* 96
RNA assay test, 74
Rock Island County Health Department, 16
Rodriguez, Felicia, 124
Rosa, personal story, 256
Roseland Christian Health Ministries, 69
Roseland Community Hospital HIV Clinic, 69, 101
Rothas, Edward, 44-47
RPA (Refugee and Repatriate Assistance), 220, 221
RTIs. *See* nucleoside analogues
Rucker, Terry, 118, 182
Rush Hospice Partners, 264
Rush Presbyterian–St. Luke's Medical Center, 69
Ryan White AIDS Drug Assistance Program, 92-93
Ryan White CARE Act Hospice Network, 262, 264

S

Safe Encounters: How Women Can Say Yes to Pleasure and No to Unsafe Sex (Whipple and Ogden), 161
safer sex. *See* sexual activities, safer
Safer SexPage (Web site), 161
Safer Sexy: The Guide to Gay Sex Safety (Tatchell), 161
"Safe Start" program, 207

saliva, HIV not transmitted through, 127
"Sam," stories and opinions, 121, 190, 232
Sandi, stories and opinions, 6, 138, 143, 169-70, 232
   on death and dying, 253
   on relationship with children, 121, 253
S&M, light, 155
San Francisco AIDS Foundation, 104, 155
saquinavir (Invirase), 83, *table* 96
schools, treatment of HIV-infected children, 112-14, 118
   legal rights, 233, 235
second opinions, as a right, 75
seizures, as symptom, 88
self-awareness, of long-term survivors, 49
self-employed people
   entitlement to SSDI, 216
   individual health insurance, 189
self-esteem, 168
self-image, 38, 116
self-love, 46, 52-53
semen, 156
Serenity House, 174
seroconversion, 162, 268
seropositive for HIV. *See* HIV-positive
service organizations, HIV/AIDS, 20-23, 56, 109, 157, 199, 224
   publications available at, 214-15
   referrals, 65, 130-31
sex talk, 155
sex toys, 155
sexual activities, 1, 44, 155-61, 177
   denial of risk from, 57-58
   discussing with doctor, 73, 76
   of homeless people, 176

   intercourse, 1, 156-57, 158
   partners, 53, 76, 138, 156-59
   safer, 129, 155-59, 166, 181
sexual assault, in jails and prisons, 177
sexually transmitted diseases (STDs), 87, 88, 89, 155, 156, 177. *See also* AIDS; HIV
   questions on health insurance forms, 190, 196
   testing women for, 72
sexual partners, 76, 138, 156-59. *See also* partners and abusive relationships, 53
Share Program, 174
Shari, stories and opinions, 52, 83, 119, 144-45, 166, 258
shelters, 27-28, 30, 176, 226-27, 229
   for domestic violence victims, 157, 176, 226
Sherman, Christopher D., 55-56
shingles (disease), 181
shortness of breath, as symptom, 6, 86, 88
short-term assistance programs, 219
short-term guardians, 246
side effects of medications, 5, 75, 84, 86
   of antivirals and combination therapies, 78-83, 254
   relief for, 99, 132-33, 136
"Silverlake Life: The View from Here" (video), 19
skin conditions
   as drug side effect, 79, 80, 83
   as symptoms, 6
skin test for tuberculosis, 72, 86
sliding scale fees, 67-70, 141, 147, 208, 210
   for hospice care, 262, 263
   for housing assistance, 225-26, 227
   long-term care facilities, 265
   for meals-on-wheels, 228

for pastoral counseling, 153-54
for substance abuse treatment, 171-74
Slocum, Michael, 35-39
Small Estate Affidavit, 245
Smith-Kline Beecham, needle-free HIV test, 127
smoking. *See* tobacco use
Snow Valley Nursing and Rehabilitation Center, 266
Social Security Administration, 188
card, 212, 218
number, 217, 21
programs, 215, 216-20, 222-23, 267 (*see also* Medicare; Social Security Disability Insurance)
Social Security Administration (Illinois), 217, 220, 267
Social Security Disability Insurance (SSDI), 198, 215, 216-18, 219, 238, 250
eligibility for food stamps, 223
eligibility for Medicare, 219
Social Security Disabled Widow/Widowers' benefits, 222
social workers. *See* case management
"Sonia," stories and opinions, 6, 36, 80, 151, 155
Southern Illinois University School of Medicine, 16, 69, 210
South Suburban Council on Alcoholism and Substance Abuse, 174
Spanish-language services. *See* bilingual services; Hispanic-Americans
"Sparky," story and opinions, 63, 198
Special Pregnant Women and Children Program (AFDC), 220, 222

"spend-down"
for MANG, 222
for Medicaid, 92
sperm
donation, 125, 165, 181
"washing," 164
spermicides, 156
spiritual journey
death and dying as, 256-59
use of credit cards to pursue, 233
spiritual support, 54, 148, 149-54
personal perspectives on, 150-52
SSDI. *See* Social Security Disability Insurance
SSI. *See* Supplemental Security Income
St. Catherine's of Genoa Catholic Worker, 174, 228
St. Clair County Health Department, 16
St. Francis Hospital of Evanston, 69
St. Joseph Hospital, 69, 101
St. Thomas Hospice, 264
Stadtlanders Pharmacy, 98, 134
stand-by guardians, 246-47
STAR Hospice, 264
Starlight Foundation, 26
state hotlines, 9-11
State Supplemental Payments, 219
Statscript Pharmacy, 98
Stavudine (d4T; Zerit), 79, *table* 96
STDs. *See* sexually transmitted diseases
Steinkopf, Deborah, 53, 117, 159, 199, 205
on caregivers, 143-44
on new medical treatments, 84-85
on survivor guilt, 260
on use of credit cards, 233
steroids, as immunomodulators, 84

Steven, stories and opinions, x, 43-44, 119
Stevens-Johnson syndrome, as drug side effect, 80
Stop AIDS
African-American Program, 22, 30, 161
Latino/a Program, 161
North Side, 160
stress, 176, 212, 243
reduction, 98-99, 129, 137
substance abuse, 43, 64, 166-70, 176. *See also* alcohol use; drug use
substance abuse programs/treatment, 22-23, 28, 64-65, 167, 171-75, 204, 209-11
at hospitals and clinics, 67, 68, 70
for people of color, 30
support groups, 39
therapy and support groups, 139, 167
12-step programs (*see* 12-step programs)
suicide attempts, 169
Sulzer Regional Library, 17
"Sun Chi: Techniques of Relaxation and Positive Imagery" (video), 19, 102
Supplemental Security Income (SSI), 215, 218-19, 223
supplemental (alternative; holistic) treatments, 56, 64, 72, 75-76, 98-103
at hospitals and clinics, 67, 69-70
personal experiences with, 83, 130, 137
use by people of color, 62
support
acknowledging need for, 38-39, 43, 49, 59, 108
from families, 41
emotional, 137-48, 176, 203
spiritual, 54, 148, 149-54

support groups, 30, 39, 42, 65, 138-48, 204, 207
   and dealing with issues of safer sex, 158
   for death and dying issues, 260-61, 262-65
   for families, friends, and caregivers, 31-32
   at hospitals and clinics, 67, 68-70
   personal experiences with, 42, 45-46
   referrals, 65, 236
   for teenagers, 39, 123, 139
survival, 3, 47-49, 60, 129
Surviving AIDS (Callen), 18
Surviving and Thriving with AIDS: Collected Wisdom, Volume Two (Callen, editor), 18
Surviving with AIDS: A Comprehensive Program of Nutritional Co-Therapy (Calloway and Whitney), 134
swallowing problems, as symptom, 6
   possible solutions, 132
swollen glands, as symptom, 6, 163
symptoms, HIV-related, 6-7, 73, 190, 253-54
   effect on nutritional needs, 131
   in infants, 162-63
   nutritional solutions to, 132-33
   of opportunistic infections, 86-88
symptoms, of food contamination, 135
syphilis, 155, 156
syringes. *See* needles, IV
systemic therapies, 88

T

"TAG" (publication), 104
tai chi, 98, 136
Take-A-Hike, 137

"Taking Charge: The HIV Planning Guide," 202
"Taking Charge as a Person of Color" (Wakefield), 57-60
Take Control: Living with HIV and AIDS (AIDS Project Los Angeles), 18
Talkline Help Lines, 11
TB. *See* tuberculosis
T-cell count(s), 2-3, 4, 48, 73-74, 78
   drug and alcohol use effects, 168, 170
   exercise effects, 136
   pregnancy effects, 162, 164
   protease inhibitors effects, 80, 83, 84
   use in diagnosing infants, 163
   and use of prophylactic treatment, 86-88
Teen Living Programs, 28
teens, 27-28, 123-24, 140-41, 153, 173
   HIV-infection in, 112-13, 123-24, 163
   publications for, 28
   services for, 22, 70, 146, 208, 228, 230
      support groups, 39, 123, 139
   stories and opinions, 53, 124, 144, 158
   telephone hotlines, 9, 11
Teens Tap AIDS Hotline, 9
Teens with AIDS Speak Out (Kittredge), 28
telling others, 51, 55-56, 107-27
   children, 121-23
   personal perspectives on, 115-21
terminal condition
   as condition for the Illinois Health Care Surrogate Act, 249
   defined for living wills, 247-48
Test Positive Aware Network (TPA; TPAN), 17, 21, 22, 60, 137, 239

   directory of clinical trials, 91
   legal clinic, 239
   publications, 19
   resources for gay men, 29
   resources for people of color, 30, 57
   suggestions for telling others, 109-10, 119
   support groups, 139, 142, 148, 254
   Web site, 31, 102, 148, 207
therapy. *See* mental health, services; support groups
"Thinking about Death" (video), 19, 267
Thomas, Franklin, 188
3TC (Epivir; lamivudine), 79, 83, *table* 95
thrush, as symptom in infants and children, 163
tingling sensations
   as drug side effect, 80
   as symptom, 88
tissue donation, 181
tobacco use, 73, 84, 129, 143, 166, 168
toilets, pets' drinking out of, 183, 184
toxoplasmosis, 79, 86, 87, 183, 184
TPA (TPAN). *See* Test Positive Aware Network
trade associations, group health insurance, 189
transmission of HIV, 1, 38, 108, 127. *See also* sexual activities
   in abuse situation, 119
   lawsuits over infection, 234
   from mother to child, 7, 74-75, 82, 162-63, 164-65
   preventive measures, 5, 7, 82 (*see also* drug use, injection equipment; sexual activities, safer)
      hygiene rules, 129, 181-82, 184

in prisons, 177-78
reinfection, 155, 177
risk of and Chicago Board of Education policy, 114
and safer sexual activities, 155-56
transportation, 233
assistance, 65, 176, 208, 224, 227, 229-30
Travelers & Immigrants Aid, 31, 228
Chicago Health Outreach, 69
Neon Street Center, 28, 228
Rafael Center, 174, 210, 228, 231
<u>Treating AIDS with Chinese Medicine</u> (Ryan and Shattuck), 102
treatment, 35, 51, 72-76, 78-106. *See also* clinical research trials; doctors; medications; supplemental treatments
discrimination in, 63, 233
Illinois Health Care Surrogate Act on, 249-50
life support/life-sustaining (*see* life support/life sustaining treatment)
making decisions on, 54-55, 56
paying for (*see* finances; medications, meeting costs)
preventive/prophylactic, 4, 6, 86-89, 163
proactive participation in by long-term survivors, 48-49, 51
running out of options, 254
and survivor guilt, 268
Treatment Alternatives for Safer Communities (TASC), 210
"Treatment Issues" (publication), 105
"Treatment Review" (publication), 105
"trial work situations," allowance for under SSDI, 217

Trinity United Church of Christ, 148, 154
TTY/TDD services
for homeless people, 176
hotlines, 8, 9-10, 16
for information, 21-22, 26-29, 32-33, 93, 98, 101, 208-11, 230-31
on clinical drug trials, 91
on food and nutrition, 136
on hospice care, 262, 264
on housing, 225, 226-28
on insurance, 194, 201, 202
on legal assistance, 238-39
on needle exchange programs, 168
on pregnancy and HIV, 162
on safer sex resources, 160
on support groups and mental health services, 147-48
on transportation, 229
for physicians, hospitals, and clinics, 66, 68-70
tuberculosis (TB), 86-87, 176, 181
skin test, 72, 86
12-step programs, 40, 167
Alcoholics Anonymous (AA), 22, 171, 227
Narcotics Anonymous (NA), 68, 167, 227
"typical-progressors," 3. *See also* people living with HIV/AIDS

U

UIC Community Outreach Intervention Project, 174, 211
ulcers in esophagus or mouth, as a drug side effect, 79
Unabridged Books (bookstore), 17
unemployment
credit protection plans, 232
disability insurance, 198
health insurance, 189, 193-95
unions

and eligibility for COBRA, 193
group health insurance, 189
Unity Hospice, 265
University of Chicago Hospitals, 69
University of Illinois at Chicago, 69, 211
Community Health Project, 70
Hospital HIV/AIDS Project, 25, 69
<u>Until the Cure</u> (Kurth), 24
urine, guidelines for handling, 181

V

vaccination (immunization), 72, 84, 181
for HIV-infected children, 163
for pets, 184
vaginal delivery for HIV-infected women, 165-66
vaginal intercourse, 1, 156
veterans
life insurance options for, 201
services for, 70, 175, 201, 228, 266
Veterans Affairs, U.S. Department of
Edward Hines V.A. Hospital, 70, 175
Medical Center–North Chicago, 70, 175, 228
Medical Center–West Side, 70
Veterans Service Division, 201, 266
veterinarians, 183-84
viatical settlements, 200-201
Vida/SIDA, 17, 31, 102
videos, 18-19, 24, 91, 102, 154, 175
on caring for infants and children, 164
on death and dying, 267
on food and nutrition, 134
on guardianship of children, 19, 240
on safer sex, 161

318 INDEX

Videx (ddI; didanosine), 4, 79, *table* 94
Viracept (nelfinavir), 83, *table* 95
viral load counts, 4, 5, 73-75, 124, 155, 162
    in children, 74, 82
    effect on of protease inhibitors, 80, 83, 84
Viramune (nevirapine), 79-80, *table* 95
viruses, 2-3. *See also* HIV
vision
    changes in as symptom, 6, 87
    insurance benefits under COBRA, 193
visitation rights, of the power of attorney agent, 248
visualization, 98
vitamins, 72, 98, 176
Vitas Corporation, 265
Vitas Innovative Hospice, 265
VNA North Hospice, 265
volunteer work, 56
vomit, guidelines for handling, 181

W

waiting periods
    for CHIP benefits, 197
    in health insurance clauses on pre-existing conditions, 189, 190, 191, 194, 196
    for Medicare based on SSDI, 219-20
    for public assistance, 212
    for SSDI, 217
    for SSI, 218
Wakefield, Steve, 57-62, 157
wasting, 130, 254. *See also* weight, loss
    antiwasting drugs, *table* 94-95
WATCH Program, 23
water
    contaminated, 135
    importance of drinking, 83, 131, 181
water sports, risk involved, 156

Way Back Inn, 174
Web sites, 11-14, 31, 97, 98, 127, 148, 202
    for information
        on case management, 207
        on clinical drug trials, 91
        on food and nutrition, 134
        on safer sex, 161
        on treatment options, 86, 102, 104, 105-6
    for legal assistance, 240
    for prisoners resources, 179, 180
weight, 130
    gain, infant's difficulty in, 163
    loss
        in children, 131
        possible solutions, 132
        as symptom, 6, 88, 116, 254
Weiss Memorial Hospital, HIV/AIDS Program, 70, 102
"Welfare" *See* AFDC; General Assistance
Wendy, stories and opinions, 122, 140, 155, 245, 246
Western Blot test for HIV, 125
Western Clinical Health Services, 175
Westside Association for Community Action (WACA), 211
West Towns Visiting Nursing Service, 211, 265
"What About My Kids?" (video), 19, 267
What's A Virus Anyway? The Kids' Book About AIDS (Fassler and McQueen), 27
When Someone You Know Has AIDS (Martelli et al), 32
white blood cells, 2. *See also* T cell count(s); T-cell count(s)
WIC (Women, Infant, and Children Supplemental Food Program), 220, 223

Will County Center for Community Concerns, 228
Will County Health Department, 16, 211
    HIV/AIDS Care Consortia, 16, 211
wills, 243, 244-47, 251-52, 254
Windy City Rainbow Alliance of the Deaf, 29
Winfield Moody Community Health Center, 70
Winnebago County Health Department, 16
"WISE Words" (Women's Information Service and Exchange) (newsletter), 24
Wolf, Harvey, 55, 76, 115, 166
women, 3, 53, 143-45. *See also* OB-GYN care; parents; pregnancy
    bookstores for, 17-18
    childbirth, 1, 7, 162, 165-66
    eligibility for WIC program, 223
    health problems specific to, 6, 72, 87, 89
    housing assistance for, 227-28, 229
    opportunistic infections, 87, 89
    services for, 22-24, 157, 160, 230, 262
        at hospitals and clinics, 67, 68
        support groups, 139, 142, 146-47, 208
Women, Infant, and Children Supplemental Food Program (WIC), 220, 223
Women Alive, 14, 23
Women and Children First (bookstore), 17-18
Women and HIV/AIDS (Bere and Ray), 24
Women and Infants Transmission Study (WITS), 23

Wood, stories and opinions, 4, 37, 80, 117
Woodlawn Organization Substance Abuse Services, 175
Worker's Compensation, and disability insurance, 198
"Work Your Body" (video), 19
WORLD (Women Organized to Respond to Life-threatening Diseases), 24
World Wide Web Sites, 12-14, 31
Wyler Children's Hospital of the University of Chicago, 26, 28, 70

X
X-rays, 72

Y
Yahoo AIDS/HIV Search Site, 14
yeast infections, 6, 72, 87
yoga, 98, 136

Z
zalcitabine (ddC; Hivid), 79, *table* 96
Zendell, Joseph, 271. *See also* Joe
Zerit (d4T; Stavudine), 79, *table* 96
zidovudine (ZDV). *See* AZT

NOTES:

NOTES:

NOTES:

ORDER FORM

I would like to order _____ copies of <u>There Is Hope: Learning to Live with HIV</u> (Third Edition).

There is a $15.00 charge for each book, including shipping and handling. Special rates for not-for-profit AIDS service organizations are available. (For more information, please call HIVCO at the number below.)

_____
Name

_____
Organization

_____
Address

_____
City/State/Zip

_____
Phone/Fax

_____ Check here if you'd like to receive regular mailings from HIVCO.

_____ Check here if you'd like membership information.

_____ My check is enclosed.   Amount enclosed $_____

_____ Please charge my credit card.

Circle one: VISA   MasterCard

Card number: _____

Expiration date: ____ / ____

Signature: _____

Please send your completed form and payment to:
HIVCO
1471 Business Center Drive, Suite 500
Mt. Prospect, IL 60056
847-391-9803
847-391-9826—FAX